Neuroscience-Enhanced Artificial Intelligence for Cybersecurity

Shafiq Ul Rehman
https://orcid.org/0000-0003-2266-218X
Kingdom University, Bahrain

IGI Global
Scientific Publishing
Publishing Tomorrow's Research Today

Vice President of Editorial Melissa Wagner
Director of Acquisitions Mikaela Felty
Director of Book Development Jocelynn Hessler
Production Manager Mike Brehm
Cover Design Jose Rosado

Published in the United States of America by
IGI Global Scientific Publishing
701 East Chocolate Avenue
Hershey, PA, 17033, USA
Tel: 717-533-8845 | Fax: 717-533-7115
Website: https://www.igi-global.com E-mail: cust@igi-global.com

Library of Congress Cataloging-in-Publication Data

LCCN: 2025041871 (CIP Data Pending)
ISBN13: 9798337350127
Isbn13Softcover: 9798337350134
EISBN13: 9798337350141

British Cataloguing in Publication Data
A Cataloguing in Publication record for this book is available from the British Library.

Table of Contents

Detailed Table of Contents

Neurocriminology explores the biological, neurological, and psychological underpinnings of criminal behavior, offering a science-based alternative to traditional sociological theories. It examines how brain structure, genetics, and environmental influences contribute to antisocial and violent tendencies. Abnormalities in areas like the prefrontal cortex and amygdala are linked to aggression, impulsivity, and lack of empathy. Technologies like fMRI and PET reveal brain deficits in offenders. Neurotransmitter imbalances, such as low serotonin and dysfunctional dopamine, also play a role. Studies, including on the MAOA "warrior gene," highlight how genetic traits interact with childhood trauma. Neurocriminology informs legal processes, emphasizing crime prevention, rehabilitation, and ethical integration into justice systems. While rejecting biological determinism, it underscores a biopsychosocial model essential for a modern, humane approach to criminal justice.

This chapter explores the integration of Artificial Intelligence within judicial systems under the emerging concept of "Smart Criminal Justice." It examines how AI can streamline legal processes, enhance decision-making, and uphold ethical accountability in the digital era. By linking cognitive aspects of human judgment with AI-driven reasoning, the chapter highlights parallels between legal decision-making and neuroscience-inspired intelligence models. It further discusses how ethical

reducing operational risks, and offering a strong means of protecting contemporary digital infrastructures.

Traditional cybersecurity models cannot keep up with current threats and our increasingly complicated digital landscape. This article proposed a potential hybrid architecture that could unify neuroscience technology, artificial intelligence (AI), and blockchain. Neuroscience allows for biometric identification in real-time through brain-computer interfaces (BCIs) or electroencephalography (EEG). AI provides the effective usage of adaptive defense, behaviour profiling, and autonomous detection. Blockchain provides secure transparency, decentralisation, and an immutable ledger. This architecture relationship uses a tri-layer system of sensing (neuro data), intelligence (AI analytics), and ledger (blockchain security). Real-world use cases include BCI-controllable devices, AI-driven energy management systems (smart grids), and federated learning in healthcare. There are still latency, privacy, and scalability hurdles that need to be overcome, but with the advent of quantum computing and advanced neural interfaces, positive opportunities for overcoming challenges exist.

The computational design of neuromorphic architecture represents a new era of computing that mimics the human brain's neural networks to achieve superior efficiency and faster task execution. This chapter explores advanced neuromorphic system architectures, emphasizing synthetic neurons and synapses that unify memory and processing units to minimize latency and reduce energy consumption. Notable examples include Intel's Loihi and IBM's TrueNorth chips, each showcasing distinct design philosophies and applications. The discussion highlights innovations in

Preface

The accelerating convergence of neuroscience and artificial intelligence (AI) marks a profound shift in how cybersecurity challenges are understood, anticipated, and mitigated. As digital infrastructures become increasingly complex, adaptive, and human-centered, traditional rule-based and purely data-driven security mechanisms are proving insufficient against cognitively sophisticated adversaries, insider threats, and socially engineered attacks. *Neuroscience-Enhanced Artificial Intelligence for Cybersecurity* responds to this challenge by advancing an interdisciplinary perspective that integrates insights from brain science, cognitive psychology, ethical governance, and advanced AI architectures to reimagine cybersecurity as an intelligent, adaptive, and explainable socio-technical system.

This volume is grounded in the recognition that cyber threats are not merely technical phenomena but are deeply intertwined with human cognition, behavior, emotion, and decision-making. By drawing inspiration from neural processes such as attention, learning, memory, affect, and plasticity, neuroscience-enhanced AI offers new paradigms for anomaly detection, behavioral analysis, predictive risk management, and trustworthy automation. At the same time, the deployment of such systems raises critical ethical, legal, and governance questions that demand rigorous scholarly engagement.

Edited with contributions from researchers and practitioners across computer science, neuroscience, law, education, and engineering, this book presents a coherent and forward-looking exploration of brain-inspired intelligence for cybersecurity. The chapters collectively emphasize explainability, human oversight, and ethical accountability, rejecting technological determinism in favor of a biopsychosocial and human-centric approach. The volume is intended for academics, graduate students, cybersecurity professionals, AI researchers, and policymakers seeking to understand and shape the next generation of intelligent cyber defense systems.

CHAPTER OVERVIEW

Chapter 1, ***Neurocriminology: The Brain Behind Crime,*** establishes the biological and neurological foundations of antisocial and criminal behavior. By examining brain structures, neurotransmitter systems, genetic predispositions, and environmental interactions, this chapter provides a scientific lens for understanding malicious behavior. Its insights offer a conceptual bridge between human criminality and cybercrime, underscoring the relevance of neuroscience to prevention, rehabilitation, and ethical justice frameworks.

Chapter 2, ***Smart Criminal Justice: Cognitive and Ethical Foundations for Trustworthy AI Systems,*** extends this perspective into judicial and legal domains. It explores how AI can augment legal decision-making while aligning with cognitive principles and ethical safeguards. The chapter frames "Smart Criminal Justice" as a model for building trustworthy, secure, and accountable AI systems—principles that are directly transferable to cybersecurity governance.

Chapter 3, ***Affective Computing and Neuro-Symbolic Intelligence in the Protection of Digital Learning Ecologies,*** reframes educational cybersecurity through a neurocognitive lens. Integrating affective computing, behavioral biometrics, and neuro-symbolic AI, the chapter demonstrates how cognitive load, emotion, and vigilance influence vulnerability in digital learning environments. It offers a human-in-the-loop, ethically grounded roadmap for securing educational ecosystems.

Chapter 4, ***Integrating AI and Neuroscience for Cyber Threat Detection and Response,*** examines biologically inspired AI models for adaptive and proactive cyber defense. Drawing parallels between cognitive processes and machine intelligence, the chapter reviews neural network architectures, hybrid models, and real-world case studies that enhance anomaly detection, behavioral analysis, and response accuracy while addressing privacy and explainability concerns.

Chapter 5, ***Neuro-Symbolic AI and Behavioral Intelligence: Towards Explainable Cybersecurity Mechanisms,*** focuses on the critical need for transparency and accountability in advanced security systems. By combining neural learning with symbolic reasoning and behavioral profiling, the chapter presents explainable frameworks that improve detection accuracy and reduce false positives, particularly in insider threat and phishing scenarios.

Chapter 6, ***Neuro-Symbolic Architectures for Cognitive Threat Detection,*** advances a brain-inspired system capable of identifying subtle social engineering and behavioral anomalies. Modeling attention, memory, bias, and emotional states, the proposed architecture demonstrates how adaptive sensing, reasoning, and decision-making can strengthen defenses against psychologically driven cyberattacks.

Chapter 7, ***Neuroscience-Enhanced AI for Real-Time Behavioral Anomaly Detection in Cybersecurity,*** addresses the limitations of static intrusion detection systems. Inspired by neural plasticity, working memory, and affective neuroscience, this chapter presents real-time architectures for identifying insider threats, zero-day exploits, and social engineering attempts through deviations in behavioral patterns.

Chapter 8, ***Integrating Predictive Analytics with AI for Cybersecurity Risk Management*****,** shifts the focus from reactive defense to proactive risk anticipation. By merging predictive analytics, machine learning, and risk intelligence, the chapter outlines adaptive models for forecasting attack vectors, managing vulnerabilities, and reducing operational risk in dynamic digital environments.

Chapter 9, ***Hybrid Systems Combining Neuroscience, AI, and Blockchain for Secure Environments*****,** proposes a tri-layer architecture that integrates neuro-biometric sensing, AI-driven intelligence, and blockchain-based trust. Through real-world use cases, the chapter illustrates how decentralized, transparent, and adaptive systems can enhance security across critical domains while acknowledging challenges in scalability and privacy.

Chapter 10, ***Neuromorphic Computing Architecture, Leading Chips, Hardware Innovations, and AI Integration*****,** explores the hardware foundations of brain-inspired computing. Focusing on neuromorphic chips, programming frameworks, and emerging memory technologies, this chapter highlights how energy-efficient, low-latency architectures can support real-time AI-driven cybersecurity, particularly at the edge and within IoT ecosystems.

Chapter 11, ***The Digital Corpus Callosum: Establishing Governance for Neuro-Enhanced AI Security*****,** concludes the volume by addressing governance and oversight. Introducing a layered framework that integrates ethical, technical, and operational controls, the chapter provides a blueprint for aligning autonomous Neuro-AI systems with human values, accountability, and long-term societal trust.

Together, these chapters present a comprehensive and multidisciplinary foundation for neuroscience-enhanced AI in cybersecurity. The book argues that the future of cyber defense lies not only in faster algorithms or larger datasets, but in intelligent systems that understand, adapt to, and ethically coexist with the human mind.

Shafiq Ul Rehman
Kingdom University, Bahrain

Chapter 1
Neurocriminology: The Brain Behind Crime

Harshini R.
https://orcid.org/0009-0004-2854-8876
Gujarat University, Ahmedabad, India

Dipak Kumar Mahida
https://orcid.org/0000-0003-1299-4623
Gujarat University, Ahmedabad, India

Kiran R. Dodiya
https://orcid.org/0009-0001-9409-7303
Gujarat University, Ahmedabad, India

Kapil Kumar
Gujarat University, Ahmedabad, India

Ankita Patel
Gujarat University, Ahmedabad, India

ABSTRACT

Neurocriminology explores the biological, neurological, and psychological underpinnings of criminal behavior, offering a science-based alternative to traditional sociological theories. It examines how brain structure, genetics, and environmental influences contribute to antisocial and violent tendencies. Abnormalities in areas like the prefrontal cortex and amygdala are linked to aggression, impulsivity, and lack of empathy. Technologies like fMRI and PET reveal brain deficits in offenders. Neurotransmitter imbalances, such as low serotonin and dysfunctional dopamine, also play a role. Studies, including on the MAOA "warrior gene," highlight how genetic traits interact with childhood trauma. Neurocriminology informs legal processes,

DOI: 10.4018/979-8-3373-5012-7.ch001

emphasizing crime prevention, rehabilitation, and ethical integration into justice systems. While rejecting biological determinism, it underscores a biopsychosocial model essential for a modern, humane approach to criminal justice.

INTRODUCTION

Neurocriminology is a field that researches the biological, psychological, and neuroscience by combining the insights from sociology that contribute to crime. Neurocriminology is a complex discipline studying the association of criminal behaviour with neurological, innate, and how well the brain works. In the 19th Century, Cesare Lombroso's controversial theories, the Modern advancement in research has built a firm scientific ground that exposure to redisposition in Neurobiological factors and brain abnormalities in the brain contribute to criminal behavioural tendencies. The modern neurocriminology offers a cutting-edge, integrative brain imaging, neurochemistry and physiological studies to reveal the correlation between brain structure and function with reference to particular studies in the prefrontal cortex, amygdala and criminal actions. It challenges the idea that crime is solely a social construct and how factors can vary, such as hereditary trauma, social context and brain injury. The studies involving twins, adoptees, have uncovered complex and compelling evidence that factors such as aggression and impulsive behaviour predispose individuals caused abnormalities in the amygdala, and reduced functional activities of the prefrontal cortex. The symbiosis between nature vs nurture seems crucial, while the factors like childhood abuse, lead exposure and poor nutrition also play a miserable role. From other criminological perspectives, which look at behaviour, cognition, and motivation factors independently, the neurocriminological perspective uniquely looks at the brain as the central convergence point. The new and expanding literature on neurocriminology poses intricate moral and legal conundrums pertaining to legal culpability and the punishment and prevention of criminal behaviour. The more we understand the structure of violence, the more we have to balance the proliferation of our technology with the social responsibility we owe to violence aggressors when we identify, contain, and possibly modify their behaviour.

Definition and Scope of Neurocriminology

Adrian Richard Raine & Andrea Lynn Glenn: "Neurocriminology means bringing together neurosciences with criminology. It studies what brain structures and functions are related to what forms and levels of delinquency and the legal and illegal uses of such information." (Glenn & Raine, 2014a).

Colleen Marie Berryessa & Adrian Richard Raine: "Neurocriminology seeks to apply principles, methods, and insights garnered from the field of neuroscience to the study of what causes crime, as well as how to predict best, prevent, and manage criminal behaviour and its consequences." (Berryessa & Raine, 2017).

Nathan Evan Anderson, Charles Henry Allen, and Kent Alan Kiehl: "Neurocriminology is an integrative perspective that draws on neuroscience and related biological sciences to understand crime, antisocial behaviour, and violence—emphasising how genetics, culture, pathology, and environment influence the brain and behaviour." (Anderson et al., 2024).

Figure 1 depicts the intersection of neuroscience and criminology, highlighting how brain structures and neural pathways relate to behavioural responses relevant to criminal behaviour.

Figure 1. This illustration depicts the intersection of neuroscience and criminology.

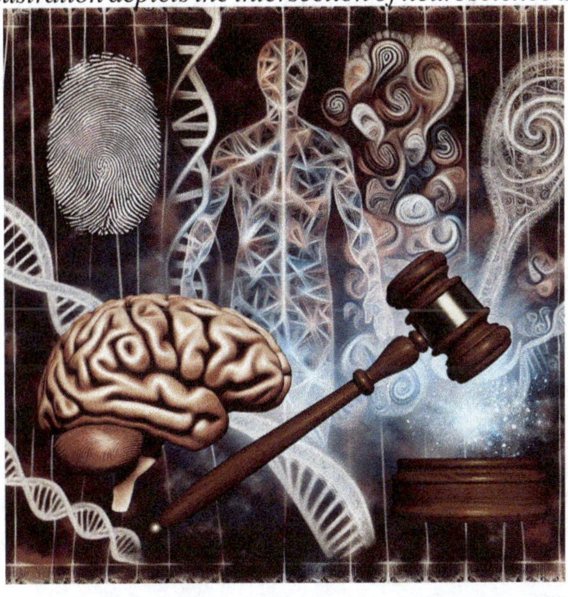

Historical Perspectives on Crime and Neuroscience

The modern specific advancements. Early criminological perspectives of 19th-century Italian Psychiatrist Cesare Lombroso speculated that criminal behaviour was deep-rooted in biological irregularities, including brain defects (Savopoulos &

Lindell, 2018). Lombroso's debatable theories influenced phrenology, proposing that physical traits and brain structure could predict criminal predispositions. His work laid the underpinning for biological positivism, which shifted the emphasis from crime itself to the offender's biological and psychological characteristics. ("Cesare Lombroso and the Origins of Criminology: Rethinking Criminological Tradition," 2005). Current neuroscience has been lingering on these ideas, utilising cutting-edge technology like EEG, fMRI, and PET scans to explore the association between brain function and criminal behaviours. Study related structural brain abnormalities, such as impairment to the prefrontal cortex or limbic system, to impulsivity, aggression and violent tendencies. For example, cases like Charles Whitman's violent action due to a brain tumour highlight how physiological factors can affect behaviour. (Glenn & Raine, 2014b).

The emerging field of neurocriminology fits in neuroscience with criminology to better understand criminal responsibility, recidivism and prevention methods. This method challenges meeting traditional notion of free will by emphasising how biology and environmental factors form behaviour. Neuroscience also describes legal practices through "neurolaw", which scrutinises the implications of brain science and culpability and passes judgments. While promising, this incorporates rising ethical concerns about determinism and justice in criminal accountability. (Aharoni et al., 2013) .

The Role of the Brain in Criminal Behaviour

The brain plays a pivotal role in significant criminal behaviour, with research importance in how structural and functional aspects can predispose individuals to antisocial actions. Two key reasons often associate are the prefrontal cortex and the Amygdala. (Anderson et al., 2024).

The prefrontal cortex, in charge of executing functions like decision making, impulse control, and moral reasoning, is recurrently linked to criminal propensities. Damage or underdeveloped in this part can weaken judgement and self-control, foremost to impulsive and aggressive behaviour. For example, individuals with prefrontal deviations often struggle to estimate consequences for consistent emotions and trade-offs commonly linked with vicious crimes. (Anderson et al., 2024).

The amygdala, part of the limbic system complex in emotional processing, also plays a substantial role. Abnormalities in the amygdala are connected with compact empathy and heightened aggression. Research has shown that individuals with smaller or less activity of Amygdalae may revelation psychopathic traits such as impulsivity and lack of remorse, which can contribute to criminal behaviour. (Anderson et al., 2024).

Elsewhere, structural issues, "neurochemical imbalances" relating to serotonin and dopamine, further stimulate behaviour. Low serotonin levels are linked to increased impulsivity and aggression, despite the fact that dopamine dysregulation can drive thrill-seeking and reward-seeking actions, hypothetically leading to criminal acts. (Anderson et al., 2024)..

Despite the fact that these neurobiological factors can increase the probability of criminal behaviour, they are not deterministic. Environmental impacts, personal choices, and social conditions also play a crucial role. Considering the brain's engagement provides valuable perceptions for prevention and rehabilitation strategies. However, it must be cohesive with across-the-board psychological and societal contexts. (Anderson et al., 2024).

Table 1. Major brain regions and their corresponding crime-related behaviours

Region	Function	Associated Behavior
PFC	Executive control	Impulsivity, risk-taking
Amygdala	Emotional reactivity	Aggression, reduced empathy
Striatum	Reward pathway	Sensation-seeking, compulsive acts

NEUROBIOLOGICAL BASIS OF CRIMINAL CONDUCT

Criminal behaviour correlates with certain neurobiological factors that pertain to certain arrangements of the brain and its genetics. In particular, the prefrontal cortex and the amygdala, which are responsible for controlling impulses and emotions, respectively, tend to have noticeable structural and functional deficiencies among offenders. On the other hand, the striatum is believed to possibly have increased activity and growth in individuals who possess antisocial traits and or have a low level of self-control, and is associated with the reward processing (Yang & Raine, 2009). Environmental factors collude with the genetic factors that explain 40 to 60% of the variance pertaining to antisocial behaviour. Impulsivity and aggression are increased by neurochemical factors (such as low serotonin and or dopamine). These factors, in addition to the social environment, are best described as predictors of criminal behaviour (Raine, 2008).

Brain Areas Connected with Aggression and Violence

The ventrolateral ventromedial hypothalamus (VMHvl) and the additional brain portion with aggression control are focally concerned with aggression-related brain components. VMHvl engages in predatory aggression and, from mouse studies, VMHvl is active anterior to predatory attacks (Hashikawa, Falkner, & Lin, 2017)). The control of impulse and decision making is concerned with the prefrontal cortex (PFC). More specifically, the dorsolateral (dlPFC) and the orbitofrontal areas are the most influential, whereas lesions of the PFC are correlated with response inhibition deficits, positive aggression and implicit violence attitudes. The Amygdala is the brain structure that is augmented in aggressive individuals and is principally in charge of threat recognition and control of emotions, and is, at the same time, with the PFC, in control of emotions. A significant portion of PFC in aggressive individuals is atrophic. This is connected with the podus subdivision of today's control. The superior temporal gyrus and the temporoparietal junction are acknowledged and are iso/volumetrically linked to the borderline of mydi violence. These constructios are linked to crude violence, and the temporoparietal junction is iso volumetrically known. Additionally, in fractionated aggressive individuals, the prefrontal cortex is under the subordination of the striatum, and there are attenuated constructions. These constructions are neuroimaging the limbic system, indicating that the control of the cortex is predominantly over the propagation of rational aggression. (Raine et al., 2000).

Neurotransmitters and Hormonal Effects on Behaviour

Serotonin deficiency reduces prefrontal cortex control, which in turn increases impulsive and aggressive behaviour. Dopamine imbalance, which is a factor in seeking out reward, also leads to risk-taking and violent action. GABA is a calming neurotransmitter which puts the brakes on subcortical action; we see increased aggression when GABA activity goes down. Also, it has been found that testosterone plays a role in dominant and responsive aggression, which, in particular, we see a lot of in competitive settings (Seo et al., 2008). Oxytocin, which is mostly known for its role in social bonding, can also be seen to increase aggression toward out-groups in stressed states. Vasopressin, which is tied to territory issues, does, in fact, in a study increase aggression(De Dreu, 2012). Alcohol plays a role by its effect on the prefrontal cortex, which it impedes, and also by what it does to the amygdala, which it heightens, thus increasing violence. We see that neurochemical imbalances, along with environmental factors like stress, play a role in the development of aggression by, in large perturbing the brain's regulation(Carré & Olmstead, 2015). As shown in Figure 2, trauma has a significant impact on brain development, particularly affecting regions responsible for emotional regulation, memory, and decision-making, and Figure 3 presents a classification of childhood trauma based on nature and severity, illustrating how various forms of abuse and environmental stressors contribute to long-term psychological outcomes.

Figure 2. Impact of Trauma on Brain Development

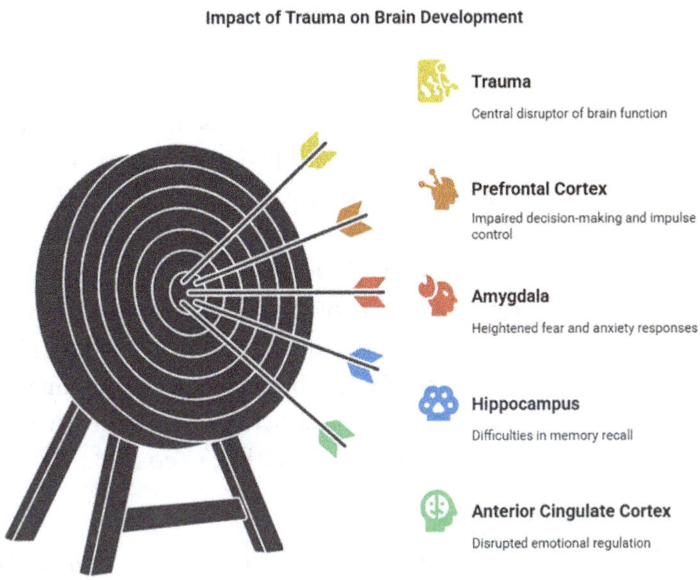

Figure 3. Classification of childhood trauma based on nature and severity.

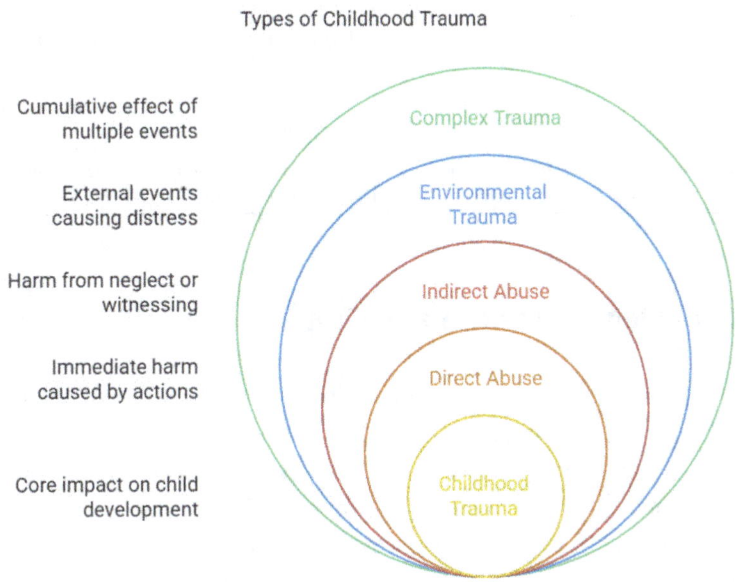

Genetic and Epigenetic Factors in Criminality

Research reports that between 40 and 60% of what we see in anti-social traits is hereditary, which we see play out via genes like MAOA, which is involved in serotonin processing. Also, it is noted that low activity forms of MAOA L, when coupled with child trauma, increase the chance of violent outbursts. Also, we see those epigenetic changes in stress-related genes like FKBP5 play a role in how the environment plays into genetics' role in increased aggression after trauma. Also, there is the case of COMT, which we see play a role in impulsive behaviour, in which CDH13 mutations are associated with ADHD and violent crime. However, it is also true that these genetic predispositions do not work in a vacuum -- they play out in the context of psychosocial issues like abuse or neglect, which in turn play a role in criminal behaviour. Also, we see that from substance abuse or trauma brought on epigenetic changes that in turn modify neural structures, which in turn change what sets off aggressive responses (Verhoeven et al., 2012), (Yeo et al., 2017)

Table 2. Key Genetic/Epigenetic Markers and Their Interaction With Environmental Factors

Gene / Marker	Environmental Moderator	Effect on Risk
MAOA-L (Low-activity variant)	Childhood abuse, maltreatment	Strongly increases aggression and violent behaviour when paired with early trauma.
COMT (Val158Met)	Stress, low socioeconomic status	Increases impulsivity and weak executive control
FKBP5 (Epigenetic methylation)	Early-life trauma, chronic stress	Heightens emotional dysregulation and aggression due to altered stress-response
CDH13	ADHD symptoms, social adversity	Associated with antisocial traits and violent offending
5-HTTLPR (Short allele)	Stressful life events	Increased aggression/anxiety due to impaired serotonin regulation

The Role of Mental Disorders in Crime

Conduct disorder and antisocial personality disorder (ASPD) are the most common disorders linked to aggression and often are the result of prefrontal-amygdala undercontrol. Amygdala dysfunctions with a lack of empathy are associated with instrumental violence, also known as psychopathy. Aggression may occur in other violent conditions, such as schizophrenia, during psychotic episodes, because of sheer paranoia or hallucinations, although most sufferers are nonviolent. In combination with substance abuse, PTSD increases reactivity to aggression due to heightened amygdala activity and diminished control from the prefrontal cortex (PFC). Interventions rely heavily on ADHD and intermittent explosive disorder (IED), which is characterised by impulsivity and serotonin deficiencies, which causes more aggression. Addressing neurobiological factors with psychosocial contexts is essential for effective treatment, as mental illness alone rarely explains criminal activity. (Raine & Marek, 2013), (Goodkind et al., 2015).

COGNITIVE AND EMOTIONAL DEFICITS IN OFFENDERS

Unscrupulous acts stem from diminished activity in the prefrontal area of the brain, which is vital for control of impulses and decision-making. The emotional disentanglement due to the amygdala–prefrontal disconnect reduces empathy and increases aggression. Underlying criminal acts like substance abuse stem from a dopamine imbalance in the striatum, which drives risk-taking and addictive behaviour. Address these deficits with behavioural cognitive strategies to improve self-control and recidivism. (Chamberlain & Sahakian, 2007).

Impulsivity and Decision-Making Deficits

Offenders often commit impulsive and bad decisions due to a problem in the brain's prefrontal cortex. The dorsolateral PFC plays a key role in planning and controlling our actions. Reduced levels of grey matter in the area are associated with impulsive aggression and poor assessment of risk and its consequences. Offenders often engage in delay discounting, choosing immediate rewards over long-term outcomes as a result of weak PFC regulation of limbic regions such as the amygdala and striatum. Tests that ask people to stop doing something or change how they do something find it hard. Offenders frequently distort their thinking, such as by downplaying the harm their behaviour causes or justifying it. Environmental triggers, such as substance abuse, worsen PFC hypoactivity and judgment impairment caused by these deficits. Different kinds of cognitive interventions focus on regulating and improving related skills to help reduce re-offending (Bechara, 2005).

Emotional Dysregulation and Lack of Empathy

Criminals frequently show lower affective empathy, as evidenced in studies where they have a diminished emotional response to others' suffering using emotion-related videos. Convicts and offenders participate in research, and the outcome usually shows reduced affective empathy, which exhibits a reduced response to sadness due to one's condition. Dysregulation of the amygdala-prefrontal circuits causes problems with the regulation of emotions, which produces excess aggression when stress or frustration overcomes cortical control (Decety & Jackson, 2004). People with psychopathy may be able to understand other people's intentions (cognitive empathy), but they are unlikely to feel much compassion or remorse for others. Experiencing failure of affective empathy, which is associated with dysfunction of the inferior frontal gyrus and anterior insula, makes that happen. Sex offenders, for instance, may not feel guilty, as they cognitively distort reality (e.g., blame the victim). Low serotonin level influences emotional dysregulation due to the loss of control over violent impulses. Therapies that focus on feeling and empathy-building can deal with these deficiencies (Blair, 2005).

Risk-Taking Behaviour and Addiction

An offender's tendency to take risks is due to the hyperactivity of the striatal reward pathways and dopamine dysregulation. These phenomena intensify the offender's sensation-seeking and impulsive choices. Many criminals abuse substances, which makes them take risks. This is because drugs further disable the PFC, while enhancing striatal dopamine release. Studies on delay discounting show that offenders prioritise risky and immediate rewards because of insufficient PFC-striatal connectivity. Environmental factors that include trauma and peer pressure will further entrench maladaptive behaviour and also normalise risk-taking behaviour, both at home and on the street. Crimes (like stealing to get drugs) happen due to compulsive reward-seeking, which is a direct result of brain changes that take place in the mesolimbic pathway. Using approaches that combine cognitive remediation (eg, boosting executive function) and addiction treatment (eg, contingency management), the brain and behaviour that underpin risk-taking are each treated. (Volkow et al., 2003), (Chamberlain & Sahakian, 2007).

THE INFLUENCE OF EARLY LIFE EXPERIENCES

Experiencing trauma as a child harms how the brain develops. Maltreatment causes a surge in cortisol, damaging the hippocampus and negating stress control. Being poor makes things worse by limiting nice experiences, causing bad behaviour. Brain training at a young age to heal trauma may be helpful in crime prevention. (Anda et al., 2005).

Childhood Trauma and Brain Development

Childhood trauma such as abuse, neglect or household dysfunction disrupts key brain development, especially in areas that govern emotion and behaviour. People with a high ACE have reduced grey matter volume in a part of the brain called the prefrontal cortex that controls impulse control and decision-making. Due to this, they are impaired in their ability to control themselves. The amygdala may become hyperactive, leading to aggressive and fearful behaviours. When stress occurs in childhood, this causes the cortisol levels to be elevated, which damages the hippocampus. The change in structure makes you more compelled to do something without thinking, and increases harm and defects. (Anda et al., 2005).

The Impact of Abuse, Neglect, and Socioeconomic Factors

As a result of maladaptive stress responses, people who suffer from physical abuse are more likely to be aggressive. On the other hand, emotional neglect causes difficulty feeling empathy and forming social bonds. Poverty makes things worse. It makes people go to the wrong schools and lose their health can use crime to cope. Research indicates that people from poorer backgrounds are overrepresented in crime. Factors arising from poverty, such as parental instability, compound the impacts of ACEs on people. Neglect refers particularly to physical neglect, which is greatly associated with recidivism because it disrupts attachment and self-worth, and this pushes people to take risks. (Farrington, 2005).

The Role of Parenting and Environmental Stressors

Parenting that is inconsistent and/or harsh will undermine a secure attachment. This can result in attachment disorder and a lack of empathy. Being exposed to domestic violence treatment teaches children that violence is a way to solve conflicts and that crime is normal behaviour. Experiencing violence in the community and police involvement in childhood further entrenches anti-social behaviour through added trauma and reduced trust. Environmental stressors and the substance abuse of caregivers obstruct child nurturing, along with the exclusion of these children from school. The combination of these factors enhances their risk of delinquency. To break this cycle, timely interventions that enhance parenting quality and environmental stability matter (Margolin & Gordis, 2000).

NEUROCRIMINOLOGY AND VIOLENT OFFENDERS

People who commit violent crimes have unique biological abnormalities, including problems with the amygdala and the prefrontal cortex. Psychopaths have less grey matter in the anterior cingulate cortex linked to instrumental aggression. Offenders of sexual crimes often show striatal hyperactivity and orbitofrontal dysfunction. The latter induces an irresistible urge or compulsion to act. Based on this reasoning, it is possible to plan a neurofeedback intervention to improve emotional regulation. (Shamay-Tsoory et al., 2010).

Serial Killers and Psychopathy: Brain Abnormalities

Serial killers and psychopaths seem to have neurobiological traits that set them apart from normal people. For example, there are some noticeable structural abnormalities in the brains of serial killers. These areas control our ability to prevent such actions, feel empathy, and process fear. Malfunctions of this system are noted for the lack of remorse, instrumental type of violence, and poor emotional regulation. Brain abnormalities like cavum septi pellucidi maldevelopment are linked to serious criminality and aggression. Functional neuroimaging reveals low levels of glucose metabolism in the prefrontal cortex and low levels of activity in the amygdala during moral decision-making, which could explain the lack of feeling guilt and lack of feeling empathy. Psychopaths' damage to their posterior cingulate and angular gyrus disrupts social cognition, self-awareness (Shamay-Tsoory et al., 2010).

Mass Shooters and Terrorism. Neurological Perspectives

People who do mass shootings often have hyperactive limbic systems paired with PFC hypoactivity, leading to poor threat assessment and impulsive aggression. Studies involving brain imaging show that a person suffering from violent outbursts is likely to show raised subcortical activity due to a high reaction to emotion. Certain environmental causes (social isolation, trauma), along with neurochemical imbalance (low serotonin, high dopamine), can worsen the violence which seeks reward. Research did not find the so-called "terrorist brain" profiles. However, some argue that cognitive rigidity and aggression linked to group identity may result from impaired frontal-limbic connectivity and consequential inability for rational decision making. (Dom et al., 2018).

Neurocriminology of Sexual Offenders

Sexual predators present with OFC dysfunction, which in turn causes issues with impulse control and reward processing. Amygdala prefrontal disconnect, which we see in these offenders, also causes low empathy and high in predatory behaviour. At the same time, we see hypersexuality related to striatal hyperactivity and dopamine dysregulation. Also, we see that cognitive distortions like victim blaming in these patients present with reduced ACC activity, which in turn impairs error identification and guilt. We have neurobiological interventions like neurofeedback and cognitive behavioural therapy, which we use to target these issues in an effort to reduce recidivism. (Raine et al., 1994).

CASE STUDIES

Notorious Criminal Cases Analysed Through Neurocriminology

The study of neurocriminology has shed light on unique and damaging instances like the one involving Phineas Gage. In 1848, Phineas Gage's prefrontal cortex (PFC) was injured and with that injury came an alteration in his brain. He used to be a responsible worker, but after his injury, he became impulsive, aggressive, and transformed into a sociopath. He is one of the main examples of brain-behaviour links being present and not absent, showing evidence of the Gage phenomenon. Donta Page was a borderline sociopath murderer, and, in his case, childhood trauma mixed with abuse was deadly. Combine that with meagre glucose metabolism in the PFC, and we get a chronic angry man who is regularly violent. His prefrontal lobe dysfunction, along with his environment, predisposed him to violence. Whitman, who infamously shot people in the Texas Tower in 1966, had a brain tumour compressing his amygdala. This part of his brain was crucial to explosive violence. Edward Rulloff was a transitive killer active in the 19th century. Rulloff underwent post-mortem brain research, inferring physical characteristics of morality to violence, trying to attempt the path of modern neurocriminology. It was conducted with markers of neurocriminology still not present. It is astonishing how ultimately we all receive solutions from the strangest places, such as the examples of Jeffrey Dahmer and Issei Sagawa. Their torment and the social control and strain paradigms are also to be mindful of the more basal, primal bio components of neurophysiopathy abstention and sociopathy of the closed urges deprivation neurology. These exemplars amplify the interaction of brain pathology with the social and executive systems of the PFC and amygdala, trauma inflicted upon the individual, and the MAOA genotype-poverty as criminal behaviour. Determinism and the absence of moral and legal accountability are the paradigms to be addressed. (Rigoni et al., 2010).

Brain Imaging Evidence in Criminal Trials

Brain imaging, with instruments like PET scans and fMRI, has become an integrated part of evaluating a person's culpability. In the case of Donta Page, there was impulsiveness as a factor, which in his case was explained by reduced ventral PFC glucose metabolism. He was not exonerated of his guilt, however. Adrian Raine studied 41 murderers in 1994 and found that they had prefrontal hypoactivity, amygdala incompetence, which made his statement on emotional regulation impairment harder to dispute. Contemporary research on homicide offenders has shown losses of grey matter in the orbital frontal cortex and anterior temporal lobes, differentiating them from non-homicidal offenders. While the courts are still careful, it is already established that using imaging techniques, such as temporal lobe epilepsy, mitigates the punishment. These techniques can also establish the defence of 'the crime was not committed with free volition', which commonly undermines personal responsibility. Landmark cases such as Anthony Battaglia came up with the idea such as using MRI scans to detect lies, which many deem does not provide sufficient reliability. Neuroimaging's role in trials highlights tensions between neurobiological determinism and legal responsibility, emphasising the need for interdisciplinary collaboration to balance science and justice. (Raine et al., 1994).

ADVANCES IN NEUROSCIENTIFIC TECHNIQUES

High-resolution fMRI and AI-derived brain-age estimation are sharpening crime analysis. Hypoactivity in prefrontal regions and hyperactivity in the striatum, based on fMRI studies, correlate with impulsivity in offenders. 90% accurate and free from human error, fMRI-based lie detection outperforms polygraphs, yet has not received legal acceptance due to its reliability. BCIs for intent detection threaten Fifth Amendment rights; instead must be coded ethically. (Tortora et al., 2020). Figure 4 visualises brain activation and neural signal transmission, offering insight into how specific areas of the brain process stimuli that may influence aggressive or antisocial behaviour.

Figure 4. Visualisation of brain activation and neural signal transmission.

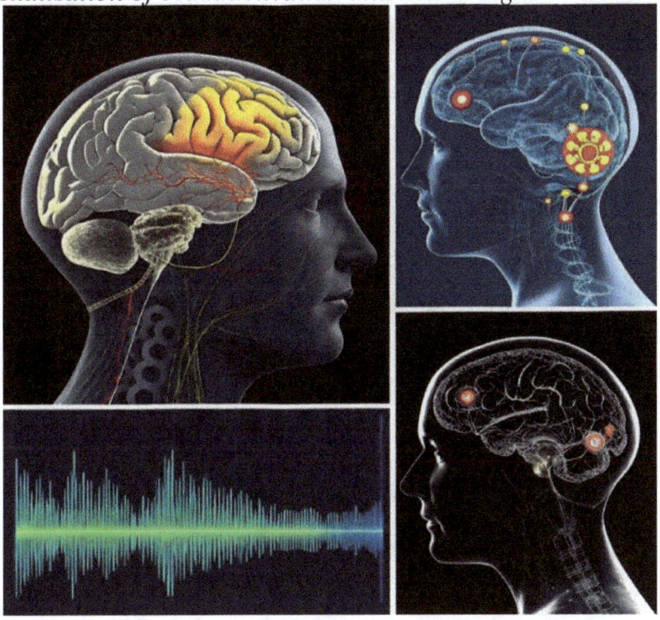

Neuroimaging: fMRI, PET Scans, and EEG in Criminal Behaviour Studies

There is a connection between reduced prefrontal cortex (PFC) activity, impaired impulse control and decision making, and violent offending, as determined by functional MRI (fMRI). PET scans of the brain in psychopaths also demonstrate amygdala dysfunction, which accounts for the absence of fear and empathy. Structural MRI (sMRI) shows less grey matter in the orbital frontal cortex and anterior temporal lobes of homicide offenders, which is a difference that sets them apart from non-violent criminals. Abnormal brain wave activity, like the irregular theta waves associated with aggression, is what the EEG registers in impulsive people. These are some of the ways we can quantify a neural risk factor (e.g., PFC-amygdala dysregulation) and some of the ways we can customise a cognitive-behavioural therapy intervention. Figure 5 (Nilawati et al., 2024) shows the brain's various violent tendencies by comparing the structural, functional, and electrical components of the brain through the use of fMRI, PET, and EEG technology.

Figure 5. Comparative imaging of brain activity using fMRI, PET, and EEG.

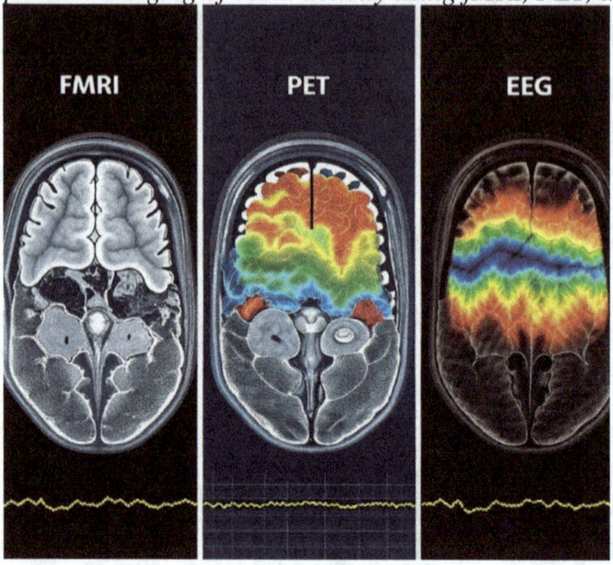

Lie Detection and Polygraphy: Neuroscientific Perspectives

Although they also measure physiological stress (e.g., heart rate), their accuracy (~70%) has been debated due to the number of false positives. An fMRI plan that uses the anterior cingulate cortex and ventrolateral brain activity associated with deception may give 90% accuracy, compared to polygraphs. However, says Wong, fMRI has a hard time telling lies from self-interested decisions without algorithmic tweaking. Courts have continued to be wary: in the case of Anthony Battaglia, fMRI lie detection was said to be unreliable for the purposes of law. The ethical issues remain around misuse as a "brain defence" to avoid accountability. (La Tona et al., 2020), (Schauer, 2010). The standard setup of a polygraph test, as shown in Figure 6, illustrates how physiological responses are monitored to assess deception during forensic interviews and investigations.

Figure 6. Standard setup of a polygraph (lie detector) test.

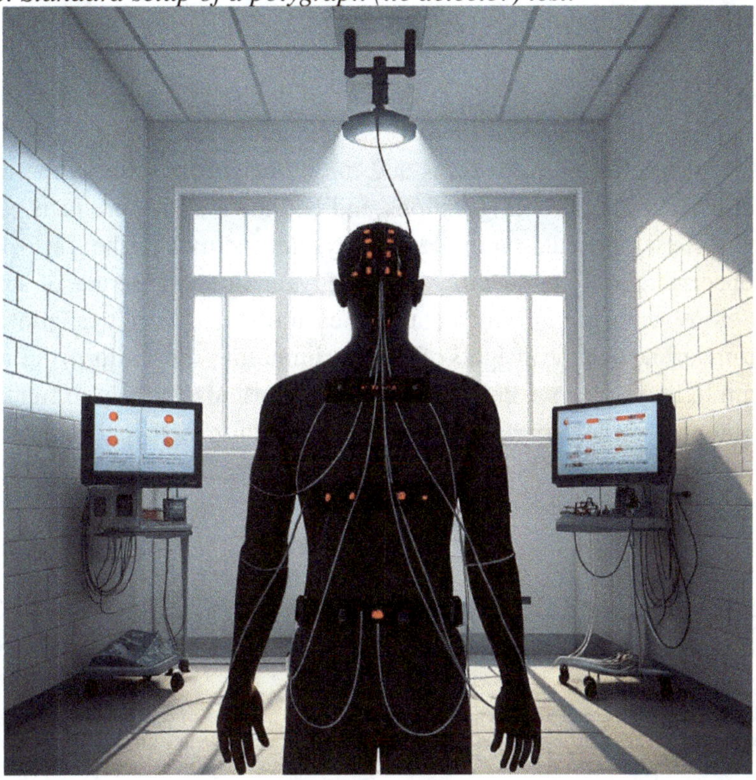

Brain-Computer Interfaces and Criminal Intent Detection

Rendering neural signals actionable: BCIs are typically used twofold, first to determine a person's intent via neural decoding, such as with EEG-based "brain fingerprinting", which detects hidden knowledge. Some systems analyse activity from the PFC and the parietal lobe to predict premeditated behaviour; however, precision is limited. Legal discussions focus on self-incrimination risks, as BCIs could sidestep verbal testimony and infringe upon Amendment V. Still experimental, BCIs underscore the tension between neuroscience's promise as the best bet for preventing crime and its perils to cognitive liberty. (Poldrack et al., 2020; Van Veen et al., 2001).

LEGAL AND ETHICAL CONSIDERATIONS OF NEUROCRIMINOLOGY

Neurocriminology studies the convergence of the Neurosciences and law. There is currently a palpable interest from theorists and practitioners alike in the possible links between specific brain patterns and the propensity to offend, the rationale being that certain neural configurations and activities might produce particular behaviours. These particular activities, in my view, stimulate the most pertinent ethical concerns relating to social responsibility, equity and the use of science in Courts. Before venturing into the details of each of these activities, allow me, of course, to underline that the insights of Neurocriminology must inform the activities that pertain to these case studies. However, they must also adhere to fundamental rights pertaining to due process and the negative right to self-incrimination. Only then can a compatible equilibrium be achieved between society's claim to public safety and justice (Kraft & Giordano, 2017).

Table 3. Ethical and Legal Considerations When Using Neurodata in Justice Settings

Issue	Risk Description	Recommended Safeguards / Policy Options
Privacy & Cognitive Liberty	Brain imaging and neurodata may reveal mental states, personal traits, or unintended information; risk of compelled brain data collection.	Strict data-protection laws prohibit forced neuroimaging, treat neural data as highly sensitive, and require judicial warrants and a narrow scope.
Informed Consent	Offenders may feel pressured to consent to neurointerventions, imaging, or testing in exchange for reduced sentences.	Ensure voluntary consent; provide independent legal/medical counselling; ban coercive plea-based neurointerventions.
Bias & Discrimination	AI/neuro-risk algorithms may reinforce racial or social bias, risk of unfair profiling or predictive sentencing.	Transparent algorithm auditing; bias testing; integrate social-context variables; restrict use for punitive decisions.
Determinism & Reduced Responsibility	Courts may overinterpret neural abnormalities as excusing guilt or predicting future dangerousness.	Judicial guidelines clarifying limits of neuroevidence; expert testimony standards; emphasise non-determinism.
Coercion in Rehabilitation	Neurotechnologies (TMS, medication, neurofeedback) may be mandated without proper safeguards.	Clear ethical frameworks, allow opt-out, prioritise therapy over punishment, and periodic oversight committees.

The Use of Neuroscience in Criminal Trials

More recently, both defence attorneys and prosecutors have begun to utilise neuroscience in the courtroom, presenting evidence such as functional MRIs, EEGs, or genetic evidence. One such example is the legal issue of evidence admissibility: a judge applying the Daubert or Frye standards must decide whether the scientific technique in question is sufficiently reliable and a preaching consensus exists in the scientific community before it can be presented to the jury. As an example, evidence of a functional MRI which demonstrates a decrease of activity in the prefrontal cortex (which controls impulse regulation) may be admitted as evidence of a legal diminishing of the defendant's mental capacity, which could serve to lower a defendant's legal consequences. (Jones & Shen, 2012).

However, courts must be vigilant against undue reliance on "neuromyths." Brain scans can be persuasive to laypeople, but they rarely have the precision required of an individual-level proof of causation. There needs to be clear jury instructions to judges and juries that a neural anomaly does not prove Mens rea. To prevent misleading the fact-finder, expert witnesses should ground their testimony in lay language and clear state limitations and error rates. (Jones & Shen, 2012).

Neuroevidence also raises privacy concerns, both from an ethical standpoint as human cognition is involved and from practical considerations when such information is given to others. Mandating that a defendant undergo brain imaging can conflict with the Fifth Amendment privilege against self-incrimination, at least if the imaging results were used as testimonial evidence. (Jones & Shen, 2012).

Likewise, utilisation of predictive biomarkers in pretrial evaluations may yield profiling or discriminatory bail decisions. (Jones & Shen, 2012) .

In the end, the role of neuroscience in the courts needs to be a happy medium: It should bring something to bear on the court's search for truth without violating procedural due process. Establishing clear rules of procedure for expert qualifications, for the chain of custody of neural data and for judicial gatekeeping is necessary to ensure that frontier science supports rather than subverts justice. (Kraft & Giordano, 2017).

The Debate on Free Will vs Determinism in Crime

Within neurocriminology exist two opposing schools of thought: free will and determinism. These supposedly opposing constructs highlight our ability to determine our actions, while the latter proposes that our behaviours are a result of the interplay between our biology, the surrounding environment, and the underlying neurophysiology. The foundation of criminal law rests on the assumption that individuals have the ability to make choices and that these choices are voluntary actions. How do we determine accountability when evidence provided by neuroscience suggests that an individual has such limited choices to make because of a suboptimal brain configuration? (Urbaniok et al., 2006)

Advocates of free will argue that neuroscience illustrates a trend, rather than establishing a cause for criminal actions. For instance, a genetic variant or a lesion in a given brain region may increase the propensity for impulsivity. However, it would not necessarily lead to a justification for a criminal act. The law upholds that individuals, except in the case of complete exoneration through duress or insanity, maintain moral and legal accountability. The insanity defence outlined in the Model Penal Code stipulates that, in such cases, the individual must have had a significant lack of ability to grasp the concept that what they were doing was wrong (Urbaniok et al., 2006)

In response to the comments from advocates of free will, if the actions of the brain ultimately result in behaviour, then the justification for retributive justice should also be questioned, and, to some extent, this would be correct. Determinism suggests that such behaviours are pre-determined, and that the range of choices available to an individual determining how they will act in a given situation is in itself severely limited.

Why punish people for decisions that are not really theirs? This line of thought encourages a preventive or rehabilitative model: neuropsychological screening of at-risk individuals to identify, channel, and treat or counsel them, instead of locking them up (Urbaniok et al, 2006).

This line of thought generates ethical considerations on sentencing. A judge may conclude that a criminal's brain scan shows a high likelihood of reoffending and, in the name of societal protection, impose a longer sentence, even when that sentence punishes a person for a condition that is not within their control. Alternatively, recognising neurocognitive shortfalls may open the door to mitigation, and therefore to a reduction of sentences, but this generates a reasonable concern about public safety (Hirstein, 2022).

A good bridge between free will and determinism will require an understanding of how law must recognise the impact of biology on human conduct, without losing sight of the fact that the law must also consider that individuals are, of course, responsible for their decisions. A society that seeks the most judicious application of this new knowledge about the human condition in the courtroom will require a social contract guided by the law, clear definitions of mental responsibility, and a partnership between the life sciences and the law (Hirstein, 2022).

The Ethical Implications of Neuroscience: A Case Study

The rise of mainstream neurotechnology, of deep-brain stimulation, neurofeedback training, and pharmacological modulation, now enables the prospect of targeting the prevention and treatment of criminal behaviour. The ethical implications of attempting to persuade a larger segment of the population to consent to what are being called neurointerventions are, if anything, more profound (Tesink et al., 2023).

I believe the first suggestion must be informed consent, a defendant who has been offered the alternative of prison to be provided with the possible consequences of personality changes, cognitive changes or other unknowns (Tesink et al., 2023). Courts and doctors have a responsibility to manage the risk of voluntariness from a vulnerable person with the possible benefit of a plea deal, as this may reject real consent (Tesink et al., 2023).

Next, there is the medicalisation of crime, the reclassification of some antisocial practices as a neural and behavioural disorder. This may decrease the stigma associated with diminished responsibility, but this is the slippery slope in which the medical model of antisocial neurological practices is dominant (Lara, 2023).

Finally, there is a real danger of exacerbating a social inequity. 'highly promoted and developed in economically affluent practices' cutting-edge technological treatment are in contrast to the rest of the population (Tesink et al., 2023).

Lastly, concerns must be addressed regarding the ethics of such changes. If it is possible to decrease aggression or increase empathy through neural modulation, would we be removing the real self? If we consider the moral enhancement of someone, the question of ethics becomes more complex. Should we, with the assistance of technology, shift an individual's behaviour toward the socially acceptable, even if we do it with their consent? (Lara, 2023)

In conclusion, to act responsibly with the proposed potential of neuroscience must be controlled. Access to any such incentive must be equitable with the purpose of monitoring the result. It must be made clear in law which side of the law would apply to such treatment protocols so that public safety is assured, and individuals remain unhindered.(Lara, 2023).

NEUROCRIMINOLOGY IN CRIMINAL JUSTICE AND REHABILITATION

Neurocriminology makes the justice system aware of brain functioning, and thereby the consideration of risk assessment and damage control. Changes to brain structure, e.g. smaller prefrontal cortex, and genetic predisposing factors, e.g. CDH13, allow us to detect individuals at risk. TMS and neurofeedback, both neuromodulation techniques, may help rehabilitate offenders by regulating connectivity in the amygdala-prefrontal circuit. Nonetheless, ethical issues of coercion in prison-based interventions require frameworks which protect autonomy and equity. (Harms et al., 2017).

Predicting Criminal Behaviour Using Neuroscience

Neuroscience can identify neurobiological risk factors for criminal behaviour, but there are ethical and practical challenges. MRI and other structural neuroimaging techniques are primarily used to illustrate abnormality in brain structures, such as reduced prefrontal cortex (PFC) volume, amygdala dysfunction, which correlates with aggressive and impulsive behaviours. Studies using functional MRI (fMRI) show that violent offenders have low activity in the part of the brain that makes decisions. Genetic markers such as MAOA-L variants increase the risk for aggression when combined with childhood trauma. Epigenetic changes like methylation of FKBP5 mediate stress responses.(Verhoeven et al., 2012). Abnormal theta waves, when detected on EEG, may indicate impulsivity in high-risk individuals. (Harms et al., 2017).

However, predictive models face limitations. A positive result for a biological condition may stigmatise an individual. Neuroplasticity and environment limit deterministic claims. Current tools do not yet generate precise forecasts of who will commit a particular crime. This is an ethical concern in itself, as pre-emptive policing may discriminate against various social groups. For example, models trained on recidivism-related data generally capture the biases present. The legal system struggles with how to balance public safety with individual rights, such as using neurodata for parole. Even as neuroscience improves the stratification of risk, the incorporation of psychosocial assessments is essential to prevent the reduction of criminality to biology.(Reyes & Amador, 2009).

Neurological Interventions for Criminal Rehabilitation

Using neurointerventions to reduce re-offending by modifying biological contributors to crime is becoming popular. Medicines such as SSRIs reduce aggression, while medicines that reduce sex drive (e.g. cyproterone acetate) suppress any sex urges in offenders. Using techniques like transcranial magnetic stimulation (TMS) and deep-brain stimulation (DBS) to regulate PFC-amygdala connectivity can help improve impulse control. Neurofeedback helps offenders control their brain activity and learn to manage emotions better and develop empathy. (Tesink et al., 2023).

Table 4. Neurorehabilitation Techniques and Their Targets with Ethical Notes

Intervention	Neural Target	Ethical Considerations / Notes
TMS (Transcranial Magnetic Stimulation)	Prefrontal cortex (impulse control, emotion regulation)	Moderate evidence; risk of coercion in prisons; must ensure voluntary consent.
DBS (Deep Brain Stimulation)	Amygdala, ventral striatum (aggression circuits)	Experimental; highly invasive; major consent concerns; not suitable as a sentencing alternative.
SSRIs / Pharmacotherapy	Serotonin pathways affecting aggression & impulsivity	Strong evidence; risk of forced medication; requires medical monitoring & informed consent.
CBT (Cognitive Behavioural Therapy)	Prefrontal cognitive networks for decision-making & empathy	strong evidence; low ethical risk; must avoid coercive framing and ensure fair access.
Neurofeedback	PFC–amygdala connectivity (self-regulation circuits)	Moderate evidence; privacy issues with neural data; participation must remain voluntary.

Studies that examine populations with ethical concerns regarding consent (especially where there are power imbalances) are more likely to be criticised than studies that examine populations without ethical concerns. Danish studies highlight the need to reflect on how psychiatric treatments can devolve into custodial forms of control. X faces concerns regarding under-medicalisation that can accompany forms of over-medicalisation, where the problem is approached from a biological perspective rather than. Some advocates of Argument One suggest that neurorehabilitation as a form of therapy could be a moral imperative to counter the dehumanisation that occurs during incarceration and, more broadly, to provide equitable access to adequate therapeutic interventions. It is necessary to have more stringent control and more multidisciplinary approaches, incorporating mechanisms of rehabilitation that are not violative of human rights (Lara, 2023).

Risk Assessment and Prevention Strategies

Neuroscience-informed risk assessments consider neurobiological and psychosocial dimensions to update and enhance predictions about recidivism. Integrated systems utilise fMRI, genetic, and cognitive testing to pinpoint individuals requiring specific intervention strategies and risk management (so that they can be fully targeted). For instance, specific biomarkers of impulsivity can identify individuals who may benefit from cognitive behavioural therapy focusing on PFC (dys)function and empathy training. Significant early intervention and trauma-focused strategies neuroplastically engage adolescents, steering their development along more positive paths (Mulyadi et al., 2024).

Strategies must also address structural inequities: poverty and trauma increase neurobiological risk, underscoring the need for risk-reducing policies that tackle stressors like housing instability. Community-based neurorehabilitation - for example, mindfulness-based programs - provides non-intrusive, yet effective, strategies for emotional dysregulation. On the other hand, untempered reliance on the neuro predictors can lead to biological determinism, creating the risk of overshadowing other important social equity reforms of the systems. The social equity gained from systems will be undermined, and systemic reforms will be postponed without appropriate social equity frameworks for systems that respect privacy and social autonomy, and refrain from punitive, pre-crime level predictions. Social equity, justice and legislative frameworks must be centred on the positive social equity gained, restorative justice, and active rehabilitative justice (Gavazzi et al., 2008).

Neurocriminology hopes to refine the accuracy of risk assessment tools for predicting and preventing crime using machine learning and new technologies in neuroimaging (particularly in the prefrontal cortex) and in genetics (particularly the MAOA-L variant), A minial sample population challenges the efficacy of machine learning fueled algorithms, and risk stratification is to be improved. A more precise neuro ethical framework is needed to address the infringement of cognitive liberty. The possible rehabilitation of individuals with neurodevices and CRISPR technologies is controversial as self incrimination and privacy in a digital world are paramount. Predictive modeling suffers from a lack of large data sets, and the incorporation of new protective measures is needed. Future research will be able to create new protective measures (Tortora et al., 2020).

The Potential of AI and Neurocriminology

AI will most likely reshape neurocriminology by making predictions and personalized approaches more accurate than ever before. Machine learning techniques that evaluate neuroimaging data like fMRI and PET scans can detect aggression, impulsivity, and psychopathy-linked markers. For example, some studies have enhanced the prediction of recidivism by using neural combustions such as the anterior cingulate cortex (ACC) activity and brain-age measures alongside structural and functional brain features with AI classifiers. Aharoni et al. (2013) have proven that people with low ACC activation during the NC task have a doubled arrest risk, bringing the spotlight on its prospects as a neurocognitive predictor. (Aharoni et al., 2013). Delfin et al. (2019) have shown, albeit unsuccessfully, that adding cerebral blood flow measurements to traditional risk models improves predictive power in forensic psychiatric populations. (Delfin et al., 2019).

AI allows neuroprediction through treatment outcome or criminal behavior prediction using brain data. An illustration would be machine learning classifiers predicting treatment success from ERP or fMRI scans using brain connectivity networks. However, some models have small sample sizes and are inappropriately fitted (overfitting) to data, which impedes them from being broadly applicable. Future work must focus on the development of large scale neuroimaging data sets with standardized procedures to enhance the algorithms used to make predictions. There are AI ethics concerns like unfair bias in algorithms, privacy concerns, or discrimination that arise and require the creation of policies that foster accountability and justice concerning these issues with AI risk classifiers. Merging psychosocial data with neurobiological data could help AI provide precise rehabilitation by addressing neural deficits like prefrontal-amygdala connectivity using targeted neurofeedback or neuromodulation.(Tortora et al., 2020).

Table 5. AI-Based Neuroprediction: Applications, Data Inputs, Performance Limits, and Ethical Risks

Application	Data Inputs Used	Performance / Current Limits	Bias & Privacy Concerns
Recidivism Prediction	fMRI (ACC activity), structural MRI, behavioral tests, machine-learning classifiers	Moderate accuracy; small datasets; risk of overfitting; not reliable at individual level	May reinforce racial/ socioeconomic bias; sensitive neural data at risk of misuse
Violence Risk Assessment	Brain-age biomarkers, connectivity maps, and EEG/ERP patterns	Promising but inconsistent; results vary across populations; not courtroom-ready	Potential profiling; unequal error rates across groups; privacy intrusion
Treatment Response Prediction	fMRI connectivity, ERP signals, neurocognitive task data	Can predict CBT/ medication outcomes in small samples; lacks generalizable evidence	Use of brain data without consent; risk of coercion in therapy decisions
Deception Detection / Lie Prediction	fMRI activation patterns, reaction-time tasks	Accuracy remains questionable; vulnerable to countermeasures; not admissible legally.	Violates cognitive liberty; high risk of compelled self-incrimination
Early Identification of At-Risk Individuals	Genetic variants (e.g., MAOA), early-life data, and neurodevelopmental markers	Low robustness; ethically contentious; risk of labelling minors	Creates deterministic bias; may trigger pre-emptive policing; high privacy threat

The Role of Neuroethics in Crime Prevention

Neuroethics looks at the issues of what is right and wrong in the application of neuroscience to criminal justice, which in turn balances public safety and individual rights. We see in this field great issues of cognitive liberty, which is the protection of choice against the use of brain manipulation technologies, and also that of biogenetic determinism, which puts at play that criminal action is a result of biology.(Sententia, 2004). Also, we note that the use of AI in brain prediction may end up stigmatising people based on their brain data and, in that process, may also put into practice system-wide bias, which is large against underprivileged groups. (Farah, 2012).

Ethical structures must be put in place to ensure informed consent for neurotechnologies such as brain-computer interfaces (BCIs) and also prevent their use in punitive settings. Poldrack et al. (2018) report on the need for best practices in predictive modelling, which in turn will help prevent misinterpret of correlation as cause. Also, in the field of Neuroethics, we see a push for what they term rehabilitative justice, which is to say we should put forward interventions that repair neural function (for example, cognitive behavioural therapy for prefrontal deficits) before we reach for punishment. Also, we see out of the emerging guidelines a stress on the collaboration between neuroscientists, ethicists, and policy makers to address issues like pre-emptive incarceration based on neuro-predictive risk score. (Aggarwal & Ford, 2013).

Emerging Technologies and Their Applications in Forensic Science

Thanks to neuroimaging developments like high-resolution fMRI, we are starting to get a good idea of which neural circuits are involved in aggression and impulse control. AI-based brain age estimation allows for better risk stratification in people who exhibit neurodevelopmental delays. Wearable devices which can monitor brain electrical activities (e.g. EEG headset) in real time can help monitor the stress or emotional state of parolees. (Harju et al., 2025).

Scientists are testing BCIs to uncover concealed knowledge and decode intent behind crimes because of neuro-signalling(Pustilnik, 2013). The use of such evidence forensically raises Fifth Amendment concerns, as brain data may circumvent self-incrimination. The use of CRISPR in epigenetic editing could theoretically change the expression of certain stress-response genes linked to criminal behaviour. One such gene is FKBP5. However, the approach comes with safety and ethical hurdles. (Yeo et al., 2017).

Predictive policing algorithms that combine neurodata and geospatial analysis can prevent crime but may reinforce racial or other biases. Future directions include neuroprognostic tools for rehabilitation, which use VR-based empathy training, targeting the pathways between the amygdala and the prefrontal cortex. Cooperation must drive these technologies towards equity and rehabilitation, not surveillance (Blitz, 2017).

CONCLUSION

The integration of neurology, genetics, psychology, and sociology pioneers the field of study. It focuses on several aspects of criminal behaviour. Neurocriminology analyses behaviours related to impulsivity, aggression, and poor decision-making. There is a focus on brain structures, including the prefrontal cortex, amygdala, and striatum. The construction of these structures contributes to the aforementioned behaviours. Neurotransmitter systems that are paired with one's genetic makeup, epigenetics, and the environment are also examined. Crime, as we refer to it, is characterised as a product of complex, biopsychosocial interactions.

The use of the technique is not only in forensic science and in the criminal process, but also in rehabilitation, which poses some ethics issues and identifies probable risks as well. Evidence, including studies of brain imaging, has served and continues to serve the strong assertion of not only the existence of diminished responsibility, but also the biological basis of aggression. However, some caution with respect to the court system as well as to courts' use and interpretation of the evidence is unavoidable, because there is a dominant use of determinism in the interpretation. Likewise, the application of neurofeedback and transcranial magnetic stimulation aimed at the treatment of certain neurological disorders is widening the scope of offender rehabilitation, which poses some ethics concerns with respect to autonomy, coercion, and so-called unacceptable disparity, and therefore, caution must be exercised.

Looking ahead, the potential of artificial intelligence and machine learning in improving predictive analytics pertaining to crimes is boundless. On the other hand, the ethics of mental autonomy, privacy, and the potential for bias embedded within the algorithms exercised in analytics require ample multijurisdictional regulatory discourse. The controversial technologies, particularly brain-computer interfaces and editing of genes, are highly desirable; nevertheless, they may place at risk the already insufficient access to some basic rights and may further complicate the existing social inequalities if not properly guided by ethical principles.

When and how should justice be served when reconciling with classical philosophical dilemmas and the field of criminology, considering the nature of punishment? Involuntary manifestations of behaviour are determined by the underlying biological makeup of the individual, thus raising the question of the moral and social responsibility of the individual in criminology neuroscience integration. In focusing on subordinate neurobiology, crime prevention policy, crime social rehabilitation, and reintegration approaches are away from punishment.

In establishing a field and an obligation, the balance between the application of modern scientific thinking and the respect for the individual from the social point of view cannot be maintained. An interdisciplinary, beyond the disciplines of law and criminology, modern criminology will be able to bring justice from a neurobiological perspective and integrate it with a social justice perspective and modern rehabilitation.

REFERENCES

Aggarwal, N. K., & Ford, E. (2013). The Neuroethics and Neurolaw of Brain Injury. *Behavioral Sciences & the Law*, *31*(6), 789–802. DOI: 10.1002/BSL.2086;CTYPE:STRING:JOURNAL

Aharoni, E., Vincent, G. M., Harenski, C. L., Calhoun, V. D., Sinnott-Armstrong, W., Gazzaniga, M. S., & Kiehl, K. A. (2013). Neuroprediction of future rearrest. *Proceedings of the National Academy of Sciences of the United States of America*, *110*, 6223–6228. DOI: 10.1073/pnas.1219302110

Anda, R. F., Felitti, V. J., Bremner, J. D., Walker, J. D., Whitfield, C., Perry, B. D., Dube, S. R., & Giles, W. H. (2005). The enduring effects of abuse and related adverse experiences in childhood: A convergence of evidence from neurobiology and epidemiology. *European Archives of Psychiatry and Clinical Neuroscience*, *256*(3), 174. DOI: 10.1007/S00406-005-0624-4

Anderson, N. E., Allen, C. H., & Kiehl, K. A. (2024). A neurocriminological perspective on violence. In *Handbook of Gun Violence* (pp. 423–441). Elsevier., DOI: 10.1016/B978-0-323-95272-9.00019-X

Bechara, A. (2005). Decision making, impulse control and loss of willpower to resist drugs: A neurocognitive perspective. *Nature Neuroscience*, *8*(11), 1458–1463. DOI: 10.1038/NN1584

Berryessa, C. M., & Raine, A. (2017). Neurocriminology. In *The Routledge Companion to Criminological Theory and Concepts* (pp. 78–82). Taylor and Francis., DOI: 10.4324/9781315744902-18

Blair, R. J. R. (2005). Applying a cognitive neuroscience perspective to the disorder of psychopathy. *Development and Psychopathology*, *17*(3), 865–891. DOI: 10.1017/S0954579405050418

Blitz, M. J. (2017). *The Fifth Amendment: Self-Incrimination and the Brain*. 59–79. https://doi.org/DOI: 10.1007/978-3-319-50004-1_4

Carré, J. M., & Olmstead, N. A. (2015). Social neuroendocrinology of human aggression: Examining the role of competition-induced testosterone dynamics. *Neuroscience*, *286*, 171–186. DOI: 10.1016/j.neuroscience.2014.11.029

Chamberlain, S. R., & Sahakian, B. J. (2007). The neuropsychiatry of impulsivity. *Current Opinion in Psychiatry*, *20*(3), 255–261. DOI: 10.1097/YCO.0B013E3280BA4989

De Dreu, C. K. W. (2012). Oxytocin modulates cooperation within and competition between groups: An integrative review and research agenda. *Hormones and Behavior*, *61*(3), 419–428. DOI: 10.1016/J.YHBEH.2011.12.009

Decety, J., & Jackson, P. L. (2004). The functional architecture of human empathy. *Behavioral and Cognitive Neuroscience Reviews*, *3*(2), 71–100. DOI: 10.1177/1534582304267187

Delfin, C., Krona, H., Andiné, P., Ryding, E., Wallinius, M., & Hofvander, B. (2019). Prediction of recidivism in a long-term follow-up of forensic psychiatric patients: Incremental effects of neuroimaging data. *PLoS One*, *14*(5), e0217127. DOI: 10.1371/JOURNAL.PONE.0217127

Dom, G., Schouler-Ocak, M., Bhui, K., Demunter, H., Kuey, L., Raballo, A., Frydecka, D., Misiak, B., Gorwood, P., & Samochowiec, J. (2018). Mass violence, radicalization and terrorism: A role for psychiatric profession? *European Psychiatry : the Journal of the Association of European Psychiatrists*, *49*, 78–80. DOI: 10.1016/J.EURPSY.2018.01.001

Farah, M. J. (2012). Neuroethics: The ethical, legal, and societal impact of neuroscience. *Annual Review of Psychology, 63*(Volume 63, 2012), 571–591. https://doi.org/DOI: 10.1146/ANNUREV.PSYCH.093008.100438/CITE/REFWORKS

Farrington, D. P. (2005). Childhood origins of antisocial behavior. *Clinical Psychology & Psychotherapy*, *12*(3), 177–190. DOI: 10.1002/CPP.448;WGROUP:STRING:-PUBLICATION

Gavazzi, S. M., Yarcheck, C. M., Sullivan, J. M., Jones, S. C., & Khurana, A. (2008). Global risk factors and the prediction of recidivism rates in a sample of first-time misdemeanant offenders. *International Journal of Offender Therapy and Comparative Criminology*, *52*(3), 330–345. DOI: 10.1177/0306624X07305481;PAGE:STRING:ARTICLE/CHAPTER

Glenn, A. L., & Raine, A. (2014a). Neurocriminology: Implications for the punishment, prediction and prevention of criminal behaviour. In *Nature Reviews Neuroscience* (Vol. 15, pp. 54–63). https://doi.org/DOI: 10.1038/nrn3640

Glenn, A. L., & Raine, A. (2014b). Neurocriminology: Implications for the punishment, prediction and prevention of criminal behaviour. In *Nature Reviews Neuroscience* (Vol. 15, pp. 54–63). https://doi.org/DOI: 10.1038/nrn3640

Goodkind, M., Eickhoff, S. B., Oathes, D. J., Jiang, Y., Chang, A., Jones-Hagata, L. B., Ortega, B. N., Zaiko, Y. V., Roach, E. L., Korgaonkar, M. S., Grieve, S. M., Galatzer-Levy, I., Fox, P. T., & Etkin, A. (2015). Identification of a common neurobiological substrate for mental Illness. *JAMA Psychiatry*, *72*(4), 305–315. DOI: 10.1001/JAMAPSYCHIATRY.2014.2206

Harju, H., Tuisku, J., & Nummenmaa, L. (2025). *Shared brain basis of aggression in clinical, forensic, and healthy samples: A meta-analysis.* https://doi.org/DOI: 10.1101/2025.02.17.638609

Harms, M. B., Birn, R., Provencal, N., Wiechmann, T., Binder, E. B., Giakas, S. W., Roeber, B. J., & Pollak, S. D. (2017). Early life stress, FK506 binding protein 5 gene (FKBP5) methylation, and inhibition-related prefrontal function: A prospective longitudinal study. *Development and Psychopathology*, *29*(5), 1895–1903. DOI: 10.1017/S095457941700147X

Hashikawa, Y., Hashikawa, K., Falkner, A. L., & Lin, D. (2017). Ventromedial hypothalamus and the generation of aggression. *Frontiers in Systems Neuroscience*, *11*, 94. Advance online publication. DOI: 10.3389/fnsys.2017.00094

Hirstein, W. (2022). Neuroscience and Normativity: How Knowledge of the Brain Offers a Deeper Understanding of Moral and Legal Responsibility. *Criminal Law and Philosophy*, *16*(2), 327–351. DOI: 10.1007/S11572-021-09600-W/METRICS

Jones, O. D., & Shen, F. X. (2012). Law and Neuroscience in the United States. *International Neurolaw: A Comparative Analysis*, 349–380. https://doi.org/DOI: 10.1007/978-3-642-21541-4_19

Kraft, C. J., & Giordano, J. (2017). Integrating brain science and law: Neuroscientific evidence and legal perspectives on protecting individual liberties. *Frontiers in Neuroscience*, *11*(NOV). Advance online publication. DOI: 10.3389/FNINS.2017.00621

La Tona, G., Terranova, M. C., Vernuccio, F., Lo Re, G., Salerno, S., Zerbo, S., & Argo, A. (2020). Lie Detection: fMRI. *Radiology in Forensic Medicine: From Identification to Post-Mortem Imaging*, 197–202. https://doi.org/DOI: 10.1007/978-3-319-96737-0_18

Lara, F. (2023). Neurorehabilitation of Offenders, Consent and Consequentialist Ethics. *Neuroethics*, *16*(1), 1–15. DOI: 10.1007/S12152-022-09510-1/METRICS

Margolin, G., & Gordis, E. B. (2000). The effects of family and community violence on children. *Annual Review of Psychology*, *51*, 445–479. DOI: 10.1146/ANNUREV.PSYCH.51.1.445

Mulyadi, M., Fernando, Z. J., Putra, P. S., & Anditya, A. W. (2024). Unleashing Justice's Future: The Dawn of Neuro-Cognitive Risk Assessments (NCRA) in Transforming Rehabilitation. [Indonesian Journal of Criminal Law Studies]. *IJCLS, 9*(1), 61–86. DOI: 10.15294/IJCLS.V9I1.50152

Nilawati, S., Amri, S., Hasanah, N., Saodah, S., Juliati, J., & Sapnita, S. (2024). Unraveling emotional regulation through multimodal neuroimaging techniques. *BrainBridge: Neuroscience and Biomedical Engineering, 1*(1), 1–26. DOI: 10.35335/A0CFDA08

Poldrack, R. A., Huckins, G., & Varoquaux, G. (2020). Establishment of Best Practices for Evidence for Prediction: A Review. In *JAMA Psychiatry* (Vol. 77, pp. 534–540). American Medical Association., DOI: 10.1001/jamapsychiatry.2019.3671

Pustilnik, A. C. (2013). Neurotechnologies at the Intersection of Criminal Procedure and Constitutional Law. *The Constitution and the Future of Criminal Justice in America*, 109–134. https://doi.org/DOI: 10.1017/CBO9781139108034.011

Raine, A. (2008). From Genes to Brain to Antisocial Behavior. *Current Directions in Psychological Science, 17*(5), 323–328. DOI: 10.1111/J.1467-8721.2008.00599.X

Raine, A., Buchsbaum, M. S., Stanley, J., Lottenberg, S., Abel, L., & Stoddard, J. (1994). Selective reductions in prefrontal glucose metabolism in murderers. *Biological Psychiatry, 36*(6), 365–373. DOI: 10.1016/0006-3223(94)91211-4

Raine, A., Lencz, T., Bihrle, S., LaCasse, L., & Colletti, P. (2000). Reduced prefrontal gray matter volume and reduced autonomic activity in antisocial personality disorder. *Archives of General Psychiatry, 57*(2), 119–127. DOI: 10.1001/ARCHPSYC.57.2.119

Raine, A., & Marek, W. K. (2013). The anatomy of violence: The biological roots of crime. In *American Journal of Forensic Psychology* (Vol. 31, pp. 67–71). https://doi.org/DOI: 10.1080/10511253.2018.1445334

Reyes, A. C., & Amador, A. A. (2009). Qualitative and quantitative EEG abnormalities in violent offenders with antisocial personality disorder. *Journal of Forensic and Legal Medicine, 16*(2), 59–63. DOI: 10.1016/J.JFLM.2008.08.001

Rigoni, D., Pellegrini, S., Mariotti, V., Cozza, A., Mechelli, A., Ferrara, S. D., Pietrini, P., & Sartori, G. (2010). How Neuroscience and Behavioural Genetics Improve Psychiatric Assessment: Report on a Violent Murder Case. *Frontiers in Behavioral Neuroscience, 4*, 160. DOI: 10.3389/FNBEH.2010.00160

Savopoulos, P., & Lindell, A. K. (2018). Born criminal? Differences in structural, functional and behavioural lateralization between criminals and noncriminals. In *Laterality* (Vol. 23, pp. 738–760). Routledge., DOI: 10.1080/1357650X.2018.1432631

Schauer, F. (2010). Neuroscience, lie-detection, and the law: Contrary to the prevailing view, the suitability of brain-based lie-detection for courtroom or forensic use should be determined according to legal and not scientific standards. *Trends in Cognitive Sciences, 14*(3), 101–103. DOI: 10.1016/j.tics.2009.12.004

Sententia, W. (2004). Neuroethical Considerations: Cognitive Liberty and Converging Technologies for Improving Human Cognition. *Annals of the New York Academy of Sciences, 1013*(1), 221–228. DOI: 10.1196/ANNALS.1305.014

Seo, D., Patrick, C. J., & Kennealy, P. J. (2008). Role of serotonin and dopamine system interactions in the neurobiology of impulsive aggression and its comorbidity with other clinical disorders. *Aggression and Violent Behavior, 13*(5), 383–395. DOI: 10.1016/J.AVB.2008.06.003

Shamay-Tsoory, S. G., Harari, H., Aharon-Peretz, J., & Levkovitz, Y. (2010). The role of the orbitofrontal cortex in affective theory of mind deficits in criminal offenders with psychopathic tendencies. *Cortex, 46*(5), 668–677. DOI: 10.1016/j.cortex.2009.04.008

Tesink, V., Douglas, T., Forsberg, L., Ligthart, S., & Meynen, G. (2023). Neurointerventions in Criminal Justice: On the Scope of the Moral Right to Bodily Integrity. *Neuroethics, 16*(3), 1–11. DOI: 10.1007/S12152-023-09526-1/METRICS

Tortora, L., Meynen, G., Bijlsma, J., Tronci, E., & Ferracuti, S. (2020). Neuroprediction and A.I. in Forensic Psychiatry and Criminal Justice: A Neurolaw Perspective. *Frontiers in Psychology, 11*, 493506. DOI: 10.3389/FPSYG.2020.00220/BIBTEX

Urbaniok, F., Hardegger, J., Rossegger, A., & Endrass, J. (2006). Neurobiologischer determinismus: Fragwürdige schlussfolgerungen über menschliche entscheidungsmöglichkeiten und forensische schuldfähigkeit. *Fortschritte der Neurologie-Psychiatrie, 74*(8), 431–441. DOI: 10.1055/S-2006-944237

Van Veen, V., Cohen, J. D., Botvinick, M. M., Stenger, V. A., & Carter, C. S. (2001). Anterior Cingulate Cortex, Conflict Monitoring, and Levels of Processing. *NeuroImage, 14*(6), 1302–1308. DOI: 10.1006/NIMG.2001.0923

Verhoeven, F. E. A., Booij, L., Kruijt, A. W., Cerit, H., Antypa, N., & Van der Does, W. (2012). The effects of MAOA genotype, childhood trauma, and sex on trait and state-dependent aggression. *Brain and Behavior, 2*(6), 806–813. DOI: 10.1002/BRB3.96

Volkow, N. D., Fowler, J. S., & Wang, G. J. (2003). The addicted human brain: Insights from imaging studies. *The Journal of Clinical Investigation, 111*(10), 1444–1451. DOI: 10.1172/JCI18533

Yang, Y., & Raine, A. (2009). Prefrontal structural and functional brain imaging findings in antisocial, violent, and psychopathic individuals: A meta-analysis. *Psychiatry Research: Neuroimaging*, *174*(2), 81–88. DOI: 10.1016/j.pscychresns.2009.03.012

Yeo, S., Enoch, M. A., Gorodetsky, E., Akhtar, L., Schuebel, K., Roy, A., & Goldman, D. (2017). The influence of FKBP5 genotype on expression of FKBP5 and other glucocorticoid-regulated genes, dependent on trauma exposure. *Genes Brain & Behavior*, *16*(2), 223–232. DOI: 10.1111/GBB.12342

Chapter 2
Smart Criminal Justice Cognitive and Ethical Foundations for Trustworthy AI Systems

Dana Alrumaihi
https://orcid.org/0009-0004-9939-6339
College of Law, Kingdom University, Bahrain

Omar Fakhri Abdulrazak Al-Hadi
https://orcid.org/0000-0002-4982-9384
College of Law, Kingdom University, Bahrain

Shafiq Ul Rehman
https://orcid.org/0000-0003-2266-218X
Kingdom University, Bahrain

ABSTRACT

This chapter explores the integration of Artificial Intelligence within judicial systems under the emerging concept of "Smart Criminal Justice." It examines how AI can streamline legal processes, enhance decision-making, and uphold ethical accountability in the digital era. By linking cognitive aspects of human judgment with AI-driven reasoning, the chapter highlights parallels between legal decision-making and neuroscience-inspired intelligence models. It further discusses how ethical and data security safeguards in judicial AI systems can inform the development of trustworthy, resilient, and human-centered cybersecurity frameworks.

DOI: 10.4018/979-8-3373-5012-7.ch002

1. INTRODUCTION

Considering the technological advancements, countries are rapidly progressing toward enhancing technical capabilities across all sectors. Artificial Intelligence (AI) stands as one of the most prominent precursors of the Fourth Industrial Revolution. Therefore, it is the responsibility of nations to advance toward technologically developed sectors. The judiciary sector, however, remains among the most lagging fields due to its unique characteristics, resulting in a general reluctance to incorporate AI tools in legal proceedings. Over the years, access to justice has required navigating a complex system of procedural routines that lack efficiency and speed.

Today, the presence of AI in all sectors has become essential due to its significant role in keeping pace with the rapid technological leap occurring globally, especially within the judiciary. Consequently, studying the experiences of technologically advanced countries becomes imperative.

1.1 Importance of Research

The significance of studying smart criminal justice lies in its relevance to several areas, most notably the global advancements in AI. Given the breakthrough in this specific field, transitioning the judicial system from traditional to smart has become inevitable. Delving into this topic allows for the automation of legal processes, enhancement of judicial information systems, and extraction of patterns that aid in crime prediction and prevention. This contributes to easing court workloads by limiting proceedings to high-priority cases and ensuring judgments are issued with greater precision, efficiency, and speed—at lower costs.

Furthermore, the study of smart criminal justice plays a role in improving legal systems by addressing legislative gaps and enhancing operational efficiency, thereby ensuring better access to justice. Hence, it is incumbent upon legal professionals and legislators to integrate the law within AI structures to pioneer modern legal frameworks.

1.2 Research Problem

One of the main issues this study aims to address is the overcrowding of courts with non-critical cases, which results in procedural delays and entrenched legal bureaucracy, leading to wasted effort and time. Moreover, the current judicial system struggles to keep up with emerging crimes, such as cybercrimes and information crimes—phenomena born of the digital age—due to their transnational nature and the difficulty in proving and attributing them to specific perpetrators. Therefore, tackling these crimes requires a judicial system equipped with advanced data analysis capabilities and digital evidence processing.

1.3 Research Questions

- How can AI tools be employed in the judicial system?
- What are the ethical challenges associated with AI's role in issuing judicial rulings, and how can they be mitigated?
- What is AI's role in achieving criminal justice? Is there harmony between human input and technology?
- How can we balance technological reliance with human interaction in legal processes?
- How can we prevent AI from becoming authoritarian and from affecting justice in a negative manner?
- What impact might smart systems have on defense rights and judicial principles?

2. NATURE OF SMART CRIMINAL JUSTICE

The concept of smart criminal justice systems from ongoing research in technology that aim to improve the judicial processes and to transform the legal sector from traditional to modern AI – Based systems.

Figure 1 below depicts the recent literature emphasizing the following areas:

Figure 1. Smart criminal justice systems

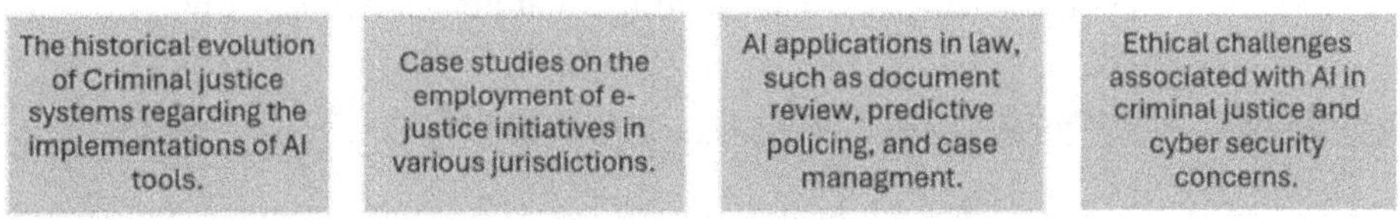

By examining these aspects', the literature suggests a robust framework for understanding that would help ease the traditional legal system into smart criminal justice system, which is inevitable in this current era as it is essential because cybersecurity faces a major challenge with regard to artificial intelligence, which by its very nature evolves, making it difficult to keep up with these development.

This is precisely why we need these research studies, because they provide vision on how to integrate smart criminal justice system into Cybersecurity, which is crucial for several reasons:

- This process will enhance the efficiency of law enforcement with advanced technologies.
- proactive threat detection, as this system can identify potential cyber threats before they occur.
- Achieving public safety and trust within the community.
- Adaptability to Emerging threats as Cyber threats are constantly evolving.
- Improved data management, more effective evidence achieving.

2.1 Understanding Smart Criminal Justice

Achieving smart criminal justice requires a comprehensive understanding of criminal justice itself. The goal is to align the litigation system with smart justice concepts by incorporating AI tools, particularly through e-justice or virtual courts. This section is divided into four subsections, beginning with the definition of smart criminal justice.

Definition of Smart Criminal Justice

Criminal justice generally refers to the practices and systems used to deter criminals and reduce crime through legislation and penalties. Traditionally, this occurs within a rigid system involving report preparation, documentation, litigation, appeals, and court hearings. This traditional model results in wasted time and resources, delayed proceedings, and case backlogs that compromise timely justice. The judiciary, a key pillar of the state, has significantly lagged in adopting technology, which has negatively impacted judicial efficiency and accessibility. In contrast, smart criminal justice emphasizes speed, efficiency, and technological integration. It seeks to digitize judicial procedures using AI, establishing what are known as "smart courts."

E-litigation and Smart Courts

E-litigation is defined as: "Using modern communication technologies in litigation—partially through electronic means or fully through online courts—to handle legal proceedings." (Al-Shar'ah, 2020). This definition focuses on the tools and benefits of e-litigation but lacks depth regarding how smart litigation works and what safeguards are required.

A more comprehensive definition would be:

"A smart judicial system where all litigation procedures—from filing to judgment execution—are carried out through secure, official AI applications. These include storing case files, generating rulings from databases, and issuing executable judgments based on predefined criteria. This system aims to revolutionize

traditional processes, establishing centralized legal databases for streamlined, automated justice delivery." (Al-Marzouqi, 2021).

Benefits of Smart Criminal Justice

- Time Efficiency: Automating routine judicial tasks saves valuable time.
- Enhanced Data Use: AI allows the creation of legal databases, integrating statutes, rulings, appeals, and case data.
- Complex Case Focus: By offloading routine matters, legal professionals can prioritize complex or urgent cases.
- Improved Decision-Making: AI systems can process large datasets quickly and with high accuracy, aiding in legal analysis and reducing court overload.

2.2 Legal Personality of Artificial Intelligence

The term "legal personality" in general refers to the eligibility to acquire rights and bear duties or obligations. It is divided into natural and juridical personalities. Natural personality applies to humans, where a person acquires legal personality at birth and retains it until death. Juridical personality, on the other hand, is the capacity granted to entities such as companies and institutions to acquire rights and bear responsibilities, enabling them to achieve the purposes for which they were established.

Accordingly, we raise the following question: Where does Artificial Intelligence fall in terms of legal personality? What are the ethical challenges associated with AI's involvement in issuing judicial decisions? And how can these challenges be avoided?

Diverging Legal Opinions

Legal opinions vary significantly on this matter, and many scholars are cautious, given the ethical dilemmas it presents.

To answer this question, we must explore some viewpoints from legal doctrine:

Pro-AI Legal Personality: Some legal scholars and experts support granting legal personality to AI entities. They argue that doing so would allow these systems to possess legal rights and obligations, which would be beneficial for the development and expansion of AI technologies. It would also enhance accountability for any harm caused by AI systems.

Against AI Legal Personality: Opponents argue that AI has not yet reached a level of intelligence equivalent to or surpassing human intelligence—particularly the ability to make autonomous decisions. Therefore, it is impossible to grant AI full legal personality, whether in terms of legal capacity to act or to be held liable.

This position is supported by French scholars Bourgeois-M and Loiseau-G, who warned about the serious risks involved (Al-Dajjah, 2024).

Their concerns center on the future consequences of creating such entities, as regulating and controlling them would be extremely difficult.

Our Perspective

In our view, AI systems have reached an extremely advanced stage in this technological era. Contrary to the pro-personality stance, we believe that AI systems already demonstrate autonomous decision-making with minimal human intervention. This is clear evidence of how AI tools are now competing with humans across various fields. However, this does not mean that we support granting AI entities full legal personality. Rather, we emphasize the need for careful regulation and control.

Due to the unique nature of artificial intelligence, it is proposed that its legal personality should be hybrid, combining aspects of both natural and juridical personality:

AI may be granted limited rights akin to those held by natural persons, such as a digital nationality to enable international legal accountability. However, AI would not receive human-specific rights like marriage, divorce, or the right to life—these are inherently human and non-transferable. Simultaneously, AI may be granted certain juridical privileges, such as an independent financial liability. This would allow courts to impose fines or require compensation from AI entities if damage occurs due to their actions. Certain legal principles, especially those relating to civil and criminal liability, could be modified to suit the complex nature of AI entities.

Ethical Challenges Arising from AI in Judicial Decision-Making

Discussing the legal nature of AI leads us to the second part of the main question:

What are the ethical challenges associated with AI in the process of issuing judicial rulings? And how can they be avoided?

To answer this, we must reiterate the judiciary's inherent privacy and sensitivity. Thus, the use of AI in judicial systems raises serious concerns, especially when it comes to issuing final and just rulings, which is the core of our discussion.

Primary Ethical Challenges Identified by Legal Scholars:

- Legal Accountability
- Loss of Human Touch
- Bias
- Errors in Judgment

Key Question: How Can We Avoid These Challenges and Prepare for an AI-Driven Judiciary?

Firstly, it is crucial to define accountability clearly and develop precise mechanisms to handle potential AI errors. This is essential to protect innocent individuals who may fall victim to unjust rulings issued by AI systems.

Secondly, it is necessary to integrate human involvement in the judicial process. A human touch adds the essential moral and emotional perspective needed for just rulings. Maintaining human oversight ensures that AI remains a tool, not a replacement, for judges and legal professionals, and this is precisely why human-in-the-loop governance is essential.

Lastly, successful implementation of AI in the judiciary demands ongoing evaluation of AI performance and continuous monitoring of AI-based rulings to minimize ethical risks, as autonomous decision system using AI can without any doubt rise the ethical challenges such as bias and accountability gaps.

For this purpose, The OECD AI principles are based of five main values that can reduce the risks that might arise when employing artificial intelligence tools in the legal system. The guide was adopted by the organization for economic Co-operation and development in 2019, endorsed by G20 and 42 other countries, and was reaffirmed by UNESCO Convention, as it addresses many ethical issues regarding AI usage sensitive and high-stake environment.

2.3 The Role of Artificial Intelligence in Achieving Criminal Justice

Modern research has shown that the artificial intelligence in the judicial system has increased massively, As the evolution of AI started in the Mid-20th century, In the 1950s to be specific as the seed of the concept of AI was on the hands of Alan Turing and Jhon McCarthy. With that the concept of AI "thinking machines" was born, in this stage the concept was a mere idea, Until the 1970s in which the idea of AI became more than just a though and was translated to tangible algorithms.

The Figure 2 below shows the timeline in which AI was born, – as a concept – as well as the evolution of artificial intelligence and its employment in the legal system …

Figure 2. Evolution of Artificial Intelligence timeframe

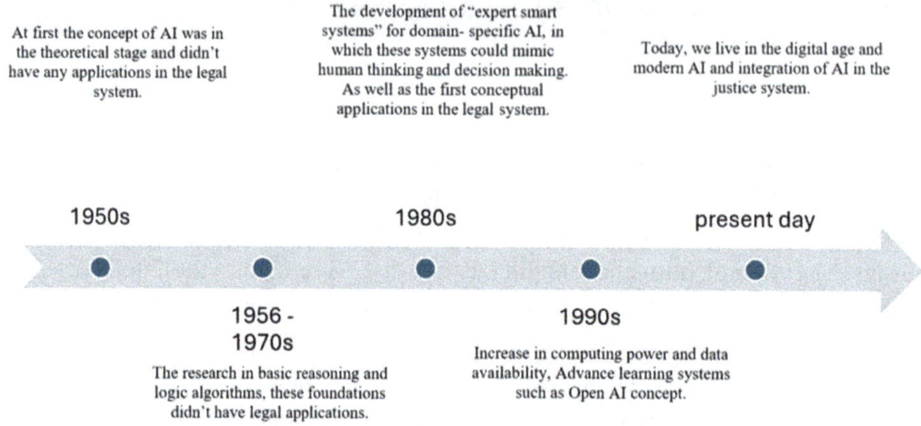

The University of Southampton published an article (University of Southampton, 2025) regarding the growing demand for AI Skills on criminal justice. The article presents the most in-demand AI skills employed in criminal justice such as data analysis and predictive modeling, Natural language processing (NLP), computer Vision and biometrics, Automation and workflow optimization, and ethical AI development. Artificial Intelligence (AI) plays a central role in achieving criminal justice. It serves as an effective tool to enhance the efficiency of legal procedures, criminal investigations, and the judicial system as a whole.

The article explored the role of AI systems in the criminal justice as well, some of these implementations are policing and crime prevention which is already used to help identifying criminals and to predicate possible criminal behavior in the future. As well as emergency response, forensic analysis, administrative tasks, cybersecurity and digital crime, and probation and rehabilitation.

As aforementioned, the judicial field lacks technological advancement, making a fundamental transformation essential. The role of AI in serving criminal justice can be outlined as follows:

A. Crime Prediction

In United States of America, predictive algorithms are used to support the judiciary and reduce pressure on the judicial system. In some states, police departments have adopted predictive algorithms to develop strategic force distribution across areas by analyzing crime statistics and geographic coordinates.

B. Digital Evidence Processing

AI also plays a vital role in processing digital evidence, enabling judges to analyze crime data and the context of incidents more efficiently, thus facilitating faster rulings with less effort. This also aids defense attorneys by providing easier access to previous judgments to support their cases.

Moreover, digital evidence analysis supports investigations by:

- Interpreting how crimes were committed,
- Evaluating the likelihood of crime by a suspect,
- Identifying key links and drawing logical inferences.

C. Enhancing Efficiency and Speed of Legal Procedures

AI significantly improves legal procedure efficiency by allowing legal professionals to focus on technical and practical aspects, while automating repetitive tasks. These include:

- Routine litigation processes,
- Accessing legal principles,
- Searching judicial precedents.

This automation reduces delays and simplifies complex judicial procedures. Undoubtedly, improve efficiency directly facilitates access to justice. Practical Applications in Countries Using AI in Criminal Justice.

Several countries have adopted AI applications that promote criminal justice, as presented in Figure 3 below:

Figure 3. AI applications for smart criminal justice

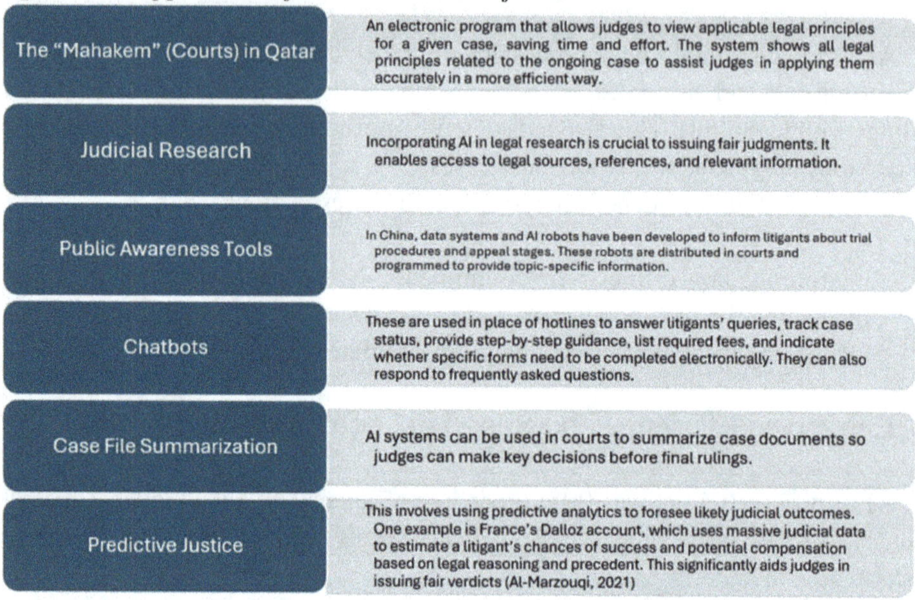

3. PRACTICAL APPLICATIONS OF ARTIFICIAL INTELLIGENCE IN THE JUDICIAL FIELD

After delving into AI concepts and its role in achieving criminal justice, it is important to review the experiences of countries that have pioneered AI implementation in the judicial sector. Doing so allows us to stay abreast of global developments and benefit from these examples.

In this section, we explore practical applications of AI in the judicial field. We will present various countries' experiences in using AI tools across the judiciary's key components.

This section is divided as follows:

- AI Judge (Robot Judge)
- AI Prosecutor (Robot Prosecutor)
- Electronic Notary
- AI Lawyer (Robot Lawyer)

3.1 The Robot Judge

Judges form the core of the litigation system. Given their pivotal role in delivering justice, it is crucial to provide them with all possible tools to reach judicial truth and issue rulings efficiently. This can be achieved by incorporating AI tools into judicial processes—especially for routine cases that do not require court appearances—thereby increasing judgment quality and case resolution speed.

3.1.1Virtual Magistrate Project – USA (1995)

A notable initiative was the Virtual Magistrate Project, launched by the American Arbitration Association (AAA) in 1995. This project introduced online arbitration dispute resolution through computer networks.

The U.S. Federal Rules of Civil Procedure, Article 34(a), endorsed this by allowing: *"Electronically stored information, including writings, graphs, photographs, sound recordings, or any data stored on electronic media, to be presented as sources of information, either directly or through translation, in court proceedings." Every U.S. state organizes electronic litigation procedures differently, including how to handle announcements, payments, file submissions, and document exchanges. However, all agree on adopting electronic means in litigation. Some states have expanded to include comprehensive digital court operations (Al-Marzouqi, 2021)*

3.1.2 China – Virtual Courts and Smart Judiciary

In December 2019, China announced that millions of legal cases are now decided by Virtual Courts, which include non-human (AI-powered) judges.

These courts allow litigants to:

File cases online, conduct digital court hearings, Resolve disputes in intellectual property, e-commerce, finance, product liability, and certain administrative areas. For example: In Beijing, the average case duration is 40 days, with hearings lasting about 37 minutes 80% of litigants are individuals; 20% are entities. 98% of rulings are accepted without appeal.

This judicial transformation included publicizing court rulings via official platforms, enabling case filing, real-time updates, and even digital evidence submission based on judicial requests or party demands. AI systems filter out unreliable evidence and detect data inconsistencies. Publishing verdicts online increases transparency and builds public trust in the judiciary system (Shaheed & Mahdi, 2024).

3.1.3 Estonia – AI for Small Claims

Estonia implemented AI judges for small claims disputes, such as contract claims under €7,000. This limitation is considered prudent, as it avoids replacing human judges entirely—something impractical due to AI's limitations (Lo, 2021).

Even if AI systems can make autonomous decisions, can we truly guarantee fair rulings from a robot judge?

This concern arises because AI judges rely on static databases and legal texts. While this may work for civil courts, it is unacceptable in criminal courts, where judicial discretion is key and decisions aren't limited to written submissions. Thus, Estonia's limited implementation is commendable. While we encourage AI integration in judiciary systems, caution is essential when applying these modern technologies into our courts.

3.2 The Robot Prosecutor

Today, robots have reached an advanced stage in the legal field in several countries, among them China, where a group of researchers at the Chinese Academy developed a robot to serve as a criminal investigator. This robot can charge suspects based on a massive collection of data, including judicial precedents and criminal profiles, which allows it to accurately classify and describe crimes, and match them to perpetrators through verbal descriptions of facts and analytical processing of this data.

Furthermore, China has introduced interactive humanoid robots to perform police patrol duties on the streets. For instance, robots known as PM01, developed by Engine AI, were seen wearing police vests and walking alongside police officers in the city of Shenzhen. These robots interact with pedestrians, shake hands with them, and respond to voice commands, as reported by a Chinese online news outlet. The PM01 robot was launched in December 2024 and is distinguished by its fast movement, interactive screen, and open-source platform that allows global developers to enhance its capabilities through secondary development.

The field of investigation can be divided into two categories of tasks. The first category involves general tasks, which are mostly routine procedures within criminal investigations, such as documenting the progress of investigations, recording statements and surveillance, writing reports, and adding them to the case file.

The second category includes complex tasks that requires deep understanding and legal expertise. These fall under the specialized skills of investigators, such as analyzing crime scenes, evaluating and comparing the credibility of evidence, and assessing the importance of witness testimony based on a nuanced understanding of human behavior and emotional responses, something robots are fundamentally incapable of comprehending. Such duties require psychological tactics, interpreting suspects' or witnesses' reactions, interacting with officers, and ultimately identifying the perpetrator—all of which are core elements of the work of the investigators and are currently beyond the scope of robotic capabilities.

Therefore, we believe that AI can be employed in the routine and administrative aspects of the investigative process. However, it must not extend to complex or human-sensitive tasks. This is essential to safeguard criminal justice and preserve the integrity of investigations.

3.3 The Electronic Notary

One of the most prominent international experiences in this field is the initiative launched by the Administrative Judiciary Court in the Sultanate of Oman, which, on January 22, 2022, inaugurated a new electronic website along with the activation of Najir Portals. This step aimed to achieve the goals of Oman Vision 2040, particularly its strategic digital transformation plan.

The judicial system in Oman has also undergone continuous modernization to keep up with rapid developments in the digital and technological spheres. The core task of such systems lies in their use of specific software and algorithms to offer litigants a suite of judicial services that streamline the litigation process by saving time and effort.

These systems can handle routine notarial tasks, such as:

- Document authentication,
- Supervising transactions,
- Providing general legal consultations,
- Record-keeping and archiving through automation.

In December 2022, the Ministry of Justice in Egypt announced the launch of the electronic litigation platform for economic courts. This move marked the beginning of a gradual digital transformation, with the Ministry of Justice preparing the new system in cooperation with the Ministry of Communications and Information Technology and in coordination with courts of appeal (Al-Faliti, 2024).

The platform allows the use of information technology tools to submit and manage electronic legal cases. In the Kingdom of Saudi Arabia, we find a leading example in implementing AI applications in the judiciary. For instance, the "Najiz" platform is one of the most notable tech-based litigation platforms. It allows users to access all electronic legal services provided by the Ministry of Justice, serving individuals, business owners, and lawyers alike.

Through the platform, users can: Submit enforcement requests, File lawsuits, Present written pleadings, Check application statuses, And book hearing appointments.

A key strength of "Najiz" lies in its integration with other support entities via partner platforms such as "Khibrat", "Nafed", "Taradhi", and "Public Auctions". To gauge the success of such digital judicial platforms, we present some statistics from the "Najiz" platform:

These numbers clearly demonstrate the judiciary's ability to adapt to technological developments and embrace AI tools.

The Qatari courts also show a strong track record in facilitating judicial services through electronic systems. As part of their technological advancement, Qatar launched the "Electronic Courts Program", enabling both litigants and lawyers to: Access case data easily, respond to frequently asked questions, and reduce the number of calls and daily visitors to the courts (Bilal, 2023_b).

Similarly, the North Carolina Courthouse in the United States used Tango Technology for the same purpose, resulting in a 43% reduction in incoming calls. In New Jersey, Judge Glenn Grant tasked a technical support staff member with developing chatbot systems to enhance access to court services. Around 11,000 questions were compiled and answered using this system, which significantly improved the quality of judicial services.

This AI-based tool delivers accurate responses at a 75% success rate and is available 24/7, making it far more efficient than a human-operated system, which would face time and workload constraints (El-Din, 2024).

3.4 The Robot Lawyer

The field of legal practice is one of the most significant domains that, if enhanced and aligned with technological advancements, can greatly benefit the judicial system, and reduce procedural complexities. We recognize the importance of focusing on the role of lawyers within the broader scope of smart litigation (Bilal, 2023_a).

In the United States of America, the legal profession has embraced advanced AI technologies to support legal work—particularly the role of the lawyer. One example is the implementation of the "Robot Lawyer" project, designed to provide legal information and communicate with users in a human-like manner. This project also provides certain legal services, granting access to legal knowledge, judicial rulings, and case precedents. We can imagine the extent to which lawyers and legal advisors benefit from this technology, especially in areas such as legal research, drafting legal opinions, and reviewing case law.

Additionally, "DoNotPay" company, which offers a robot lawyer application in the United States. It specializes in online legal services and chatbot technology, providing the "Robot Lawyer" service. This application was established in 2015 by Joshua Browder and has since grown into one of the leading platforms in AI-powered legal assistance.

The lawyer Tara Vasdani, recognized as one of the 25 most influential lawyers in Canada, published an article in The Lawyer's Daily affirming that legal professionals—particularly lawyers—must utilize AI tools in their work due to their profoundly positive impact on the legal sector as a whole.

In her article, she emphasized: "In short, I reiterate and stress that the legal sector's resistance to the aforementioned changes will pose major obstacles for both lawyers and their staff. Modern judicial bodies already expect the use of legal technology tools by lawyers, students, and courts. If lawyers choose not to rise to the challenge, they risk severely disappointing their clients and incurring significant costs."

She concluded by noting that since 2017, this transformation has only accelerated, and failure to adapt may lead to falling behind in the legal profession (Vasdani, 2020)

And since this shift towards automating the judicial sector in inevitable, we must rely on robust ethical framework and regulations. In 2020, the US congress passed the artificial intelligence Future and prospects Act, which is the first federal Law related to regulating AI activities and plays a critical role in resolving cybersecurity dilemmas.

As we stated earlier, the ethics of artificial intelligence is a vital field that addresses the challenges that are associated with the development and usage of AI technologies. That is why the OECD principles are crucial when it comes to employing AI tools within the judicial system and these value-based principles are as follows:

1. Human values and fairness
2. Inclusive growth and sustainable development
3. Transparency and explainability
4. Robustness, security and safety
5. Accountability

In my opinion, these kinds of regulations can immensely provide an ethical framework that can safeguard justice and ensure public trust, and most importantly it will decrease the issues that accompanies AI usage in high-risk environment which will insure cybersecurity.

4. CYBERSECURITY IN AI-DRIVEN JUDICIAL SYSTEMS

As judicial institutions worldwide increasingly adopt AI-enabled platforms, cybersecurity emerges as a central requirement for safeguarding the integrity, confidentiality, and reliability of legal processes. AI systems in courts operate within complex digital ecosystems that include case-management platforms, biometric authentication tools, cloud-based document repositories, and predictive analytics models. This digital transformation, while beneficial, significantly enlarges the attack surface of judicial systems and introduces risks that were previously non-existent in traditional litigation processes (Smith, 2023).

4.1 Importance of Cybersecurity in Smart Justice

Cybersecurity is not merely a technical safeguard; it is a prerequisite for ensuring judicial legitimacy and preserving public trust. Compromise of judicial data—whether case files, identities of witnesses, or sensitive criminal records—can result in national security breaches and undermine the credibility of court decisions. Thus, cybersecurity functions as an ethical, procedural, and institutional imperative for AI-driven justice systems (Al-Rashid, 2022; OECD, 2019).

4.2 Emerging Cyber Threats in AI-Enabled Judicial Environments

AI-driven judicial systems face a variety of contemporary cyber threats, many of which directly target the integrity and reliability of legal processes:

- **Data breaches**, especially involving sensitive case files, witness identities, and classified documents (Marsh, 2023).
- **Ransomware attacks** capable of halting court operations or restricting access to legal repositories.
- **Deepfake evidence fabrication**, threatening the authenticity of audiovisual evidence in criminal cases.
- **Adversarial AI attacks**, in which malicious actors intentionally manipulate AI inputs to generate biased or incorrect outcomes (Goodfellow et al., 2015).
- **Insider threats**, where unauthorized system access by internal personnel compromises judicial confidentiality.

The growing sophistication of these threats requires judicial institutions to adopt proactive, multi-layered cybersecurity strategies.

4.3 Securing Digital Evidence and Ensuring Chain of Custody

Digital evidence is increasingly central to investigative and adjudicatory processes. Its judicial admissibility depends on secure handling procedures and an unbroken chain of custody. Cybersecurity therefore plays a crucial role in:

- Protecting evidence using end-to-end encryption during transfer and storage (NIST, 2021).
- Maintaining immutable audit logs that record every instance of access or modification.
- Applying digital signatures and timestamping to preserve authenticity.
- Storing evidence in secure cloud environments governed by zero-trust access policies.

Failure to maintain adequate cybersecurity controls may result in exclusion of evidence, procedural injustice, or wrongful convictions.

4.4 Cybersecurity Governance and Legal Frameworks

AI-enabled courts must operate within a comprehensive cybersecurity governance structure. IGI Global–aligned scholarship emphasizes the need for:

- Regular AI vulnerability assessments and system audits.
- National legislative frameworks defining standards for digital evidence, data protection, and cyber incident reporting.
- Compliance with recognized international cybersecurity standards, such as ISO/IEC 27001 and the NIST Cybersecurity Framework (UNESCO, 2021).
- Clear accountability and liability mechanisms when cyber incidents affect judicial processes.

Governance ensures that AI technologies enhance—rather than compromise—the principles of justice, fairness, and transparency.

4.5 Ethical Cybersecurity Principles in Judicial AI

Cybersecurity and AI ethics are interdependent in smart judicial ecosystems. The ethical use of AI requires security measures that support:

- **Transparency**, enabling courts to understand how AI-generated outputs were produced.
- **Explainability**, allowing human reviewers to identify errors possibly caused by cyber interference.
- **Human oversight**, ensuring that judges retain authority over all final decisions (OECD, 2019).
- **Mandatory disclosure** of cyber incidents that could influence case outcomes.

These ethical cybersecurity principles are central to the legitimacy of AI-driven judicial systems

5. CONCLUSION

In conclusion of this research, we are convinced that the judicial field is among those most likely to witness a significant leap in technological development, especially with the implementation of artificial intelligence tools. This is particularly evident given the Kingdom of Bahrain's continuous efforts to adopt advanced steps in line with the global AI boom across various domains.

In 2019, the Kingdom of Bahrain announced a pilot testing initiative for AI applications in the public sector, which was approved by the Center of the Fourth Industrial Revolution and the Information and eGovernment Authority. The main goal of this initiative was to develop a guideline for governments on the responsible use of artificial intelligence, in line with sustainable development goals.

Additionally, the Kingdom of Bahrain launched a national initiative in implementation of the directives of His Highness Sheikh Isa bin Salman Al Khalifa, titled "Tamkeen", which aims to train 50,000 Bahraini citizens in AI skills. This initiative is part of many other national efforts to keep pace with the global advancements in artificial intelligence.

These initiatives are strong indicators of Bahrain's potential to expand this development to include all sectors, especially the judiciary. Given the urgent need to improve the efficiency and effectiveness of the judicial system, I believe it is crucial to capitalize on this technological revolution and benefit from the experiences of countries that have already integrated AI into their litigation systems.

From the standpoint of integrating AI tools into Bahrain's judicial system, it is suggested that a governmental legal application be developed to function as a judicial robot specialized in judicial services that facilitate the litigation process for individuals, business owners, lawyers, and legal professionals.

Among the proposed functions of this robot are:

- Document authentication
- Transaction oversight
- General legal consultations
- Record-keeping
- Submission of enforcement requests
- Delivery of statements of claim
- Written pleadings
- Case status inquiries

- Scheduling court appointments

One can easily imagine the profound effect this application could have in reducing the number of court visitors and limiting the overload of non-critical cases. Moreover, this system would allow users to access all judicial services electronically via the app without the need to visit the courts or follow up in person on a daily basis.

Among the key conclusions of this research is the recognition of the importance of applying AI in the judicial field, especially after reviewing the successful experiences of various countries. There is a pressing need to alleviate court burdens and streamline complex procedures. The judiciary remains one of the few sectors that still clings to traditional methods, despite the dramatic evolution of crime and the emergence of new forms such as cybercrime and digital offenses.

Throughout this research, we observed a scarcity of scientific studies and projects that integrate AI with the legal sector. These fields demand dual expertise in both law and AI, and the rapid pace of AI development contributes to the lack of specialized projects in our region.

There is also a notable legislative gap concerning AI's legal personality and its relationship with humans, especially in terms of accountability and criminal responsibility, and the ethical dimensions of using AI in legal systems. Another observation is that this legislative and research shortfall is partly due to outdated educational curricula, which remain out of sync with technological advancements. School and university curricula must evolve to promote awareness and encourage scientific research in this area.

The practical ease of using AI in judiciary is evident, especially in routine tasks handled by judges, such as:

- Writing decisions,
- Legal analysis of cases,
- And legal research and consultation for repetitive cases.

This also extends to notaries who handle document verification and record organization, as well as other administrative and procedural aspects.

Lastly, there is an urgent societal need for AI training and awareness, especially for judges, lawyers, prosecutors, and notaries. Implementing such AI-driven projects demands continuous training to help legal professionals adapt to technological developments and keep pace with AI advancements.

One of the fundamental findings of this research is that integrating AI into the judicial system is no easy task. The legal field is highly sensitive, as it concerns people's rights and freedoms and the sovereignty of states. Therefore, any move toward AI integration must be coupled with enhanced oversight and supervision, to prevent and address potential risks stemming from AI usage.

Moreover, cybersecurity is indispensable in ensuring that AI-driven judicial systems remain secure, transparent, and trustworthy. As the justice sector undergoes rapid digital transformation, robust cybersecurity frameworks are essential for safeguarding judicial credibility, protecting digital evidence, and maintaining ethical decision-making practices. Incorporating cybersecurity into legislative, procedural, and technological reforms is therefore a critical prerequisite for achieving secure smart criminal justice systems.

5.1. Recommendations

- We recommend the establishment of a legal framework that incorporates artificial intelligence as a supporting tool for those working within and benefiting from the judicial system. This can be achieved by enacting legislation and regulations that facilitate the integration of AI in legal practice. These laws should define the ethical standards for AI use and ensure that judicial decisions remain accurate and fair.
- We recommend developing AI applications that house judicial databases to enable AI systems to offer legal services. These services should include scheduling court sessions, receiving lawsuits, handling enforcement requests, processing written memos and oral pleadings, and responding to inquiries. This would help reduce courtroom congestion caused by routine requests and enable judges to review materials before scheduled hearings, thereby streamlining the litigation process.
- We emphasize the need for ongoing human oversight and supervision over all AI tools implemented in the legal field. This is critical to ensure a balanced relationship between humans and AI systems. Moreover, it is essential to establish safeguards to guarantee that final decisions and rulings remain in the hands of human judges. This is especially important because the legal system is inherently sensitive and demands consistent human involvement in decision-making processes.

REFERENCES

Al-Faliti, S. A. (2024). *The Impact of Using Artificial Intelligence on the Litigation System in the Courts of the Sultanate of Oman and the Arab Republic of Egypt: Between Reality and Hope*. Scientific Research, Al-Zahraa College for Girls.

Al-Marzouqi, A. A. (2021). *Electronic Litigation (Smart Litigation) and Electronic Litigation (Smart Judiciary): A Comparative Study of the Legislation of the United Arab Emirates with Some Arab and Foreign Systems*. University of Sharjah Journal of Legal Sciences.

Al-Shar'ah, H. A. (2020). *Electronic Litigation and Electronic Courts*. Dar Al-Thaqafa for Publishing and Distribution.

Bilal, F. B. (2023). *Smart Litigation in Qatari Courts: Between Reality and Hope. A Comparative Study*. Supreme Judicial Council.

Bilal, F. B. (2023). The Role of Artificial Intelligence in Promoting Effective Justice Before the Judiciary. A Comparative Study with the Legal and Judicial Systems in the State of Qatar. Master's Thesis, Qatar University.

El-Din, R. E. (2024). *Artificial Intelligence and the Judicial System: Global Experiences. Scientific Research*. Mansoura University.

Goodfellow, I., Shlens, J., & Szegedy, C. (2015). Explaining and harnessing adversarial examples. *International Conference on Learning Representations (ICLR)*.

Lo, D. L. (2021). Can AI replace a judge in the courtroom? UNSW. Sydney. https://www.unsw.edu.au/newsroom/news/2021/10/can-ai-replace-judge-courtroom

Marsh, T. (2023). Deepfakes and the challenge to evidentiary integrity in modern courts. *International Review of Digital Forensics*, *11*(3), 120–138.

NIST. (2021). *Digital Identity Guidelines (NIST Special Publication 800-63-3)*. U.S. Department of Commerce, National Institute of Standards and Technology.

OECD. (2019). *OECD Principles on Artificial Intelligence*. Organisation for Economic Co-operation and Development.

Smith, J. (2023). Cybersecurity implications of AI adoption in judicial institutions. *Journal of Law. Technology & Ethics*, *5*(2), 66–89.

UNESCO. (2021). *Recommendation on the Ethics of Artificial Intelligence*. United Nations Educational, Scientific and Cultural Organization.

University of Southampton. (2025). *The growing demand for AI skills in criminal justice*. Southampton Online. https://www.online.southampton.ac.uk/blog/growing-demand-ai-skills-criminal-justice [Accessed 10 Dec 2025].

. Vasdani, T. V. (2020). Robot Justice: China's use of Internet Courts, The Lawyer's Daily, LexisNexis, Canada. lasted visited: 28/April/2025

Chapter 3

Affective Computing and Neuro-Symbolic Intelligence in the Protection of Digital Learning Ecologies:

Cybersecurity Infrastructures for Didactic Systems

Ashraf Alam
https://orcid.org/0000-0001-6178-1187
Alliance University, Bengaluru, India

ABSTRACT

This chapter reframes educational cybersecurity as a neurocognitively orchestrated socio-technical control regime rather than a peripheral IT safeguard. It integrates Cognitive Load Theory, dual-process reasoning, predictive processing, and neuro-ergonomics with affective computing, behavioral biometrics, and neuro-symbolic AI to explain how workload, vigilance, affect, and habit loops shape susceptibility to phishing, extortion, and configuration drift in digital learning ecologies. Brain-inspired anomaly detection, continuous authentication, and explainable risk analytics are embedded within human-in-the-loop governance, role-specific competency frameworks, and equity centric policy architectures. A staged implementation roadmap aligns identity fabrics, telemetry pipelines, federated learning, and impact audits with cost risk modelling and data protection mandates, yielding a globally relevant blueprint for neuro-intelligent, ethically constrained cyber defenses that preserve autonomy, inclusion, and instructional continuity.

DOI: 10.4018/979-8-3373-5012-7.ch003

1. INTRODUCTION

1.1 Problematizing Cybersecurity in Digitally Mediated Learning Ecologies

Digitally mediated learning now constitutes a planetary infrastructure where learning management systems, video conferencing platforms, assessment portals, and content repositories form a continuous cognitive environment for more than a billion learners. At the height of recent global school closures, close to 1.6 billion students across roughly 190 countries experienced abrupt migration to remote or hybrid formats, which accelerated platform adoption, widened device heterogeneity, and multiplied integration dependencies. This reconfiguration did not simply digitize existing classrooms, it generated complex socio-technical ecologies where identity, content, and assessment flow across institutional, commercial, and national boundaries. Within these ecologies, cybersecurity failures immediately manifest as pedagogical breakdowns, data breaches involving sensitive learner records or research outputs, and interruptions to examinations and accreditation timelines. The problem space therefore cannot be framed as a narrow technical concern, but as a systemic vulnerability within the global architecture of education that directly conditions access, continuity, and equity.

1.2 Key Constructs in Affective Computing and Neuro-Symbolic Cyber Defense

The conceptual terrain of affect-aware cyber defense in education is anchored in several interlocking constructs. *Affective computing* refers to computational systems that sense, infer, and modulate human emotional and physiological states, using signals such as pupil diameter, facial micro-expressions, heart rate variability, and interaction rhythms (Vijaya & Ramesh, 2025; Singh, 2025; Alam, 2022). *Behavioral biometrics* conceptualize identity as a stable yet context-sensitive pattern of motor and perceptual signatures, including keystroke dynamics, mouse trajectories, and touchscreen gestures, which can support continuous authentication without intrusive tokens. *Neuroadaptive cybersecurity* denotes architectures that infer latent cognitive states such as workload, vigilance, and fatigue, then adjust authentication friction and alerting intensity accordingly. *Neuro-symbolic intelligence* integrates data-driven neural models with symbolic policy representations, enabling systems that both learn from telemetry and remain aligned with institutional rules for access, assessment integrity, and data handling. These constructs converge within *didactic systems* where interfaces, algorithms, and governance mechanisms jointly shape how learners and educators encounter risk and protection.

1.3 Theoretical and Epistemic Frameworks for Neurocognitive Cybersecurity

A coherent neurocognitive approach to educational cybersecurity rests on several foundational theories. *Cognitive Load Theory* explains how finite working memory resources are partitioned among intrinsic, extraneous, and germane demands, which directly modulates the capacity to scrutinize authenticity cues in email, portals, and messaging interfaces. *Dual-process reasoning* distinguishes rapid, heuristic decision pathways from slower, analytic evaluation, clarifying why urgency and authority framings can override deliberation under time pressure. *Predictive processing* conceptualizes perception and action as continuous attempts to minimize prediction error relative to internal generative models, suggesting that subtle anomalies in domain names, certificate banners, or login patterns may remain undetected when they do not strongly violate learned expectations (Tekin & Dener, 2025; Siddique & Jahankhani, 2024; Alam, 2023a). Socio-technical systems theory, distributed cognition, and *activity systems* perspectives together frame educational cybersecurity as the emergent outcome of interactions among tools, rules, roles, and community norms rather than as an isolated IT function. These frameworks provide the epistemic scaffolding for the chapter.

1.4 Guiding Questions, Conceptual Propositions, and Boundary Conditions

The chapter is organized around a set of guiding questions that translate abstract theory into designable propositions. One central question concerns how cognitive load, attentional fragmentation, and affective arousal modulate susceptibility to phishing, credential misuse, and configuration errors within routine academic workflows. A second question addresses how multimodal telemetry, including keystroke variance, cursor intermittency, gaze dispersion, and low channel neurophysiology, can be transformed into ethically acceptable indicators of latent risk without collapsing into surveillance. A third question examines how *neuro-symbolic governance* can align adaptive detection with legal norms, children's rights frameworks, and academic freedom. The core propositions assert that cognitive and affective states are predictive of cyber risk, that hybrid neuro-AI architectures can anticipate and mitigate this risk in real time, and that participatory, explainable security cultures are necessary to maintain legitimacy. Boundary conditions include minimal network hygiene, baseline platform interoperability, and institutional commitment to privacy-preserving design.

1.5 Structure, Scope, and Contributions of the Chapter

The chapter advances a narrative review that is conceptual and design oriented rather than empirical, synthesizing constructs from neuroscience, affective computing, behavioral biometrics, cybersecurity engineering, educational technology, and governance studies. Section 2 characterizes the contemporary threat landscape and its cognitive-behavioral determinants within educational ecologies, culminating in a compact taxonomy in Table 1 that links attack modalities to neurocognitive vulnerabilities and mitigation levers. Section 3 elaborates the neuroscience and affective foundations of cyber risk and resilience, mapping brain systems, psychophysiological indicators, and learning mechanisms to specific defensive affordances. Section 4 details neuro-AI architectures and behavioral biometric mechanisms appropriate for didactic systems, while Section 5 foregrounds human-in-the-loop governance, explainability, and digital literacy as necessary complements. Section 6 translates these ideas into implementation roadmaps, economic reasoning, and policy-ethical templates. Section 7 concludes by synthesizing implications for global educational governance, signaling research priorities, and articulating a normative trajectory where neuro-intelligent cybersecurity becomes an enabler of trust, continuity, and inclusion in digital learning ecologies.

2. CYBER THREAT LANDSCAPE AND COGNITIVE VULNERABILITY IN EDUCATIONAL ECOLOGIES

2.1 Multilayered Threat Taxonomies in K–12 and Higher Education

Contemporary educational networks constitute stratified attack surfaces where threats propagate simultaneously across infrastructure, identity, and data governance layers. At the macro level, universities, colleges, and schools report incident prevalences that in some jurisdictions exceed four fifths of institutions, with universities in certain national systems approaching near universality of reported breaches within a single year, while primary and secondary institutions display lower yet still structurally significant exposure. K–12 environments globally exhibit incident frequencies that approximate or exceed one confirmed cyber event for every operative school day, with sectoral telemetry in some federated monitoring regimes recording on the order of fourteen thousand security events and more than nine thousand confirmed incidents across only a few thousand institutions within an eighteen-month window. Within this ecology, volumetric attacks such as distributed denial of service, credential stuffing, ransomware campaigns, data exfiltration, and platform compromises interlock, so that no single technical control can be treated as a sufficient barrier. Table 1 later distils this multiplex threat space into a concise matrix that explicitly couples threat modality to cognitive and affective vulnerabilities.

2.2 Micro-Level Attack Vectors for Social Engineering, Phishing, and Platform Exploitation

At the micro level of interaction, threat actors increasingly privilege human-centric attack vectors that exploit the semiotics of academic communication rather than purely protocol vulnerabilities. High fidelity phishing and impersonation messages mirror institutional tone, typography, and workflow semantics, referencing grade release, scholarship confirmation, timetable changes, conference travel, or examination logistics in order to commandeer the heuristics of ordinary academic correspondence (Rios-Campos et al., 2024; Alam, 2023b; Saikia et al., 2023). Generative language models and synthetic media pipelines now enable adversaries to fabricate persuasive emails, instant messages, and even voice or avatar representations that reproduce local idioms and administrative phrases with disquieting precision. Within learning management systems, malicious payloads can be embedded in ostensibly benign resource links, collaborative document invitations, and third-party tool launches, while misused announcement channels and course messaging spaces serve as amplifiers. Sectoral assessments suggest that human targeted vectors such as phishing, malvertising, and credential harvesting account for a majority share of impactful incidents, with human focused exploits surpassing purely technical ones by roughly half again in some K–12 aggregates, a pattern that underscores the cognitive architecture of risk documented in Table 1.

2.3 Cognitive, Behavioral, and Socio-Cultural Determinants of Susceptibility

Susceptibility within these digital pedagogical ecologies arises from structured interactions among cognitive architecture, learned behavioral routines, and socio-cultural norms. Within *dual-process reasoning* frameworks, fast, heuristic decision streams dominate when learners and staff triage overflowing inboxes, messaging feeds, and platform notifications under deadline pressure, while slow, analytic evaluation is reserved for tasks explicitly framed as complex. *Cognitive Load Theory* clarifies that intrinsic challenges of disciplinary content, accumulated extraneous frictions from cluttered interfaces or authentication obstacles, and limited residual germane capacity jointly constrain scrutiny of subtle authenticity cues such as sender domains or certificate anomalies. Social identity and authority gradients within schools and universities further amplify risk, since individuals in lower power positions may experience heightened compliance pressure when communications appear to originate from deans, principals, supervisors, or funding bodies (Perez et al., 2026; Shiwlani et al., 2024). Cultural norms around politeness, rapid responsiveness, and reputational anxiety compound these effects, particularly for first generation students and international scholars who perceive email etiquette and institutional legitimacy as high stakes. The structured mapping in Table 1 aligns specific threat modalities with dominant cognitive and socio-cultural triggers in order to support more discriminating intervention design.

2.4 Educational Risk Ecologies, Heterogeneity, and Contextual Modulation

Educational risk ecologies display pronounced heterogeneity across governance regimes, resource endowments, and technological baselines. Under-resourced public schools in many regions operate with aging hardware, shared devices, minimal segmentation, and constrained specialist support, which magnifies the consequences of commodity malware and credential reuse, while affluent institutions manage complex hybrid estates that interweave high performance clusters, commercial cloud platforms, and extensive third-party integrations, thereby generating intricate trust boundaries and misconfiguration opportunities. Rural schools with intermittent connectivity lean heavily on offline caching, portable media, and ad hoc local networks, which introduces distinct attack surfaces compared to urban campuses immersed in continuous high bandwidth connectivity (Xavier et al., 2025; Sheikhbahei & Ari, 2024). Cross-border research consortia and transnational education programs impose further complexity, since data must traverse heterogeneous regulatory spaces with divergent expectations of encryption, logging, and breach notification. Inequities in digital literacy and language confidence intersect with these structural factors, resulting in patterned vulnerability among particular cohorts such as younger learners, individuals who rely on assistive technologies, and staff with limited exposure to contemporary cyber hygiene constructs. Within this stratified landscape, Table 1 operates as a compact risk cartography that relates institutional typologies and cognitive profiles to specific threat vectors.

2.5 Multilayered Cyber Threats and Cognitive-Behavioral Vulnerabilities across Educational Contexts

Within this conceptual scaffolding, a tabular synthesis can compress the multifaceted threat landscape into a tractable analytic artefact that links attack modalities to neurocognitive dynamics and actionable mitigations. Table 1 is structured to foreground the co-variation between technical vectors, pedagogical disruption patterns, dominant cognitive-affective triggers, temporally contingent exposure windows, and the most salient cognition-aware defensive levers. Each row condenses a canonical threat class into minimal yet semantically saturated descriptors that permit rapid comparison across modalities while preserving conceptual richness. This matrix does not function as a static checklist, but as a dynamic schema through which policy makers, digital learning technologists, and institutional risk stewards can align investments and interventions with the specific vulnerabilities that emerge from cognitive architecture and academic temporality rather than treating all attack types as equivalent.

Table 1. Cyber Threats and Cognition-Sensitive Vulnerability

Threat Modality and Vector	Pedagogical and Operational Impact	Dominant Cognitive-Affective Trigger	High-Risk Temporal Context in Education	Priority Cognition-Aware Mitigation Lever
Phishing-Driven Credential Harvesting	Covert account takeover, silent grade manipulation, hijacked submissions, privacy breaches for learner records	Heuristic trust in institutional logos, authority deference, scarcity anxiety, automatic link activation habits	Admission offers, fee deadlines, examination timetables, scholarship notifications, high volume email bursts	Load-synchronized warning cues, simplified mail clients, spaced micro-simulations, *dual-process* priming, friction for irreversible clicks
Ransomware and Extortion Campaigns	Encrypted learning platforms, disrupted classes, inaccessible research datasets, emergency reversion to paper workflows	Acute loss aversion, catastrophic imagination, panic-driven compliance, tunnelled problem framing	Term breaks, grading periods, registration peaks, calendar moments with high dependency on digital systems	Segmented backups, *prospect theory* informed communication, rehearsed offline contingencies, calm explanatory dashboards, constrained privilege escalation
Distributed Denial of Service Saturation	Inaccessible portals, failed online examinations, delayed submissions, reputational erosion, crisis messaging overload	Perceived chaos, helplessness, affective contagion, attribution confusion about personal error versus systemic failure	Synchronous online examinations, real-time lectures, live-streamed events, high profile institutional announcements	Traffic scrubbing, exam-tolerant scheduling, redundant access channels, prebriefed expectations, *predictive processing* of likely outage patterns

continued on following page

Table 1. Continued

Threat Modality and Vector	Pedagogical and Operational Impact	Dominant Cognitive-Affective Trigger	High-Risk Temporal Context in Education	Priority Cognition-Aware Mitigation Lever
Data Exfiltration and Leak Coercion	Exposure of sensitive research, personal identifiers, behavioural telemetry, undermined trust, regulatory sanctions	Shame anticipation, reputational fear, moral injury, overestimation of adversary omniscience	Large-scale data consolidation, migration to cloud platforms, mergers of student information systems, major research consortium activities	Encryption with institutional key custody, minimised retention, transparent breach protocols, *information governance* literacy, narrative framing that reduces panic
Configuration Drift and Shadow Integration	Latent privilege escalation, orphaned accounts, unmonitored tools, inconsistent policy enforcement across courses	Illusion of continuity, habituated clicking through consent prompts, underestimation of compound risk, optimism bias	Rapid pivot to new tools, emergency remote teaching, local integration of third-party applications, high staff turnover	Automated configuration baselines, sunset policies, *socio-technical systems* mapping, faculty onboarding with cyber hygiene, periodic consent renewal prompts

Table 1 illustrates that each threat class is not only a technical phenomenon, but also a structured interaction between external adversarial intent and internal cognitive-evaluative dynamics. Phishing-driven credential harvesting weaponises trust heuristics and urgency perceptions, whereas ransomware amplifies loss aversion and catastrophic risk framing. Distributed denial events disrupt perceived reliability and induce affective contagion among learners, which can persist long after service restoration. Data exfiltration and leak coercion destabilise identity and reputational security, often producing psychological sequelae for staff whose research or communications have been exposed. Configuration drift and shadow integrations exemplify slow forming vulnerabilities that accumulate through local improvisations and legacy residues rather than deliberate malfeasance. By framing mitigation levers in explicitly cognition-aware terms such as load-synchronised prompts, narrative reframing, and socio-technical cartography, the table aligns with the broader argument that educational cybersecurity must be designed through a neurocognitive lens.

3. NEUROSCIENCE AND AFFECTIVE FOUNDATIONS OF CYBER RISK AND RESILIENCE

3.1 Cognitive Load, Working Memory, and Attentional Bottlenecks in Education

Cyber behaviour in digital classrooms is constrained by the finite capacity of working memory and the partitioning of resources postulated by *Cognitive Load Theory*. Intrinsic demands arise from disciplinary problem solving, extraneous demands accumulate from cluttered interfaces, multiple overlapping notification streams, and opaque authentication rituals, while germane resources must sustain schema construction and metacognitive monitoring (Pazouki et al., 2022; Alam, 2023c; Zahm et al., 2022). When extraneous load swells, learners and staff increasingly rely on heuristic shortcuts, such as automatic acceptance of institutional branding or habituated clicking on routine links, rather than analytic scrutiny of subtle anomalies in addresses or certificate banners. Attentional bottlenecks, described by *selective attention* and *bottleneck* models, become acute in multiwindow learning environments where video conferencing, chat, shared documents, and assessment portals compete for visual and cognitive bandwidth. Under such conditions, low salience security cues are easily filtered out as noise. Later, Table 2 systematises these dynamics by mapping specific cognitive mechanisms to digital interaction markers and corresponding cyber-defensive design levers.

3.2 Affective, Neuroendocrine, and Social-Neuroscience Mechanisms of Risky Compliance

Cyber decision making in educational milieus also emerges from the interplay of affective appraisal, neuroendocrine modulation, and socially embedded cognition. High stakes assessments, funding milestones, and progression decisions trigger arousal profiles governed by cortisol and catecholamine dynamics that reshape the balance between prefrontal executive control and limbic urgency signalling (Nagar et al., 2022; Kumar et al., 2025). Within such states, the *affect heuristic* compresses complex risk evaluations into rapid, valence laden judgments, so that messages implying account suspension, plagiarism accusations, or scholarship loss evoke reflexive compliance behaviours. *Social neuroscience* constructs emphasise that authority representation, status hierarchies, and in-group affiliation modulate susceptibility, particularly when emails or platform prompts appear to emanate from professors, deans, or examination offices. Emotional contagion in group chats and social media streams can propagate anxiety or fatalism after visible incidents, weakening individual vigilance. The multi-level structure captured in Table 2 shows that these affective and social mechanisms are not epiphenomenal, but central determinants that can be instrumented through staging, communication framing, and affect labelling skills.

3.3 Neuroplasticity, Habit Formation, and Learning Theories for Cyber Resilience

The same neural systems that encode maladaptive cyber routines can be repurposed to scaffold durable resilience when educational design aligns with *neuroplasticity* principles. Habit loops theorised in *habit formation* models reveal how repeated cue routine reward cycles consolidate automatic responses, such as reusing passwords or immediately opening attachments from familiar names (Merat & Almuhtadi, 2024; Alam & Mohanty, 2022; Liv & Greenbaum, 2023). However, *reinforcement learning* constructs indicate that variable ratio rewards, timely feedback, and explicit reward prediction errors can gradually rewire these loops toward secure behaviours, for instance through micro acknowledgements for correct reporting or safe refusals. *Spacing* and *interleaving* principles from learning sciences suggest that brief, varied, temporally distributed micro-simulations of deceptive messages, embedded directly within routine coursework, support long term retention of discriminative heuristics without generating fatigue. As Table 2 articulates, neuroplastic mechanisms connect directly to designable levers such as graded challenge, reflective debriefing, and explicit metacognitive framing, which together promote internalisation rather than superficial compliance.

Table 2. Neurocognitive Mechanisms, Learning Stressors, and Cognition-Aware Cyber Levers

Neurocognitive Mechanism	Dominant Neural-Physiological Substrate	Prototypical Educational Stressor	Observable Digital Interaction Marker	Primary Cyber-Defensive Design Lever
Cognitive Load and Working Memory	Frontoparietal control networks, limited-capacity buffers, effortful maintenance processes	Concurrent deadlines, complex assignment portals, multi-tab resource navigation	Rapid context switching, shallow dwell on alerts, error prone form completion	Interface decluttering, task chunking, staggered prompts, *germane-load* oriented training
Selective Attention and Vigilance	Sensory gating circuits, thalamocortical pathways, vigilance regulation systems	Video lectures with parallel chats, proctored remote exams, synchronous collaboration	Narrow fixation fields, missed certificate warnings, inattentional omission of anomalies	Salient cue accentuation, notification batching, *signal detection* threshold tuning, visual hierarchy redesign
Affective Arousal and Stress Reactivity	Limbic salience networks, hypothalamic–pituitary–adrenal axis, autonomic arousal channels	High stakes grading events, disciplinary notices, financial-aid uncertainty	Impulsive clicking, rushed credential entry, bypass of secondary checks	Cooling delays, consequence transparent messages, *affect-labelling* micro-skills, low threat alternative actions
Habit Automation and Procedural Routines	Basal ganglia loops, procedural memory systems, dopaminergic reinforcement pathways	Daily logins, repetitive resource downloads, routine mail triage	Autopilot link activation, reused passwords, unreflective acceptance of requests	Default secure pathways, *habit loop* restructuring, variable ratio reinforcement, unobtrusive nudges
Predictive Modelling and Expectation Management	Hierarchical generative models, prediction error signalling, predictive coding hierarchies	Stable course layouts, repetitive platform aesthetics, consistent communication patterns	Failure to register subtle deviations in domains, unnoticed spoofed layouts	Diverse exemplars of safe patterns, *predictive-processing* informed anomaly cues, occasional benign perturbations
Social Cognition and Norm Internalisation	Medial prefrontal regions, mirror systems, norm encoding circuits	Peer group messaging, faculty announcements, cohort-wide policy broadcasts	Conformist uptake of unsafe practices, herd ignoring of alerts, socially driven risk taking	Peer modelling, *social proof* for secure behaviour, ambassador programmes, cooperative reporting norms

Table 2 reveals that each neurocognitive construct supplies at least one controllable parameter that can be modulated through instructional and technical design. Cognitive load can be engineered by simplifying authentication flows and suppressing non-essential prompts during acute workload peaks, whereas attentional allocation can be shaped by elevating the visual salience of a small subset of security critical cues and suppressing low value distractors. Affective arousal can be tempered through carefully scripted language that emphasises supportive remediation rather than punitive sanction, thereby reducing threat induced tunnel vision. Habit automation can be redirected by aligning the most effortless pathway with the most secure action, transforming friction from security into friction for insecurity. Predictive modelling can be harnessed by periodically exposing learners and staff to controlled variations in safe layouts and messages, strengthening sensitivity to deviations. Social cognition can be leveraged by making secure behaviour visible, aspirational, and collectively recognised rather than purely individual and invisible.

3.4 Integrative Neurocognitive Models of Cyber Behavior in Digital Classrooms

Integrative frameworks, such as *predictive processing* and *active inference*, provide powerful lenses through which the complex cyber behaviour of learners and educators in digital classrooms can be understood as continuous attempts to minimise expected loss under uncertainty (Loaiza et al., 2022; Mitchell et al., 2025). Within these constructs, clicking on links, ignoring warnings, or reporting anomalies are modelled as actions that update internal generative models of what constitutes normal institutional communication. When interfaces, messages, and routines remain highly predictable, minor deviations that indicate compromise may generate insufficient prediction error to breach the threshold for conscious inspection. Conversely, environments that are saturated with false alarms or inconsistent cues drive calibration drift, in which agents gradually learn to discount alerts altogether. The alignment achieved in Table 2 implies that effective educational cyber defence requires orchestrated interventions across load, attention, affect, habit, and social norms, so that the composite generative model that learners and staff hold about "how secure interaction feels" becomes congruent with institutional safeguards rather than in tension with them.

3.5 Neuroergonomics, Psychophysiological Telemetry, and Real-Time Educational Cyber Scaffolds

The field of *neuroergonomics* integrates psychophysiological telemetry with human-computer interaction design, and offers a prospective substrate for real-time cyber scaffolding in learning environments. Metrics such as pupil diameter variability, blink rate, gaze entropy, heart rate variability, and electrodermal activity can index transitions between focused engagement, overload, and fatigue during platform use

(Leider & Li, 2025; Alam & Mohanty, 2023; Kritika, 2025c). When interpreted through the mechanistic schemas summarised in Table 2, these signals can inform adaptive risk controls that raise authentication thresholds only when individuals are in vulnerable states, such as during prolonged sessions or immediately before submission deadlines, while deferring non-essential alerts to cognitive troughs. For such architectures to remain legitimate in education, telemetry must be processed locally when feasible, obfuscated into abstract state estimates, and governed by stringent consent, purpose limitation, and retention constraints. In this configuration, neurophysiological signals do not become instruments of surveillance, but resources for finely tuned, low friction, neurocognitively congruent protection.

4. NEURO-AI ARCHITECTURES AND BEHAVIORAL BIOMETRICS FOR EDUCATIONAL CYBER DEFENSE

4.1 Brain-Inspired Computational Architectures and Predictive Modelling in Didactic Infrastructures

Neuro-inspired computational architectures operationalise educational cybersecurity as a temporally structured pattern recognition and control problem, rather than as a static signature matching exercise. *Spiking neural networks* encode information in discrete temporal events that approximate action potentials, which permits highly granular modelling of authentication logs, network flows, and learning-platform interaction rhythms with energy-efficient, event-driven inference (Meghraoui & Belkhamza, 2025; Kritika, 2024). In parallel, *predictive-coding architectures* instantiate hierarchical generative models that continuously forecast expected traffic volumes, login periodicities, and resource access sequences across courses, thereby transforming deviations into explicit prediction error signals that can drive fine grained anomaly detection. Within teaching and assessment ecosystems, these mechanisms enable differentiation between legitimate surges, such as mass submission deadlines, and atypical patterns indicative of lateral movement or credential abuse. As later distilled in Table 3, such architectures must be coupled with principled uncertainty quantification and conservative control policies, so that adaptive containment actions remain proportional, reversible, and consonant with pedagogical continuity.

4.2 Neuro-Symbolic AI and Policy-Faithful Governance in Educational Cyber Regimes

Neuro-symbolic architectures fuse the representational richness of neural function approximators with the normative clarity of symbolic rule systems, thereby permitting campus security postures that are both adaptive and institutionally accountable. Neural components ingest heterogeneous telemetry from identity providers, learning management systems, collaboration suites, and research repositories, extracting latent features associated with navigation templates, discourse regularities, and resource usage trajectories (Kritika, 2025d; McCullum & Mancera, 2025; Alam & Mohanty, 2024). Symbolic layers encode *access control logics*, assessment integrity rules, data minimisation constraints, and jurisdiction-specific retention mandates in formal ontologies and temporal rule sets. Through differentiable reasoning or constraint-guided optimisation, *neuro-symbolic governance engines* can enforce invariants such as least privilege, due process, and non-discrimination while still learning from emergent behavioural patterns. This hybridisation enables automatic detection of policy violations, such as anomalous exam access or improper dataset export, while still generating human-readable rationales that can be audited by faculty committees and compliance officers. Table 3 later situates neuro-symbolic engines alongside other paradigms in terms of substrates, affordances, and inherent limitations.

4.3 Behavioral Biometrics and Multimodal Continuous Authentication in Pedagogical Platforms

Behavioral biometrics reconceptualise identity assurance in education as inference over neuromotor and perceptual idiosyncrasies, rather than over static secrets or physical tokens. Keystroke dynamics capture dwell and flight intervals, n-gram tempo signatures, and rhythm entropy during essay writing, coding tasks, and quiz completion, while mouse and touch kinematics capture curvature, jerk, and micro-correction patterns as learners navigate within course shells. These signals can support *continuous authentication* that silently verifies user legitimacy throughout a session, raising suspicion thresholds when interaction patterns deviate sharply from personalised baselines (Kabanda, 2023; Hramov et al., 2025). Within high stakes assessments, such mechanisms can supplement rather than replace more visible proctoring, thereby reducing reliance on intrusive webcams. As synthesised in Table 3, behavioural biometrics must be engineered with explicit attention to accessibility, device variability, and cultural-linguistic heterogeneity, so that neuromotor diversity and assistive-technology usage do not become proxies for suspicion or denial of service.

Table 3. Comparative Schema for Neuro-AI and Educational Biometric Mechanisms

Neuro-AI or Biometric Paradigm	Core Computational Substrate	Primary Educational Cyber Function	Key Strengths and Affordances	Principal Limitations and Precautions
Spiking-Neural Network Analytics	Event-driven spiking neurons, temporal coding, synaptic-plasticity rules	Fine grained anomaly detection in logs, flows, and interaction traces	Low latency, energy efficient inference, high temporal resolution, edge deployability	Complex training pipelines, interpretability challenges, sensitivity to encoding choices
Predictive-Coding Traffic Modellers	Hierarchical generative models, prediction-error minimisation, latent state inference	Behavioural baseline construction for logins, submissions, and resource access	Anticipatory detection of subtle drift, differentiation of expected surges from attacks	Risk of mis-specifying priors, potential overfitting to idiosyncratic institutional rhythms
Neuro-Symbolic Governance Engines	Neural feature extractors, symbolic rule bases, differentiable reasoning layers	Policy faithful access control, assessment integrity, and data handling enforcement	Human-auditable rationales, formal constraint checking, regulatory alignment	Knowledge engineering overhead, brittleness if ontologies lag evolving pedagogical practices
Keystroke-Dynamics Authentication	Temporal feature embeddings, sequence classifiers, similarity metrics	Continuous verification of learner identity during writing and assessment	No extra hardware, low friction, resilience to observation-based spoofing	Performance variability across devices, potential unfairness for atypical motor profiles
Mouse-and-Gesture Behavioral Biometrics	Trajectory analysis, jerk spectra, gesture micro-pattern modelling	Supplementary identity assurance during navigation and resource interaction	Complements keystroke features, usable on touch-first ecosystems, passive operation	Susceptible to environmental noise, influenced by input hardware heterogeneity
Hybrid Multimodal Risk Scoring Pipelines	Fusion architectures, ensemble learners, probabilistic calibration layers	Session-level risk estimation, trigger for step-up authentication and review	Robustness through redundancy, tunable sensitivity, context adaptive thresholds	Governance complexity, need for rigorous fairness audits, risk of over-collection of signals

Table 3 highlights that no single paradigm can exhaust the design space of educational cyber defense, and that robust architectures require carefully orchestrated ensembles. Spiking-neural models and predictive-coding schemes are well suited to background anomaly detection across vast telemetry streams, while neuro-symbolic engines excel at translating institutional charters and regulatory expectations into enforceable constraints that remain intelligible to human stakeholders (Hinrichs et al., 2024; Kritika, 2025a). Keystroke and gesture biometrics offer pragmatic paths to continuous authentication without demanding expensive sensors, yet must be calibrated to avoid penalising disability, neurodivergence, or temporary injury. Hybrid multimodal pipelines provide resilience by aggregating partially independent evidentiary sources, but they also heighten the need for privacy by design, clear purpose limitation, and transparent communication about what is being inferred, when, and why, in order to sustain legitimacy among learners and staff.

4.4 Robustness, Fairness, and Evaluation Regimes for Neuro-AI Defenses

Robustness and fairness constitute non-negotiable properties of neuro-AI defences deployed in educational settings, because model errors directly affect access to learning, assessment outcomes, and professional trajectories. Robustness requires explicit confrontation of adversarial dynamics, including scripted keystroke replay, robotic cursor emulation, synthetic identity injection, and crafted log perturbations intended to bypass anomaly detectors (Fernández-García et al., 2023; Kritika, 2025b). Techniques such as adversarial training, ensemble diversification, and conservative calibration can mitigate some attack surfaces, yet must be complemented by explicit *concept-drift* monitoring as platforms, curricula, and behavioural norms evolve. Fairness auditing entails disaggregated evaluation across demographic strata, language backgrounds, disability categories, and device ecologies, with metrics for differential false positive rates, calibration disparity, and error clustering. Evaluative regimes must extend beyond conventional accuracy or area-under-curve statistics to incorporate user centred indicators such as perceived legitimacy, cognitive overhead, and help-desk burden. The paradigms catalogued in Table 3 therefore require integrated evaluation frameworks that couple statistical performance with socio-ethical impact analyses.

4.5 Systems Integration, Edge Inference, and Learning-Analytics Synergy in Cyber Defense

Effective deployment of neuro-AI and biometric mechanisms in education depends on meticulous systems integration across identity fabrics, network perimeters, learning analytics stacks, and governance workflows. Edge inference nodes embedded in endpoint clients, browser extensions, or local appliances can execute spiking-network analytics and behavioural biometric checks close to the source of interaction, minimising latency and reducing the need to transmit raw telemetry (Gkintoni et al., 2025; Faraji et al., 2024). Central risk engines can then operate on distilled features and aggregated scores, integrating them with existing learning analytics indicators such as engagement trajectories, dropout risk scores, and assessment histories, while maintaining strict logical separation between pedagogical support and security decisioning. *Privacy-preserving computation* constructs, including local differential privacy, secure aggregation, and federated optimisation, enable collective model improvement without centralising sensitive traces. Alignment with the architectural characteristics summarised in Table 3 ensures that integration choices respect both the computational affordances of each paradigm and the normative commitments of education to autonomy, transparency, and inclusion.

5. HUMAN-IN-THE-LOOP CYBERSECURITY SYSTEMS IN EDUCATION

5.1 Collegial Co-Piloting and Expert Oversight in Sociotechnical Cyber Defense

Human-centred cybersecurity in education requires *human-in-the-loop* architectures in which faculty, security professionals, learning technologists, and student representatives operate as coordinated co-pilots rather than as disconnected stakeholders. In such assemblages, automated detectors ingest telemetry and generate risk scores, yet final determinations for high impact actions such as quarantining course materials, delaying examinations, or suspending accounts are mediated through structured human deliberation (Chapagain et al., 2025; Alzahrani, 2023). Risk triage frameworks incorporate pedagogical criticality, research sensitivity, legal exposure, and student welfare as explicit dimensions, so that an anomaly involving a capstone assessment or a thesis repository receives different treatment from a low stakes discussion forum. Escalation paths and decision logs formalise who authorises which interventions, under what thresholds, and with which reversible safeguards (Chandra et al., 2025; Bormpotsis et al., 2025). These arrangements prevent opaque algorithmic veto over academic processes while still harnessing computational vigilance. Table 4 later consolidates the division of labour, explanation interfaces, and outcome indicators associated with each human role in such sociotechnical ecosystems.

5.2 Explainable Neuro-AI as a Pedagogical and Governance Instrument

Explainable neuro-AI functions simultaneously as control infrastructure and as a pedagogical artefact that shapes user mental models of risk. Instead of surfacing cryptic error codes or generic alerts, systems grounded in *explainable AI* constructs provide concise natural language rationales, confidence bands, and minimal-change counterfactuals that show how small behavioural differences would have avoided a flag. These explanations are contextualised in terms that align with academic norms, for example specifying that access was temporarily limited because the device, location, and time pattern diverged sharply from the learner's usual profile during an examination window (Dal Verne, 2023; Bhardwaj et al., 2023). For faculty and administrators, higher level dashboards aggregate these explanations into interpretable patterns, such as clusters of anomalous logins around a particular course, while preserving individual privacy. When explanations are consistently calibrated, temporally well placed, and aligned with institutional policy language, they reduce defensive cynicism and transform each alert into a micro learning opportunity that reinforces secure interaction habits. Table 4 situates explanation modalities alongside role specific competencies.

5.3 Student Participatory Vigilance, Critical Data Literacy, and Cyber Civics

Students constitute the largest and most variegated population within educational networks, and their participation as active sentinels requires intentional cultivation of *critical data literacy* and cyber civics. Instead of treating security as an external policing function, curricula embed short, scenario-based learning objects that deconstruct real phishing narratives, impersonation attempts, and misconfiguration episodes, encouraging learners to analyse the cognitive triggers and interface cues that made them plausible (Ashraf et al., 2023) (Di Salvo, 2025). Gamified challenges, cooperative capture-the-flag exercises, and reflective journalling on personal digital practices foster *participatory vigilance* in which noticing and reporting anomalies becomes a valued component of academic professionalism. To sustain inclusivity, these activities support multiple languages, assistive technologies, and diverse cultural communication styles, avoiding a monocultural model of "correct" digital behaviour (Andrade et al., 2022; Mahajan et al., 2024). As a result, students generate high quality, context rich reports that materially strengthen situational awareness for institutional defenders. Table 4 codifies how student roles, explanation channels, and feedback loops can be structured to convert this vigilance into measurable security and learning gains.

Table 4. Human Roles, Explanations, and Outcomes in Cyber Defense

Human Role in Educational Cyber Ecology	Decision and Responsibility Scope	Neuro-AI and Explanation Interfaces	Key Competencies and Literacies	Feedback and Outcome Indicators
Students and Learner Cohorts	Local anomaly recognition, self-protection actions, timely incident reporting	In context alerts, just in time rationales, personal risk dashboards	Critical data literacy, basic *threat-modelling*, metacognitive awareness of cognitive load and affect	Reduction in risky clicks, richer incident reports, improved self-efficacy in cyber tasks
Faculty and Instructional Designers	Course level configuration, assessment modality choices, escalation of suspicious patterns	Course dashboards, cohort anomaly summaries, policy linked explanations	Secure pedagogy design, *Cognitive Load Theory* informed interface judgement, fairness sensitivity	Fewer misconfigured assessments, reduced assessment disruption, higher alignment of teaching flows with security guidance
IT and Security Operations Teams	Triage, containment, infrastructure configuration, tuning of detection thresholds	Analyst consoles, model behaviour traces, calibration and drift views	*Security analytics* proficiency, adversarial reasoning, interpretive skill with neuro-AI outputs	Shorter dwell times, lower false positive volumes, improved prioritisation of critical incidents
Academic and Administrative Leadership	Strategic risk appetite setting, resource allocation, policy ratification	Executive scorecards, aggregated trend explanations, scenario projections	Governance literacy, *risk management* reasoning, ability to interpret socio-technical metrics	Coherent security roadmaps, sustained investment, reduced misalignment between policy statements and operational practice
Governance, Ethics, and Student Representation Bodies	Norm setting, oversight of fairness, consent, and accountability guarantees	Audit views, anonymised case exemplars, outcome disparity diagnostics	*Participatory design* facilitation, ethical reasoning, familiarity with accessibility and equity constructs	Lower disparity in error impacts, higher perceived legitimacy, effective adjustments to policy and design patterns

Table 4 shows that human participation in cyber defense is not monolithic, but differentiated according to institutional position, decision latitude, and literacy requirements. Students primarily exercise micro level judgment and incident reporting, yet their contribution depends on fluent interpretation of in context explanations and a grounded sense of cognitive and affective vulnerabilities. Faculty act as intermediaries between platform affordances and learner experiences, requiring fluency in secure assessment design and load aware configuration. Security operations teams must be able to interrogate and recalibrate neuro-AI models, interpreting outputs not as oracles but as probabilistic signals within broader risk reasoning. Leadership bodies require abstractions that connect metrics such as dwell time and false positive rates to strategic objectives, while governance and ethics committees synthesize evidence about fairness, consent, and accessibility into normative adjustments. Across these strata, explainability interfaces and competency frameworks coevolve, so that each human node in the system becomes both a beneficiary and a co-producer of security.

5.4 Organizational Learning, Feedback Loops, and Capacity Maturation

Educational cyber defense strengthens over time only when institutions deliberately encode experiences into *organizational learning* structures with explicit feedback loops. After significant incidents or near misses, cross functional review sessions map antecedent conditions, detection pathways, decision moments, and pedagogical consequences, then translate these insights into updated playbooks, configuration templates, and training artefacts. Active learning pipelines in neuro-AI models prioritise ambiguous cases flagged by analysts or faculty for human labelling, creating a virtuous cycle where human judgment systematically improves automated performance (Monteith et al., 2024; Alkhatri et al., 2024). Capacity maturation trajectories move from ad hoc heroic responses to codified, rehearsed, and continuously refined routines, with clearly articulated role expectations such as those summarised in Table 4. Structured reflection tools grounded in *double-loop learning* constructs encourage questioning of underlying assumptions, including risk appetite and default platform configurations, rather than merely adjusting superficial parameters. Over time, these mechanisms shift the institutional culture from reactive crisis management toward anticipatory, evidence informed resilience.

5.5 Role-Oriented Competency Frameworks and Distributed Accountability Regimes

To stabilise human participation in cybersecurity, institutions benefit from explicit, role-oriented competency frameworks and distributed accountability regimes that align incentives and expectations. Competency maps delineate the knowledge, skills, and dispositions required for each role in Table 4, from basic password hygiene and phishing recognition for students to interpretive fluency with calibration graphs and fairness diagnostics for security analysts. Professional development programmes, micro credentials, and performance review criteria then operationalise these expectations, embedding cyber stewardship into career progression rather than treating it as peripheral volunteerism (Moustafa, 2022; Ali et al., 2022). Distributed accountability frameworks clarify where responsibility lies when automated systems misclassify or when controls inadvertently disrupt teaching, ensuring that individuals do not become scapegoats for structural deficiencies. Mechanisms such as shared key performance indicators, cross departmental steering groups, and transparent reporting of incident statistics foster collective ownership of outcomes (Al Siam et al., 2025; Naeem et al., 2024). The result is an ecology in which human and machine agency interlock within a clearly articulated normative architecture, sustaining both robust protection and the educational mission.

6. IMPLEMENTATION ROADMAPS, ECONOMICS, AND POLICY-ETHICS FOR NEURO-INTELLIGENT EDUCATIONAL SECURITY

6.1 Socio-Technical Infrastructure, Platform Integration, and Data Architecture for Neuro-Intelligent Defenses

Operationalising neuro-intelligent cybersecurity in education requires infrastructural substrates that align *socio-technical systems* thinking with concrete architectural blueprints. Identity fabrics must combine single sign-on, phishing resistant authenticators, and context aware behavioural telemetry in ways that respect least privilege and granular role segmentation for students, faculty, researchers, and external collaborators. Network topologies need micro-segmented cores, encrypted internal pathways, and strategically placed sensors that can ingest event streams from endpoints, learning platforms, and cloud gateways without creating surveillance panopticons. Data architecture must distinguish clearly between raw interaction signals, derived behavioural features, and summarised risk indicators, with each tier governed by differentiated access controls, retention ceilings, and cryptographic protections. Integration with learning management systems, video platforms, and assessment engines should utilise open interoperability standards so that neuro-AI modules can be swapped, upgraded, or federated without brittle custom code. Throughout, *privacy by design* and *data minimisation* constructs must anchor decisions about what telemetry is truly necessary for protection, ensuring that neurocognitive insights are harvested in proportionate, purpose constrained ways.

6.2 Governance Frameworks, Legal-Regulatory Compliance, and Institutional Accountability Architectures

Governance for neuro-intelligent educational security demands a layered framework that reconciles algorithmic adaptivity with legal, ethical, and pedagogical accountability. Data protection statutes, children's rights instruments, and sector specific regulations converge on requirements for consent, transparency, purpose limitation, and robust breach handling, which must be translated into operational controls, not just policy statements. Institutions therefore need *governance char-*

ters that allocate responsibilities among data protection officers, chief information security officers, academic leadership, and independent ethics bodies, specifying decision rights for adopting, configuring, and auditing neuro-AI systems. Mechanisms such as data protection impact assessments, model risk classifications, and periodic policy reviews embed *risk governance* constructs into everyday change processes. Contractual arrangements with vendors must codify obligations around algorithmic transparency, cryptographic key custody, subcontractor visibility, and verified deletion. As Section 6.4 and Table 5 show, these governance elements can be staged across maturity phases so that even resource constrained institutions can sequence adoption in a disciplined, accountable manner.

6.3 Economic Evaluation, Risk Management, and Return on Resilience in Educational Cybersecurity

Economic reasoning for neuro-intelligent cyber defenses hinges on making risk, cost, and educational value commensurable within an explicit *risk management* and *portfolio theory* frame. Institutions must model plausible incident scenarios, such as extended platform outages, credential compromises in high stakes examinations, or exfiltration of research data, and estimate associated direct costs in remediation, legal exposure, and service credits, along with indirect costs in enrolment attrition, faculty productivity loss, and reputational damage. Against these trajectories, decision makers evaluate investment in telemetry, neuro-AI analytics, training, and governance as a portfolio of risk reducing assets whose combined effect shortens attacker dwell time and reduces incident severity. Techniques from *cost utility analysis* and *life-cycle costing* support comparison of alternatives, for instance contrasting traditional perimeter hardening with behaviour aware, neuroadaptive controls that target human error reduction. Insurance markets and funding agencies increasingly respond to demonstrable resilience practices, which means that the staged capabilities summarised in Table 5 can also function as signalling devices that attract favourable terms and collaborative opportunities.

6.4 Roadmaps, Maturity Models, and Change Management for Neuro-Intelligent Adoption

Implementation roadmaps for neuro-intelligent cybersecurity must choreograph technical deployment, institutional learning, and cultural change through phased maturity models. Rather than attempting wholesale transformation, institutions can progress through successive stages that each establish a stable baseline of capabilities, governance practices, and human competencies. Early stages focus on consolidating identity management, basic telemetry, and clear incident processes, while later stages introduce behavioural biometrics, neuro-AI analytics, and participatory oversight bodies. Change management constructs such as *stakeholder mapping*, *readiness assessment*, and *double-loop learning* underpin this trajectory, helping organisations surface latent anxieties, negotiate trade-offs, and reframe security from punitive surveillance into shared stewardship. Table 5 crystallises these phases into a compact schema that links each maturity level to core technical capabilities, governance milestones, human capital markers, and equity focused benchmarks, providing an actionable scaffold for planning and evaluation.

Table 5. Implementation Phases, Capabilities, and Governance Benchmarks

Implementation Phase for Neuro-Intelligent Security	Core Technical and Analytical Capability Set	Governance and Policy Milestones	Human Capital and Cultural Markers	Equity and Ethics Benchmarks
Initiation and Baseline Hardening	Unified identity fabric, basic logging, foundational backup, minimal anomaly alerts	Foundational security policy, breach notification protocol, role clarified incident response	Awareness campaigns, introductory training, recognition of security as shared obligation	Commitment to *privacy by design*, initial consent templates, basic accessibility safeguards
Pilot Neuro-AI and Behavioral Analytics	Limited scope behavioural telemetry, prototype neuro-AI modules, sandboxed risk scoring	Data protection impact assessment, pilot specific governance charter, vendor due diligence	Cross functional pilot team, reflective debriefs, tolerance for controlled experimentation	Explicit opt in mechanisms, exclusion of high risk cohorts, early fairness checks
Controlled Expansion and Standardisation	Integrated telemetry pipelines, calibrated behavioural biometrics, central risk engine	Formalised model governance, standard operating procedures, contract clauses for transparency	Role based competency frameworks, structured professional development, emergent security champions	Disaggregated error monitoring, accommodations for assistive technology users, published ethical guidelines

continued on following page

Table 5. Continued

Implementation Phase for Neuro-Intelligent Security	Core Technical and Analytical Capability Set	Governance and Policy Milestones	Human Capital and Cultural Markers	Equity and Ethics Benchmarks
Institutional Consolidation and Optimization	Mature neuro-AI ensembles, automated containment playbooks, federated learning for models	Standing governance committees, integrated policy stack, periodic external audits	Embedded security curricula, routine exercises, security embedded in performance evaluations	Regular fairness audits, participatory review forums, robust redress and appeal pathways
Interinstitutional Federation and Benchmarking	Cross campus telemetry sharing frameworks, federated evaluation suites, reference architectures	Sectoral agreements, shared standards, cooperative incident intelligence exchanges	Interinstitutional communities of practice, shared training artefacts, leadership coalitions	Joint equity indicators, harmonised consent norms, collaborative development of ethical baselines

Table 5 demonstrates that maturity is not defined solely by technical sophistication, but by co-evolution of governance, human capacity, and ethical reflexivity. Initiation phases are viable even for modest institutions, provided that baseline policies, communication pathways, and minimal accessibility safeguards are explicit. Pilot phases treat neuro-AI and behavioural analytics as experimental apparatus, bounded by opt in and constrained scope, which allows institutions to calibrate both performance and acceptability. Controlled expansion introduces standardisation and formal model governance, followed by consolidation, where neurointelligent defences become routine infrastructure subject to external audit and ongoing professionalisation. Federation phases recognise that threats, tools, and norms transcend institutional boundaries, inviting shared benchmarks and cooperative intelligence. Across all phases, equity is treated as a moving target that requires iterative measurement and participatory renegotiation rather than static compliance.

6.5 Equity-Centric Implementation, Stakeholder Engagement, and Ethical Pragmatics

Equity centric implementation recognises that neuro-intelligent cybersecurity can either mitigate or exacerbate existing educational stratifications, depending on how stakeholder engagement and ethical pragmatics are handled. Learners who rely on shared devices, low bandwidth connections, or assistive technologies may exhibit interaction patterns that differ markedly from those presumed by standard behavioural biometrics, which risks disproportionate false positives or service friction.

Institutions must therefore embed *inclusive design* and *disability studies* constructs into configuration decisions, ensuring alternative verification routes that do not penalise motor, sensory, or cognitive diversity. Stakeholder engagement processes that include student unions, disability offices, faculty associations, and community representatives help surface context specific harms and acceptable trade-offs. Ethical pragmatics demand that consent is meaningful, that refusals do not incur academic penalties, and that explanations of neuro-AI operations are intelligible across literacy levels and languages. When the staged governance benchmarks in Table 5 are interpreted through this equity lens, neuro-intelligent security becomes an instrument for safeguarding not only data and infrastructure, but also dignity, autonomy, and epistemic justice within global digital learning ecologies.

7. CONCLUSION

7.1 Synthesis of Neurocognitive Tenets and Cyberdefensive Praxis in Education

The preceding sections have articulated an integrated architecture in which neurocognitive constructs, affective dynamics, and computational intelligence coalesce into a coherent cyberdefensive praxis for education. *Cognitive Load Theory*, *dual-process reasoning*, *selective attention*, and *predictive processing* jointly explain why bounded working memory, fragmented vigilance, and overlearned heuristics systematically degrade judgment under academic pressure. These same constructs, when harnessed through neuroergonomic design and affect aware communication, become levers for reducing human error rather than merely diagnosing it. On the computational side, *spiking neural networks*, *predictive-coding* engines, *neuro-symbolic* governance layers, and behavioural biometrics supply a diversified repertoire of detection and authentication mechanisms calibrated to educational rhythms and constraints. Human-in-the-loop arrangements, explainable interfaces, and role specific competency frameworks embed these mechanisms within collegial institutions rather than technocratic control regimes. The result is a socio-technical configuration in which security functions as a finely tuned scaffold that preserves instructional tempo, research continuity, and institutional legitimacy while quietly attenuating adversarial opportunity.

7.2 Normative Trajectories, Cross-Sector Futures, and Research Agendas

Looking forward, neuro-intelligent cybersecurity in education can evolve along trajectories that synchronise technological sophistication with normative ambition. *Neuroadaptive* controls that regulate friction based on latent workload and affect can mature into standard features of platforms, provided that privacy preserving computation, federated optimisation, and transparent consent remain non-negotiable design axioms. Cross-sector consortia spanning schools, universities, edtech vendors, and critical infrastructure operators can stabilise interoperability standards for telemetry, tool integration, and fairness evaluation, enabling reusable reference architectures rather than bespoke silos. Research agendas must interrogate long term learning effects of affect aware training, distributional impacts of behavioural biometrics across cultures and abilities, and governance models that keep *neuro-symbolic* systems aligned with evolving rights discourses. Equally, critical scholarship grounded in *science and technology studies* and *data justice* must remain vigilant against drift toward normalised neuro-surveillance, ensuring that neurocognitive insight serves autonomy, rather than subordinating learners and educators to opaque optimisation logics.

7.3 Limitations, Boundary Conditions, and Cautions for Responsible Deployment

Several structural and epistemic limitations delineate the responsible envelope for deploying the constructs advanced in this chapter. Psychophysiological telemetry is inherently noisy, context dependent, and variably interpretable, which restricts its suitability to supportive scaffolding rather than high stakes adjudication, particularly for minors and neurodivergent learners. Behavioural biometrics and neuro-AI models are only as representative as the interaction corpora from which they are derived, so institutions operating in under resourced settings or within highly heterogeneous populations must treat imported models with principled scepticism. Economically, not all organisations possess the capacity to implement advanced telemetry and analytics, which heightens the importance of staged maturity paths, low-cost controls, and shared sectoral resources. Normatively, *inclusive design*, *proportionality*, and *epistemic justice* provide essential boundary concepts that prevent neuro-intelligent security from mutating into coercive compliance infrastructures. When these cautions are institutionalised through transparent governance, participatory oversight, and continuous reflexive evaluation, neurocognitively informed cybersecurity can function as an enabler of resilient, equitable, and trustworthy digital learning ecologies.

REFERENCES

Al Siam, A., Hassan, M. M., & Bhuiyan, T. (2025, February). Artificial Intelligence for Cybersecurity: A State of the Art. In *2025 IEEE 4th International Conference on AI in Cybersecurity (ICAIC)* (pp. 1-7). IEEE.

Alam, A. (2022). Impact of university's human resources practices on professors' occupational performance: Empirical evidence from India's higher education sector. In Rajagopal, R., & Behl, R. (Eds.), *Inclusive businesses in developing economies: Converging people, profit, and corporate citizenship* (pp. 107–131). Springer International Publishing., DOI: 10.1007/978-3-031-12217-0_6

Alam, A. (2023a). Media multitasking with M-learning technology in real-time classroom learning: Analysing the dynamics in formal educational settings for the future of E-learning in India. In *2023 2nd International Conference on Smart Technologies and Systems for Next Generation Computing (ICSTSN)* (pp. 1-6). IEEE.

Alam, A. (2023b). The secret sauce of student success: Cracking the code by navigating the path to personalized learning with educational data mining. In *2023 2nd International Conference on Smart Technologies and Systems for Next Generation Computing (ICSTSN)* (pp. 1-8). IEEE.

Alam, A. (2023c). Intelligence unleashed: An argument for AI-enabled learning ecologies with real world examples of today and a peek into the future. In *International Conference on Innovations in Computer Science, Electronics & Electrical Engineering*-2022 (Vol. 2717, No. 1, p. 030001). AIP Publishing LLC.

Alam, A., & Mohanty, A. (2022, December). Facial analytics or virtual avatars: competencies and design considerations for student-teacher interaction in AI-powered online education for effective classroom engagement. In *International Conference on Communication, Networks and Computing* (pp. 252-265). Cham: Springer Nature Switzerland.

Alam, A., & Mohanty, A. (2023, January). Learning on the move: a pedagogical framework for state-of-the-art mobile learning. In *International Conference on Data Management, Analytics & Innovation* (pp. 735-748). Singapore: Springer Nature Singapore.

Alam, A., & Mohanty, A. (2024). Integrated constructive robotics in education (ICRE) model: A paradigmatic framework for transformative learning in educational ecosystem. *Cogent Education, 11*(1), 2324487.

Ali, A., Septyanto, A. W., Chaudhary, I., Al Hamadi, H., Alzoubi, H. M., & Khan, Z. F. (2022, February). Applied artificial intelligence as event horizon of cyber security. In *2022 International Conference on Business Analytics for Technology and Security (ICBATS)* (pp. 1-7). IEEE.

Alkhatri, M., Deab, D. U., & Alzitawi, M. (2024). The role of artificial intelligence in addressing cybersecurity challenges. *International Journal of Academic Research in Business & Social Sciences, 14*(4).

Alzahrani, A. A. (2023). Using Artificial Intelligence and Cybersecurity in Medical and Healthcare Applications. *Alzahrani, AA.*

Andrade, R. O., Fuertes, W., Cazares, M., Ortiz-Garcés, I., & Navas, G. (2022). An exploratory study of cognitive sciences applied to cybersecurity. *Electronics (Basel), 11*(11), 1692.

Ashraf, M., Patterson, G., Kilhoffer, Z., Han, X., Brady, N., Rahn, A., & Yeh, T. (2023, June). Using fNIRS To Understand Adults' Empathy for Children in AI and Cybersecurity Scenarios. In *Proceedings of the 22nd Annual ACM Interaction Design and Children Conference* (pp. 630-634).

Bhardwaj, T., Upadhyay, H., Sharma, T. K., & Fernandes, S. L. (Eds.). (2023). *Artificial Intelligence in Cyber Security: Theories and Applications*. Springer.

Bormpotsis, C., Nanos, M., & Patel, A. (2025). A Neuroscience-Informed AI Framework to Decode the Complexities of Neurofinance. *IEEE Transactions on Technology and Society*.

Chandra, P., Sharma, H., & Sachan, N. (2025). Explainable and Responsible AI in Neuroscience: Cognitive Neurostimulation. *Explainable and Responsible Artificial Intelligence in Healthcare*, 27-63.

Chapagain, D., Kshetri, N., & Pokharel, B. P. (2025). AISCliteracy: Assessing Artificial Intelligence and Cybersecurity Literacy Levels and Learning Needs of Students. *arXiv preprint arXiv:2506.23321*.

Dal Verne, T. D. M. C. (2023). Artificial Intelligence, Neuroscience and Emotional Data. What Role for Private Autonomy in the Digital Market? *Erasmus L. Rev., 16*, 83.

Di Salvo, M. (2025). The Protection of Neural Rights in the Age of Neurotechnologies and AI. The Ethical Challenge for Law and Neuroscience. *Russ. J. Econ. & L., 19*, 202.

Faraji, M. R., Shikder, F., Hasan, M. H., Islam, M. M., & Akter, U. K. (2024). Examining the role of artificial intelligence in cyber security (CS): A systematic review for preventing prospective solutions in financial transactions. *International Journal (Toronto, Ont.)*, *5*(10), 4766–4782.

Fernández-García, C. E., Marín, D. V., & Velásquez, H. S. (2023). Neurohacking and Artificial Intelligence in the Vulnerability of the Human Brain: Are We Facing a Threat? In *Artificial Intelligence in Higher Education and Scientific Research: Future Development* (pp. 117–128). Springer Nature Singapore.

Gkintoni, E., Antonopoulou, H., Sortwell, A., & Halkiopoulos, C. (2025). Challenging cognitive load theory: The role of educational neuroscience and artificial intelligence in redefining learning efficacy. *Brain Sciences*, *15*(2), 203. PMID: 40002535

Hinrichs, R., Subramanian, L., Ayala, A., Endicott-Popovsky, B., & Stoll, S. (2024, November). AI-Enhanced Cybersecurity Training: Integrating Ethical Reasoning and Personalized Learning Pathways. In *Proceedings of the Future Technologies Conference* (pp. 606-622). Cham: Springer Nature Switzerland.

Hramov, A. E., Ghosh, D., Pisarchik, A. N., Pavlov, A., Stoyanov, D., Zaikin, A., & Sanjuan, M. (2025). Artificial intelligence and complex networks meet natural sciences. *The European Physical Journal. Special Topics*, •••, 1–16.

Kabanda, G. (2023). Bayesian Models in Cognitive Neuroscience. In *Artificial Intelligence and Knowledge Processing* (pp. 157–185). CRC Press.

Kritika, E. (2025a). A comprehensive study on navigating the integration of neuro-psychology and cybersecurity. *International Journal of Advanced Networking and Applications*, *17*(1), 6788–6798.

Kritika, E. (2025b). Ethical frontiers: Navigating the intersection of neurotechnology and cybersecurity. *Journal of Experimental Neurology*, *6*(1), 21–25.

Kritika, E. (2025c). Brainjacking: The cybersecurity nightmare of the future. https://www.researchgate.net/profile/Er-Kritika/publication/391858141_Brainjacking_The_Cybersecurity_Nightmare_of_the_Future/links/682ac6438a76251f22e2b799/Brainjacking-The-Cybersecurity-Nightmare-of-the-Future.pdf

Kritika, M. (2024). Neuro-driven cybersecurity: Strengthening digital defense. *London Journal of Research in Computer Science and Technology*, *24*(1), 17–26.

Kritika, M. (2025d). A comprehensive study on navigating neuroethics in cyberspace. *AI and Ethics*, *5*(1), 93–100.

Kumar, A., Rathore, P. S., Ahuja, S., & Lilhore, U. K. (Eds.). (2025). *Integrating Neurocomputing with Artificial Intelligence*. John Wiley & Sons.

Leider, A., & Li, S. (2025, February). Brain-Computer Interactions in Extended Reality with Artificial Intelligence and Cloud Computing. In *2025 Conference on Artificial Intelligence x Multimedia (AIxMM)* (pp. 51-54). IEEE.

Liv, N., & Greenbaum, D. (2023). Cyberneurosecurity. In *Policy, identity, and neurotechnology: The neuroethics of brain-computer interfaces* (pp. 233–251). Springer International Publishing.

Loaiza, F. L., Birdwell, J. D., Kennedy, G. L., & Visser, D. (2022). *Utility of artificial intelligence and machine learning in cybersecurity*. Institute for Defense Analyses.

Mahajan, S., Khurana, M., & Estrela, V. V. (Eds.). (2024). *Applying Artificial Intelligence in Cybersecurity Analytics and Cyber Threat Detection*. John Wiley & Sons.

McCullum, T., & Mancera, L. C. C. (2025). Neurotechnology Combined with Artificial Intelligence and Neurorights: A Legal Discussion. *Rev. Prop. Inmaterial*, *39*, 145.

Meghraoui, L., & Belkhamza, Z. (2025, March). Cognitive Warfare and Cybersecurity: Strategic Implications for Global Security. In *Proceedings of the 19th International Conference on Cyber Warfare and Security*. Academic Conferences and publishing limited.

Merat, S., & Almuhtadi, W. (2024, January). Innovative Application of a Sleepwalking-Based Artificial Neural Model for Cybersecurity Risk Assessment. In *2024 IEEE International Conference on Consumer Electronics (ICCE)* (pp. 1-8). IEEE.

Mitchell, A., Potter, L., Palmer, X. L., & Barnett, M. (2025, March). Exploring the Intersection of Cybersecurity, Neurocapitalism, and Biodesign. In *Proceedings of the 19th International Conference on Cyber Warfare and Security*. Academic Conferences and publishing limited.

Monteith, S., Glenn, T., Geddes, J. R., Achtyes, E. D., Whybrow, P. C., & Bauer, M. (2024). Artificial intelligence and cybercrime: Implications for individuals and the healthcare sector. *The British Journal of Psychiatry*, *225*(4), 421–423. PMID: 39308261

Moustafa, A. (Ed.). (2022). *Cybersecurity and cognitive science*. Academic Press.

Naeem, M. R., Amin, R., Farhan, M., Alotaibi, F. A., Alnfiai, M. M., Sampedro, G. A., & Karovič, V. (2024). Harnessing AI and analytics to enhance cybersecurity and privacy for collective intelligence systems. *PeerJ. Computer Science*, *10*, e2264. PMID: 39314701

Nagar, A., Kumar, T., Bhamidipati, P., & Sandhia, G. K. (2022). Cybersecurity: The Part Played By Artificial Intelligence. *NeuroQuantology : An Interdisciplinary Journal of Neuroscience and Quantum Physics*, *20*(15), 1629–1642.

Pazouki, S., Golilarz, N. A., Kazemi-Razi, S. M., & Aydeger, A. (2022, July). A self-healing cybersecurity mechanism for cyberattacks targeting artificial neural network-based human brain implants controlling smart homes. In *2022 International Conference on Electrical, Computer and Energy Technologies (ICECET)* (pp. 1-6). IEEE.

Perez, C. L., Orozco, C. M. V., & Rodríguez, I. H. (2026). General Overview Cybersecurity and Artificial Intelligence. *Reshaping Criminology with AI*, 63-90.

Rios-Campos, C., Paz, S. C. V., Vilema, G. O., Díaz, L. M. R., Zambrano, D. P. F., Zambrano, G. M. M., & Anchundia-Gómez, O. (2024). Cybersecurity and artificial intelligence (AI). *South Florida Journal of Development*, *5*(8), e4276–e4276.

Saikia, S., Athilingam, V. P., & Ahmed, F. (2023). Cybersecurity and Intraoperative Artificial Intelligence Decision Support: Challenges and Solutions Related to Ethical Issues. In *Ethical Issues in AI for Bioinformatics and Chemoinformatics* (pp. 107-118). CRC Press.

Sheikhbahei, E., & Ari, A. A. (2024). Harnessing the power of emerging digital technologies for improved sustainability and productivity in biomedical engineering and neuroscience. *Scientific Hypotheses*, *1*, 47–52.

Shiwlani, A., Hasan, S. U., & Kumar, S. (2024). Artificial Intelligence in Neuroeducation: A Systematic Review of AI Applications Aligned with Neuroscience Principles for Optimizing Learning Strategies. *Journal of Development and Social Sciences*, *5*(4), 578–593.

Siddique, R. A., & Jahankhani, H. (2024). An Investigation of Artificial Intelligence (AI) and Cybersecurity: Case of AI Integration in German Cybersecurity Strategy. In *Navigating the Intersection of Artificial Intelligence, Security, and Ethical Governance: Sentinels of Cyberspace* (pp. 123–146). Springer Nature Switzerland.

Singh, T. (2025). Neuroscience, Sociology, and Anthropology. In *Cybersecurity, Psychology and People Hacking* (pp. 73–94). Springer Nature Switzerland.

Tekin, U., & Dener, M. (2025). A bibliometric analysis of studies on artificial intelligence in neuroscience. *Frontiers in Neurology*, *16*, 1474484. PMID: 40040909

Vijaya, G., & Ramesh, K. (2025). IAS and Its Impact in Neuroscience. *Handbook of Intelligent Automation Systems Using Computer Vision and Artificial Intelligence*, 407-421.

Xavier, K. F., Subashini, K., Vijayalakshmi, P., Selvalakshmi, B., Sudhakar, G., & Pradeepa, K. (2025). Integrating Artificial Intelligence and Machine Learning for Enhanced Cyber Security in Industry 4.0: Designing a Smart Factory with IoT and CPS. *Artificial Intelligence and Machine Learning for Industry*, *4*(0), 267–286.

Zahm, W., Stern, T., Bal, M., Sengupta, A., Jose, A., Chelian, S., & Vasan, S. (2022). Cyber-neuro RT: Real-time neuromorphic cybersecurity. *Procedia Computer Science*, *213*, 536–545.

Chapter 4
Integrating AI and Neuroscience for Cyber Threat Detection and Response

Affaan Shaikh
https://orcid.org/0009-0004-7590-7456
Neuratia Labs, UAE

V. B. Aparna
https://orcid.org/0009-0000-5840-2502
Yenepoya School of Allied Health Sciences, India

Shambhavi Dogra
https://orcid.org/0009-0004-8698-1635
Christ University, India

ABSTRACT

The integration of Artificial Intelligence (AI) and neuroscience is rapidly advancing the field of cyber threat detection and response. This chapter explores how insights from neuroscience, combined with state-of-the-art AI techniques such as deep learning and neural-inspired algorithms, enhance the identification, analysis, and mitigation of sophisticated cyber threats. Drawing parallels between brain cognitive processes and cybersecurity mechanisms, the chapter examines how biologically inspired AI models improve anomaly detection, behavior analysis, and adaptive defense systems. It reviews current neural network architectures, neuro-inspired computing models, and hybrid AI systems applied to cybersecurity data such as network traffic, user behavior logs, and malware signatures. Ethical considerations, data privacy chal-

DOI: 10.4018/979-8-3373-5012-7.ch004

lenges, and explainability of AI-driven threat detection are discussed. Case studies show that combining neuroscience and AI enables adaptive, proactive cyber defenses with faster, more accurate threat detection.

1. INTRODUCTION

Over the past 20 years, cyber threats have surged drastically in both quantity and complexity (Morgan, 2020). Present day cyberattacks have evolved far beyond mere static malware signatures or even rudimentary phishing attempts. Instead, they now include advanced persistent threats (APTs), previously unknown (zero-day) exploits and highly advanced polymorphic malware that constantly morphs and changes its form to slip past conventional detection systems (Sommer & Paxson, 2010). Critical sectors, such as energy grids, transportation networks and healthcare infrastructures, are now the frequent targets of such attacks, due to their strategic importance and the potentially widespread fallout that can be caused by their compromise (Ferrag et al., 2020). According to Cybersecurity Ventures (2020), cybercrime may inflict an astonishing US $10.5 trillion in annual damages on the global economy, thus showing both the explosive growth of such attacks and the increasingly inadequate performance of traditional cybersecurity defenses (Morgan, 2020).

Standard, traditional detection methods, which employ majorly fixed rules and known signatures, proved to be insufficient while dealing with present day's fluid and complex cyber threats (Sommer & Paxson, 2010). Perpetrators have begun using machine learning methods, like adversarial AI, purposefully developing inputs that misdirect defense systems and complicate attack-identification processes (Brundage et al., 2018). This stark difference between the attackers and the defenders, wherein the attackers have evolved and continue evolving faster than those trying to fight them, necessitates the need for a change in the cybersecurity and cyber threat detection systems and the development of systems that are intelligent, proactive and continuously evolving (Nguyen & Reddi, 2021). These systems should possess the capability of not only anticipating threats but also evolving and adapting dynamically, according to the strength and complexity of the threat while simultaneously mirroring human intelligence and employing resilience in their activities to tackle emerging and evolving threats (Roy et al., 2019).

1.1. The Convergence of AI and Neuroscience in Cybersecurity Innovation

Artificial Intelligence (AI), a revolution in the field of cybersecurity, has helped bring about a dynamic change in the field through its usage in deep learning and reinforcement learning, two methods that have proven to be highly effective for crucial tasks, like pattern recognition and anomaly detection (Goodfellow et al., 2016). However, in spite of these strengths, AI faces certain limitations, such as its heavy reliance on large and well-labeled datasets and its constrained capacity for contextual and higher-level reasoning(Goodfellow et al., 2016). In order to tackle these challenges, researchers across the globe have begun to integrate principles from neuroscience into AI-based security systems (Hassabis et al., 2017).

Neuroscience provides valuable perspectives on how the human brain and biological neural networks manage information, cope with uncertainty and react flexibly to unfamiliar or unpredictable stimuli. Fundamental concepts, such as synaptic plasticity, hierarchical modes of processing and predictive coding are now being used as a base in the development of spiking neural networks (SNNs) and neuromorphic computing technologies (Hassabis et al., 2017). These approaches, which have been inspired by biology and life sciences, offer numerous advantages, such as temporal sensitivity, increased energy efficiency and adaptability, making them fit to meet the requirements of cybersecurity, a field where rapid and real-time responsiveness are crucial (Ring et al., 2019). Hybrid systems are emerging that may begin to "think" and "learn" in ways that resemble human intelligence, due the merging of cognitive models that have been derived from neuroscience with advanced AI detection techniques, while also maintaining the scalability and speed of machines (Aminu et al., 2024).

1.2. Role of Cognitive Computing in Enhancing Cyber Threat Detection and Response

Cognitive Computing, a major advancement in the field of artificial intelligence, integrates and employs not only learning but also reasoning and contextual awareness into cybersecurity threat detection (Hassabis et al., 2017). Unlike traditional machine learning approaches, which depend majorly on clean and structured data inputs, present-day cognitive systems are able to process, interpret and understand ambiguous, incomplete and even highly unstructured information and the different forms of which, which include but are not limited to user-activity patterns, unusual fluctuations in network traffic or natural language communications (Chio & Freeman, 2018). An apt example of this is IBM's Watson for Cyber Security. Watson applies natural language processing to interpret unstructured threat intelligence reports and gains insights from those reports, which are then integrated into automated defense workflows (Shah & Issac, 2018).

The three crucial contributions of cognitive computing to the field of cybersecurity are as follows:-

a) **Improved Anomaly Recognition:** By stimulating cognitive mechanisms such as memory and selective attention, these systems have been able to separate harmless irregularities from actual malicious activities and indicators of potential attacks (Pomerol, 2020).
b) **Versatile and Constantly Evolving Learning:** Similar to the brain's neuroplasticity, cognitive systems continuously refine and adjust their detection strategies as adversaries alter their attack methods, ensuring defenses remain relevant over time (Hassabis et al., 2017).
c) **Transparency and Explainability:** In contrast to the opaque, "black box" nature of many AI models, cognitive computing emphasizes interpretability. It provides justifications for why specific events or anomalies are flagged, which is essential for security professionals who must evaluate and justify responses (Gunning & Aha, 2019).

This integration of AI techniques and insights from cognitive neuroscience has helped in developing a new class of defense mechanisms, which are not only flexible, dynamic and adaptive but are also more human-like in their reasoning (Hassabis et al., 2017).

2. FOUNDATIONS OF AI AND NEUROSCIENCE IN CYBERSECURITY

2.1. Overview of AI Techniques: Deep Learning, Reinforcement Learning, and Neural Networks

A critical facet that has proven to be of great advantage in present-day cybersecurity is artificial intelligence. Deep learning and reinforcement learning models are now playing particularly important and crucial roles while acting as aids (Goodfellow et al., 2016). Deep learning uses multi-layered neural networks architectures, which are capable of uncovering complex patterns present in hierarchies and features from vast and complex datasets, which makes it extremely crucial and effective at identifying subtle and minute yet adaptive and constantly evolving cyber threats, such as polymorphic malware and sophisticated encrypted intrusions (Goodfellow et al., 2016). Variations and alternate forms of deep architectures, such as convolutional neural networks (CNNs) and recurrent neural networks (RNNs) have consistently been able to achieve impressive results in tasks like intrusion detection, with certain models even reporting accuracy rates up to and exceeding 98% on standard benchmark datasets, including CICIDS2017 (Yin et al., 2017).

Reinforcement learning (RL) aids these approaches by enabling cybersecurity systems to learn while continuously adapting and evolving and help in optimizing defense strategies in highly dynamic, evolving, volatile and unpredictable situations and environments (Nguyen & Reddi, 2021). For e.g., RL-driven intrusion detection frameworks can autonomously determine and deploy mitigation measures, such as isolating suspicious IP addresses or activating honeypot systems, thereby enhancing both response speed and operational efficiency (Chio & Freeman, 2018). Once combined, these approaches form a hybrid approach known as deep reinforcement learning (DRL), an approach that has increasingly been applied to dynamic and proactive cyber defense strategies. These systems are designed to stimulate and prompt the adaptive decision-making processes of human security analysts while simultaneously functioning at machine-scale speed (Al-Turjman, 2024).

Collectively, these neural-inspired AI approaches form the foundation for intelligent cybersecurity systems capable of continuous learning and rapid and vigorous adaptation in threatful situations, effectively bridging the gap between automated machine efficiency and human-like reasoning in threat response.

2.2. Neuroscience Concepts Relevant to Cybersecurity: Cognitive Processes, Anomaly Detection, and Adaptive Learning

The purpose of integrating neuroscience principles into cybersecurity related to the exceptional ability of the human brain to recognize patterns and make decisions in uncertain, dynamic and complex environments (Hassabis et al., 2017). Cognitive functions, such as focused attention, working memory and predictive coding, serve as important basis for the designing of AI-based defense systems that are more intelligent and context-aware (Davies et al., 2021). For e.g., just as the brain selectively filters our irrelevant sensory information to concentrate on the most important stimuli, cybersecurity systems can be structured to prioritize significant anomalies within vast, complex, dynamic and high-dimensional streams of network traffic (Davies et al., 2021).

Neuroscience also highlights the importance of adaptive learning through mechanisms like synaptic plasticity, which allows for continuous adjustment and refinement in response to new experiences. Translating this to cybersecurity, systems can dynamically calibrate their detection thresholds and strategies based on emerging attack patterns and evolving threat signatures (Roy et al., 2019). Moreover, the brain's ability to detect anomalies, especially in identifying deviations or departure from expected behavior, makes it a valuable model in offering inspiration for behavioral analytics models, which play a critical role in uncovering insider threats and previously unknown zero-day exploits. By employing these neuroscience-informed principles, cybersecurity models can evolve beyond static, rule-based classifiers into dynamic, self-refining systems capable of sustained resilience, continuous adaptation and improved long-term effectiveness (Hassabis et al., 2017).

2.3. Neural-Inspired Algorithms: Spiking Neural Networks and Neuromorphic Computing

A significant area of advancement at the intersection of artificial intelligence and neuroscience is the emergence of spiking neural networks (SNNs) and neuromorphic computing systems (Roy et al., 2019). Unlike traditional artificial neural networks that rely on continuous signal processing, SNNs transmit information through discrete spikes, resembling the temporal and event-driven signaling mechanisms observed in biological neurons (Davies et al., 2021) (see Figure 1 and Figure 2). This spike-based approach enhances energy efficiency, supports real-time adaptive responses and provides robustness in environments with high levels of noise, which are all features that are particularly advantageous for cybersecurity applications (Nguyen & Reddi, 2021). For e.g., SNNs have been successfully deployed in intrusion detection scenarios, demonstrating accuracy comparable to conventional deep networks while requiring substantially less computational power (Aminu et al., 2024).

Figure 1. AI–Neuroscience Integrated Cyber-Defense Framework

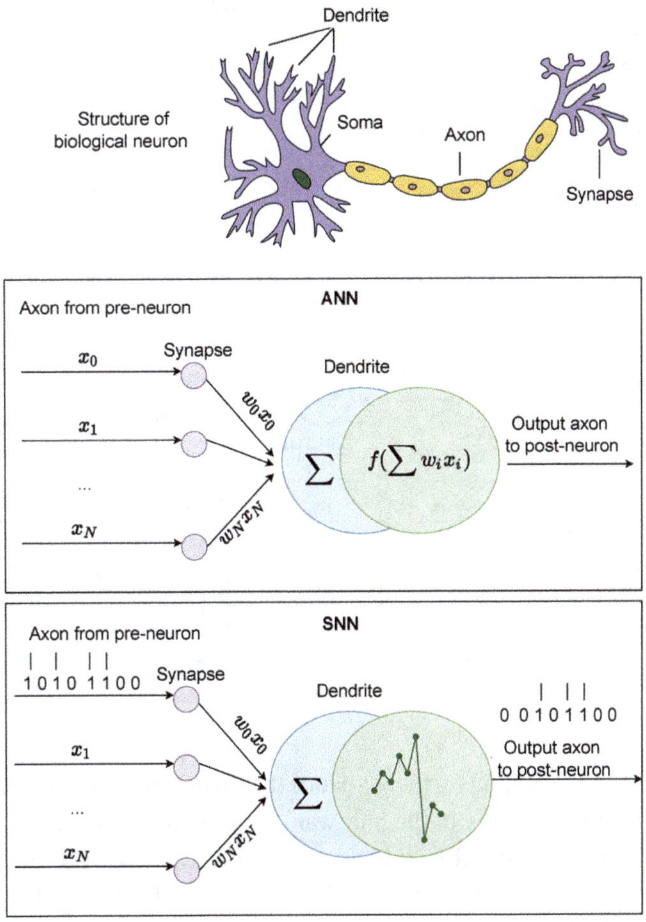

Figure 2. Spiking Neural Network (SNN) Architecture & Spike Dynamics

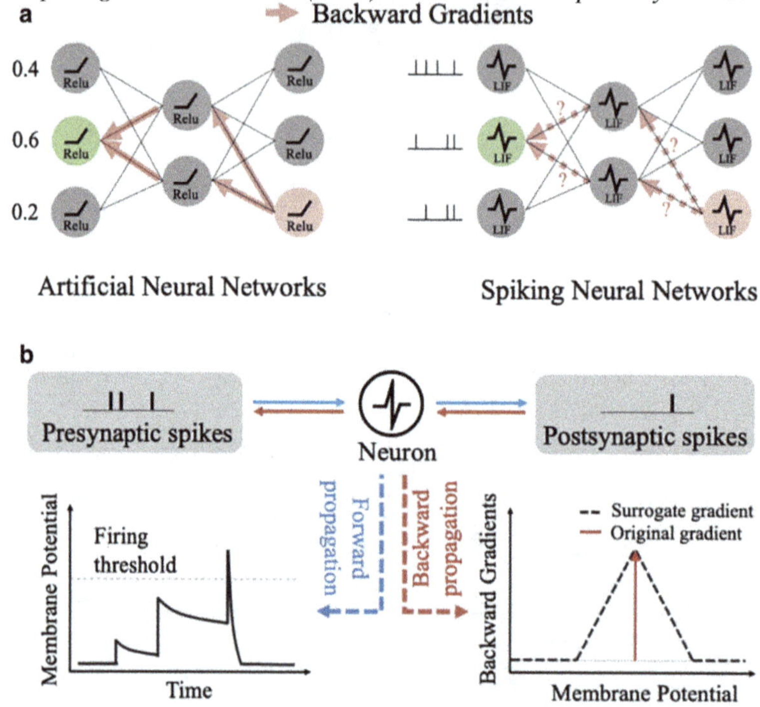

Neuromorphic computing further expands their frontier by implementing neural-inspired architectures directly at the hardware level. Platforms such as Intel's Loihi and IBM's TrueNorth exemplify this approach, offering low-power, parallel processing capabilities for cybersecurity tasks (Davies et al., 2021). These platforms are especially valuable in edge computing environments, where real-time, energy-efficient threat detection is critical (Roy et al., 2019). Recent studies indicate that neuromorphic systems can achieve classification accuracies nearly equivalent to GPU-based architectures, around 98%, while significantly reducing size, weight and energy consumption (Davies et al., 2021). This combination of efficiency and performance positions neuromorphic computing as a promising foundation for the next generation of resilient and adaptive cyber defense systems.

2.4. Public Datasets and Benchmarks for Cybersecurity AI Models

The design and assessment of AI models for cybersecurity heavily depends on publicly accessible datasets and standardized benchmarks (Ring et al., 2019). While classic datasets like KDD Cup 1999 laid the groundwork for intrusion detection research, they are increasingly regarded as outdated due to their synthetic and simplified nature (Sommer & Paxson, 2010). More contemporary benchmarks, like NSL-KDD, UNSW-NB15 and CICIDS2017, provide a higher degree of realism by encompassing modern attack types such as distributed denial-of-service (DDoS), brute-force attempts and botnet traffic (Ferrag et al., 2020).

These datasets play a critical role in enabling comparative evaluations of different AI models and establishing baselines for tasks such as anomaly detection and malware classification (Ring et al., 2019). For example, deep learning models trained and tested on the UNSW-NB15 dataset have demonstrated precision rates exceeding 95% (Ferrag et al., 2020). In addition, generative methods like Attention-GAN have been employed to augment existing datasets with synthetic attack samples, thereby enhancing model generalizability and performance in real-world scenarios (Zhou et al., 2024). The continued development and refinement of these benchmarks are crucial for validating the scalability, robustness and effectiveness of AI-neuroscience hybrid systems in cybersecurity (Roy et al., 2019).

3. APPLICATIONS OF AI AND NEUROSCIENCE IN CYBER THREAT DETECTION

3.1. Behavioral Anomaly Detection Inspired by Human Cognitive Patterns

Behavioral anomaly detection represents one of the most promising domains at the intersection of artificial intelligence and neuroscience (Hassabis et al., 2017). Drawing inspiration from the human brain's remarkable capacity to recognize deviations from anticipated patterns, AI systems can examine user activity logs and network traffic to detect unusual behaviors that might signal insider threats, advanced persistent threats (APTs) or account takeovers (Chio & Freeman, 2018). For e.g., deep learning models influenced by cognitive attention mechanisms have been applied to pinpoint atypical sequences of activity, such as irregular login times or unusual access to sensitive data, achieving detection accuracies exceeding 96% in enterprise-level datasets (Yin et al., 2017).

By integrating neuroscience concepts like predictive coding, these systems can continuously calibrate their baseline expectation, allowing them to adapt to contextual changes such as remote working conditions or evolving attacker techniques (Hassabis et al., 2017). This ongoing adaptability helps minimize false positives, which are a common shortcoming of traditional anomaly detection methods, while establishing a more resilient and responsive defense against sophisticated and behaviorally complex cyber intrusions(Nguyen & Reddi, 2021).

3.2. Intrusion Detection Systems Using Deep Learning and Neuroscience Principles

Intrusion Detection Systems (IDS) play a pivotal role in safeguarding cybersecurity and the integration of artificial intelligence with neuroscience-inspired techniques has markedly improved their accuracy and adaptability (Kolosnjaji et al., 2016). Traditional IDS solutions often struggle to detect zero-day attacks because they rely heavily on predefined signatures. In contrast, deep learning-based IDSs now employ approaches such as autoencoders, recurrent neural networks and hybrid models to identify subtle irregularities within network traffic. Research involving CNN-RNN hybrid architectures on the CICIDS2017 dataset has reported detection accuracies exceeding 98%, significantly outperforming conventional learning methods (Yin et al., 2017).

Incorporating neuroscience-inspired strategies, particularly spiking neural networks (SNNs), offers further advantages by replicating the temporal and event-driven dynamics of biological neurons (Roy et al., 2019). For example, an IDS designed using SNNs demonstrated competitive detection performance while consuming approximately 70% less energy than traditional deep learning frameworks (Davies et al., 2021). These neuro-inspired neural networks IDS models not only detect intrusions effectively but also continuously adapt to emerging patterns, emulating the brain's natural plasticity and enabling sustained, real-time resilience against evolving cyber threats (Hassabis et al., 2017).

3.3. Malware Classification and Prediction Using Neural Models

Detecting malware remains a critical area where integrating artificial intelligence with neuroscience-inspired models shows considerable promise. Traditional malware detection techniques rely on predefined signature databases, rendering them ineffective against polymorphic and metamorphic malware that continuously evolve. Deep neural networks, particularly convolutional neural networks (CNNs), have been employed to analyze malware binaries and identify patterns that are not detectable through static analysis, achieving classification accuracies up to 99% on benchmark datasets (Kolosnjaji et al., 2016).

Neuroscience-inspired approaches offer additional advantages. Spiking Neural P systems (SNP systems) simulate the spiking communication of neurons and have been successfully applied to malware detection (Song et al., 2024). These models not only classify known malware but can also predict potential mutations by modeling them as deviations in spike timing and propagation (Roy et al., 2019). This predictive capability is particularly valuable for detecting zero-day threats, where conventional systems often fall short (Nguyen & Reddi, 2021).

3.4. Phishing and Social Engineering Detection Through Cognitive Pattern Recognition

Phishing and social engineering attacks take advantage of human psychology, which makes them hard to catch using traditional rule-based systems (Baki et al., 2017). Drawing inspiration from neuroscience, AI can be trained to spot misleading patterns in language, tone, and how messages are structured (Baki et al., 2017). For e.g., Natural Language Processing (NLP) models with attention mechanisms have been successfully used to detect phishing emails, achieving accuracy rates over 97% (Basit et al., 2020).

In addition, algorithms inspired by spiking neural networks are particularly good at recognizing sequences over time. This allows AI to detect small changes in conversation flow or timing that could signal targeted attacks like spear-phishing (Song et al., 2024). By combining insights from how humans respond to persuasion with AI's ability to process large volumes of data, these approaches provide stronger protection against social engineering threats (Ferrag et al., 2020).

3.5. Comparative Performance of AI-Neuroscience Hybrid Models Versus Conventional Systems

Studies have shown that combining AI with brain-inspired models often leads to better performance in cybersecurity than traditional systems (Hassabis et al., 2017). For instance, intrusion detection systems (IDS) using neuromorphic hardware like Intel's Loihi have achieved classification accuracies around 98%, similar to GPU-based deep learning systems, but with over 80% less power consumption (Davies et al., 2021).

Additionally, spiking neural networks have demonstrated a 40% reduction in false positives compared to conventional deep learning approaches (Roy et al., 2019).

These hybrid models not only perform well but also adapt more effectively to new threats. While traditional systems may struggle with novel attack methods, neuro-inspired systems continue to learn and adjust, much like the human brain (Nguyen & Reddi, 2021).

4. AI TOOLS AND PLATFORMS LEVERAGING NEUROSCIENCE FOR CYBERSECURITY

4.1. Overview of Existing AI Cybersecurity Platforms Integrating Neuroscience Insights

Several commercial cybersecurity tools are now using AI, often incorporating ideas inspired by neuroscience, to spot threats in real time. For example, Darktrace is well-known for using unsupervised machine learning to learn the normal "patterns of life" within an organization and identify unusual activity that could indicate a cyberattack. Its Enterprise Immune System is inspired by the human immune system, mimicking neural and immune responses to continually adapt to new types of attacks (Darktrace, 2022).

Similarly, Cylance uses machine learning models trained on extensive malware datasets to detect threats before they execute, reducing the need for traditional signature-based approaches (Shah & Issac, 2018). While these platforms do not always implement direct neuroscience algorithms, their bio-inspired features, like adaptive immune-like modeling, predictive anomaly detection, and behavioral baselining clearly show that principles from cognitive science and neural systems are already being applied in commercial cybersecurity solutions (Ferrag et al., 2020).

4.2. Integration with Security Information and Event Management (SIEM) Systems

Integrating AI and neuroscience-inspired systems into existing Security Information and Event Management (SIEM) tools presents a significant challenge in cybersecurity operations (Nguyen & Reddi, 2021). SIEM platforms like Splunk and IBM QRadar collect vast amounts of security data from various sources, including logs, network traffic, and endpoints. By incorporating AI-driven anomaly detection modules within these SIEM systems, organizations can automate the initial analysis of security events, thereby reducing the workload on human analysts (Ring et al., 2019). Neuroscience-inspired approaches enhance this integration by prioritizing alerts based on their significance, similar to how the human brain focuses attention on critical stimuli (Hassabis et al., 2017). For example, combining SIEM systems with Darktrace's Enterprise Immune System has been shown to decrease false positives by over 30%, leading to faster and more accurate incident responses (Shah & Issac, 2018).

This integration represents a practical step toward the scalable deployment of cognitive cybersecurity solutions, enabling more efficient and effective threat detection and response.

Figure 3 shows the A high-level workflow diagram: raw data ingestion (logs, network traffic, user behavior) → preprocessing → AI/neuro-inspired detection engine (e.g. using SNNs / deep learning) → anomaly detection / alert generation → decision / response (e.g. quarantine, alert, mitigation) → optional human analyst / SOC integration. This visually ties together all components your paper describes (data sources, AI/neuro models, SIEM integration, response).

Figure 3. Hybrid AI-Neuroscience Cybersecurity Workflow / Pipeline

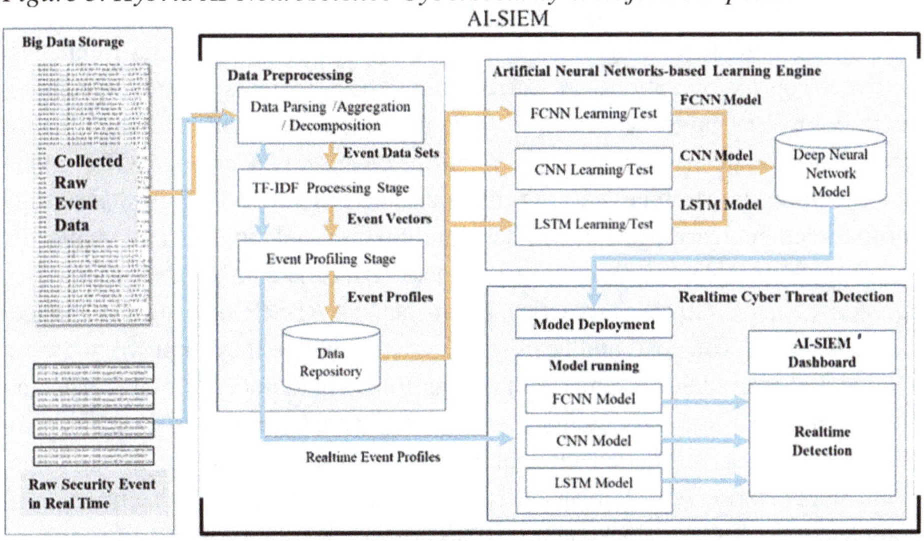

5. IMPACT ON CYBERSECURITY OPERATIONS AND INCIDENT RESPONSE

The capacity of neuro-inspired models and adaptive AI to reduce incident mean time to respond (MTTR) and mean time to detect (MTTD) has made them essential cybersecurity solutions. By applying advanced machine learning techniques, these systems support real-time intrusion detection and rapid response, which strengthens the resilience of security operations. They can process large volumes of data, such as network traffic and user activity to spot unusual patterns that may signal attacks(Rizvi, 2023). Deep learning approaches like convolutional neural network(CNN) and long short-term memory(LSTM) models have shown strong results, with CNN models reaching up to 97.3% AUC-ROC in detecting complex threats like zero-day malware and ransomware(Rishad, 2025). Real-timestream processing system have also been effective in identifying attacks such as Denial of Service (DoS) with near perfect accuracy, showing the practical use of adaptive pipeline for operational defense(Loganathan, 2018). In addition, reinforcement learning has enabled automated containment measures that reduce response time by nearly 45%(Ali, 2024), while predictive frameworks give organizations the chance to anticipate and prevent threats before they take effect(Thapaliya & Bokani, 2024). Still, adversarial attacks, high computational costs, and ethical questions around data use remain important challenges, which means that furter work is needed to make these systems more trustworthy and reliable.

Automated threat hunting and cognitive triage are also beginning to change how cybersecurity operations are carried out. These systems use algorithms to scan through very large datasets and look for suspicious patterns, which helps in reducing false positives and makes Security Operations Centers (SOCs) more efficient. Different machine learning methods, such as supervised, unsupervised, and reinforcement learning, are used here, and they are able to detect anomalies in real time and also adapt to new types of attacks (Bizzarri et al., 2024a; Ejeofobiri et al., 2024; Rishad, 2025). In practice, platforms like AI-SIEM have been applied to security data in financial and healthcare systems, where they improve malware detection and even identify samples that older tools could not (Almojel & Mishra, 2024). Cognitive triage adds another step by ranking alerts according to severity, so that analysts are not overloaded with unnecessary information and can pay attention to what matters most (Abdullahi et al., 2022; Balisane et al., 2024). In some studies, adding technologies like blockchain, IoT, and natural language processing has further strengthened predictive intelligence and widened the scale of detection (Dang et al., 2024; Jumagaliyeva et al., 2024). But even though these systems show clear improvements, problems of scalability, interpretability, and also privacy remain, which means stronger regulation and governance are still needed (Margetts, 2022; Novelli et al., 2024).

Neuro-inspired AI also has an important role in supporting analysts directly. In SOCs, analysts face high levels of alert fatigue and cognitive load, and AI can reduce this by filtering out routine alerts so that experts only focus on complex or uncertain threats. Frameworks such as Adaptive Anomaly Partitioning show how AI and analysts can interact in a smoother way, with the system taking care of repetitive tasks while the human focuses on critical ones (Hatt et al., 2024). Neuromorphic computing has also been shown to improve collaboration between human intuition and machine learning, with studies showing strong detection performance and faster decision-making (Akopyan, 2016; Pehle et al., 2022). Neurosymbolic AI is another example, because it combines neural networks with symbolic reasoning to produce outputs that are easier to interpret (Hogea & Onchis, 2024). This kind of balance is important in cybersecurity since explainability is always required (Liu et al., 2024).

Newer generative AI tools can also simplify long and complex logs into insights that analysts can use quickly . Automated triage based on studying analyst workflows has helped to lower false positives and made SOC processes more efficient (Navarro et al., 2010). At the same time, concerns remain about depending too much on automation, the possibility of bias in AI systems, and also the difficulty of interpreting AI outputs. These points show why human judgment still has to remain central in SOC operations (Hogea & Onchis, 2024).

On a broader scale, AI integration is reshaping how organizations and governments respond to cyber threats. SOCs in companies, national agencies, and even NATO exercises have started to rely on AI for detection and response. In many case studies, AI systems have shown detection rates above 95% and they have also cut down response times significantly in real-world operations (Truong et al., 2021). Hybrid CNN and LSTM models further add to this by improving detection accuracy and lowering false negatives, which directly improves SOC performance (Rishad, 2025). Platforms like SOAR take away routine processes from analysts and allow them to focus more on the urgent threats (Balisane et al., 2024; Ramakrishnan & Chittibala, 2024). Adaptive AI has also proved valuable in large-scale events such as the SolarWinds breach, where its continuous learning capacity helped improve resilience during the crisis (H. Wang et al., 2024). At the international level, this trend raises questions about standards and ethics because AI tools can be used both for defense and for offensive cyber operations(Usman et al., 2023a; Waxman, 2017). While the benefits are very clear in terms of resilience and collaboration, risks like opacity, privacy concerns, and over-dependence on automated tools continue to underline the need for human oversight and stronger governance structures ell(Lekota, 2024; Margetts, 2022; Novelli et al., 2024).

6. ETHICAL, LEGAL, AND PRIVACY CONSIDERATIONS

Data privacy remains one of the most significant ethical issues in AI-driven cybersecurity. These systems rely heavily on sensitive information such as network traffic logs, user activity records, and sometimes even biometric data. While such datasets are essential for detecting threats, they also create risk of misuse, unauthorized access, and surveillance. To address these risks, compliance with privacy-preserving methods such as Federated Learning(FL) and Differential Privacy(DP) has been introduced as a possible solution. FL allows decentralized model training across multiple devices without the need to pool raw data in a central repository, reducing exposure of sensitive information and helping organizations meet GDPR requirements(Kurupathi & Maass, 2020; Truong et al., 2021). DP works differently by adding controlled noise to dataset or model output so that individual-level data cannot be reverse-engineered, while Secure Multi-Party Computation(SMPC) supports collaborative analysis across entities without revealing private inputs(Chen et al., 2024; Yang et al., 2023). However, these methods are not without problems. FL systems remain vulnerable to attacks such as model inversion or reconstruction, where adversaries infer private data from shared parameters (Choudhury et al., 2020; Li et al., 2022).Similarly, DP often reduces model accuracy, creating a difficult trade-off between performance and privacy (Rodríguez-Barroso et al., 2020; Zhu et al., 2020). Decentralized FL also faces communication security risks, making it susceptible to adversarial interception(Chen et al., 2024). These challenges show that while privacy-preserving techniques strengthen safeguards, the balance between effective threat detection and user data protection is still an evolving concern.

Another significant problem, also known as the "black box" problem, is the inability to interpret deep learning neuro-inspired AI models. Because these systems operated in complex ways, it can be difficult for analysts to understand why certain alerts or predictions are generated. This lack of transparency creates barriers to trust, accountability, and effective action in high-stakes contexts like intrusion detection. To address this, explainable AI (XAI) has emerged as a framework for making AI decisions more transparent. By clarifying how predictions are made, XAI helps analysts interpret and validate system output(Rjoub et al., 2023). Some Intrusion Detection Systems (IDS) already incorporate XAI to provide interpretable explanations that improve analysts' confidence(Neupane et al., 2022). Neurosymbolic AI extends this by combining neural networks with symbolic reasoning, giving structured, logic-based output with fully sacrificing predictive performance(Neupane et al., 2022; Rjoub et al., 2023). Other approaches, such as Addictive Gaussian Processes(AGPs), build transparency directly into models and offer uncertainty estimates that can help reduce false positives(Kolicic et al., 2024). These developemts also connect with legal expectations like GDPR's "rights to explanation", which requires greater accountability in AI decision making(Neupane et al., 2022; Rjoub et al., 2023). Even so, the trade-off between high performance and interpretability remains a major challenge; creating explanations that are useful for both technical analysts and policymakers is still unresolved, making it clear that explainability must continue to be an active area of research.

Cross-border data sharing and the international legal framework bring additional complexity. The GDPR in Europe enforces strict standards, including extraterritorial rules that apply even to non-EU entities handling EU citizens' data. While this helps protect privacy, it also creates jurisdictional tension. For example, data transfers outside the EU are only permitted with adequate safeguards, but this often clashes with differing legal systems(Ortega Giménez, n.d.; Ryngaert & Taylor, 2020). In the US, the California Customer Privacy Act (CCPA) gives individuals greater visibility into how their data is collected and sold, though it is not as comprehensive as

GDPR, leaving regulatory gaps (Huda et al., 2024; Zwolinska, 2015). Standards such as ISO/IEC 27001 attempt to provide a global framework for information security management, but differences in national law remain(Ade Rizki Saputra, 2023). The collapse of agreements like the EU-US Privacy Shield showed how fragile cross-border mechanisms can be(Minssen et al., 2020; Ryngaert & Taylor, 2020). Cyber welfare presents additional difficulties in addition to data protection. International law, including the UN Charter and International Humanitarian Law, offers limited guidance on cyber attacks, leaving many gray areas around legality and proportionality (Pasupathieswaran M & Kapilan Bharathi G, 2024; Waxman, 2017). Ethical debates also continue over whether AI should be used in offensive cyber operations, with concerns about accountability and legality (Artzt & Dung, 2022; Timmers, 2019; Usman et al., 2023b). These issues show how legal and ethical governance struggles to keep pace with rapidly advancing technology.

Bias and accountability form another critical set of concerns in AI-driven cybersecurity. AI systems are only as reliable as the data they are trained on, and an unrepresentative dataset can introduce bias that leads to unfair outcomes. In cyber defense, this might mean disproportionate flagging of certain behaviors or groups, undermining fairness and trustworthiness (Galinec, 2023; Lloyd Booz & Hamilton, 2018).Curating varied datasets, applying fairness-aware algorithms, and employing continuous monitoring to identify skewed results are some strategies to lessen bias (Galinec, 2023; Mannes, 2020). However, accountability must be clear in order to reduce bias. Responsibility for AI decisions is often distributed across multiple actors, developers, organizations, and security analysts, all of whom play a role in ensuring ethical use (Priyanshu et al., 2024). Frameworks such as the NIST AI Risk Management Framework help define oversight responsibilities and build accountability into AI systems (Novelli et al., 2024). risk management practices that account for adversarial attacks and greater transparency are also important for building public trust. While some argue that strict regulation might limit innovation, the absence of accountability could undermine trust in AI defenses. The balance between encouraging technological progress and ensuring fairness and responsibility will be central as these systems continue to develop.

7. CHALLENGES AND FUTURE DIRECTIONS

The integration of AI into cyber threat detection still faces several critical limitations, particularly in dataset diversity, model robustness, and operational efficiency. The absence of a large and representative dataset is one of the main issues. Most existing datasets are narrow in scope and cannot capture the constantly evolving nature of cyber attacks, which often leads to overfitting and poor generalization of

AI models (Ajibuwa et al., 2023; Sarker, 2023). A similar issue exists in computational cognitive neuroscience, where dependence on limited neuroimaging datasets restricts how well models can generalize, again pointing to the need for larger and more varied data sources (Grootswagers & Robinson, n.d.). On top of this, AI systems remain highly vulnerable to adversarial attacks, where very small input changes are enough to mislead models into incorrect classifications. This makes them unreliable and exposes clear weaknesses for attackers to exploit (Fisher et al., 2024; Mathov et al., 2021; Xi, 2021). Problems with false positives and negatives are also common, which reduces trust in automated detections (Xi, 2021; W. Zhang et al., 2024). Operationally, training and deploying large models come with huge computational costs and scalability issues, making real time applications difficult (Bizzarri et al., 2024b; Sarker, 2023). The interpretability of these models is another limitation, as security teams often find it hard to understand and validate AI decisions. While solutions like adversarial training, dataset optimization, and neurosymbolic AI have shown promise(Bizzarri et al., 2024b; H. Wang et al., 2023; Zhong et al., 2022; Zou et al., 2024), overcoming these gaps is still necessary before AI can be considered fully reliable and explainable in cybersecurity

Emerging approaches in multimodal and hybrid AI are opening up new possibilities for cybersecurity by boosting detection accuracy and interpretability. Multimodal systems combine multiple types of data like network traffic, user behaviour, IoT device logs, and even social data, creating a fuller picture of the threat environment. This wider context helps in detecting complex multi-vector attacks that single-source systems often miss (Ejeofobiri et al., 2024; Hogea & Onchis, 2024; Juarez et al., 2023). Some studies show that multimodal AI has already improved prediction accuracy and responsiveness in intrusion detection systems (Bizzarri et al., 2024a; Dang et al., 2024). By combining deep learning with symbolic reasoning, hybrid AI also provides value. These neurosymbolic systems perform strongly in pattern recognition while still offering interpretable, logic-based explanations (Bizzarri et al., 2024a; Hogea & Onchis, 2024). Logic-based multimodal models are particularly useful in areas like misinformation detection, where decision transparency is crucial (Liu et al., 2024). At the same time, blockchain and Natural Language processing (NLP) are being integrated with AI to improve both security and interpretability. For example, blockchain ensures data integrity, while NLP translates model output into more understandable explanations (Dang et al., 2024; Jumagaliyeva et al., 2024). While these directions are promising, they also bring challenges, including complexity, robustness against adversarial manipulation, and ensuring that models stay interpretable enough to build user trust.

Another big challenge lies in scalability and real-time performance, especially when handling massive and high-velocity network traffic in live Security Operation Centers (SOC). In cloud and edge environments, lately and limited resources are major bottlenecks. Some new designs try to address this; for example, the NIDS model by Kim and Pak (2023) uses O(1) memory complexity to process many concurrent flows efficiently. Flexible IDS architecture built on recurrent neural networks (RNNs) also adapts to changing network conditions, improving resilience against evasive attacks (Kicho Yu et al., 2022; Zhu et al., 2020). Image-based packet analysis, which converts packet flows into two-dimensional images, has also sped up detection compared to flow-based systems, while hybrid systems such as MOVICAB-IDS combine neural networks with case-based reasoning for real-time responses(Navarro et al., 2010). Beyond algorithms, hardware-level solutions are emerging. Hyperdimensional computing (CyberHD) reduces dimensionality and latency while keeping accuracy high (J. Wang et al., 2023). Edge-based optimizations like pruning, compression, and neural architecture search (NAS) also improve speed and reduce bandwidth needs (Sander et al., 2025). Neuromimetic platforms such as SpiNNaker use event-driven computation to handle bursty traffic, while cloud control approaches enforce strict latency guarantees (Cai et al., 2021). Neuromorphic hardware, however, introduces its own scalability issues, with asynchronous circuits increasing memory and complexity. Solutions like hierarchical-mesh routing and network on chip (NoC) designs aim to improve communication efficiency (Moradi et al., 2017). Even then, usability is still a hurdle, as shown by frameworks like BrainScaleS-2, which require better software integration and faster reconfiguration (Müller et al., 2022). These approaches show progress, but the trade-off between accuracy and speed, along with integration across heterogeneous infrastructure, remains unresolved

Finally, future prospects such as neuromorphic hardware and brain-computer interfaces (BCIs) suggest that cyber defense will undergo a radical change. Neuromorphic chips like Intel Loihi and IBM TrueNorth offer low power, real-time processing that mimics biological neural networks, allowing rapid anomaly detection with high energy efficiency. TrueNorth, for instance, processes complex data streams at just 65mW, making it suitable for embedded cyber defense (Akopyan, 2016; Pehle et al., 2022). These event-driven, parallel architectures are highly adaptive to dynamic cyber threats and scalable across different environments. BCIs, on the other hand, open up the possibility of cognitive augmentation for analysts, linking brain activity directly with machines to improve decision making, situational awareness, and human AI collaboration (Moore & Col, 2013; X. Zhang et al., 2020). By integrating neurophysiological data into defense systems, resilience could be enhanced further, with frameworks adapting to the analyst's mental state in real time (Boccardi et al., 2024; Boi et al., 2016; Talanov et al., 2022). This kind of human AI teaming combines machine speed with human intuition, leading to more adaptive defense strategies (Ali, 2024). Yet these developments raise major ethical and regulatory concerns, especially regarding privacy, adversarial risks, and potential misuse in cyber warfare. As a result, strong governance, transparency, and interdisciplinary oversight will be necessary to make sure neuromorphic and BCI-based systems are deployed responsibly.

8. CASE STUDIES AND GLOBAL PERSPECTIVES

The integration of AI and neuroscience-inspired approaches in cybersecurity is not only a research topic but something that is already being applied in real-world contexts. Across industries like finance, healthcare, and defense, these systems are being tested and in some cases widely adopted, showing how they can move from theory into practice. In the financial sector, where fraud and cybercrime result in heavy losses every year, neural networks have become important for monitoring transactions and identifying suspicious activities. Studies have reported accuracies above 98% in detecting fraudulent transactions, which translates into fewer losses and better support for fraud investigators (Aryendra Dalal, 2018). Systems like AI-SIEM, which combine convolutional and recurrent neural networks, have also been used to analyze patterns in large amounts of security data, helping to detect malware that was not identified by traditional systems. Some reports show these systems reaching close to 90% accuracy in identifying previously unknown samples, which is significant because traditional models are often limited to known signatures (Rishad, 2025). In healthcare, the challenge is often around IoT-based medical devices, which are vulnerable to attacks if not properly monitored. Here, hybrid LSTM-CNN models have achieved training accuracy of 99.53% and testing accuracy of 91.42% in detecting anomalies, which is crucial for protecting sensitive patient data and keeping hospital operations safe(Almojel & Mishra, 2024). These models also integrate behavioral analytics, which gives an added level of protection against insider misuse or unusual activity(Abdullahi et al., 2022; Almojel & Mishra, 2024; Thapaliya & Bokani, 2024b). In defense and government, platforms like Darktrace show how autonomous AI can detect threats as they happen and adapt quickly. NATO cyber exercises have already applied AI-driven simulations to strengthen preparedness for large-scale threats, highlighting that these approaches can scale beyond organizations to national security (Ejeofobiri et al., 2024; Thapaliya & Bokani, 2024b). Looking across these industries, it becomes clear that neuroscience-inspired AI is starting to provide measurable improvements, but at the same time, questions of bias, data quality, and human oversight remain ongoing barriers(Aryendra Dalal, 2018).

At an organizational level, resilience is a central outcome of integrating these systems. Resilience in cybersecurity does not mean that attacks will not happen, but rather that detection is faster, response is coordinated, and recovery is shorter. AI-driven detection models such as CNNs and LSTMs have achieved high levels of accuracy, at 97.3% and 96.8% respectively, while also bringing down false positive rates (Rishad, 2025). Automated response systems make this resilience stronger. For example, the integration of SOAR platforms with SIEM systems has enabled real-time coordination of responses, reducing the time between detection and containment (Thapaliya & Bokani, 2024). Another dimension is proactive defense, where systems are not only waiting for threats to appear but are actively monitoring and adapting. The Adaptive Anomaly Partitioning Framework, for instance, can detect ransomware dynamically and continuously, catching activity before encryption takes place (Hatt et al., 2024). Other layered strategies combine continuous monitoring, threat hunting, and adaptive profiling, which allow organizations to keep pace with changing attack strategies. Reports from field deployments indicate that these systems shorten mean time to recovery and also strengthen information sharing between organizations, which is critical for building resilience at a larger scale(Ramakrishnan & Chittibala, 2024). Still, even with these advances, implementation is not simple. These tools require regular retraining, analyst upskilling, and constant updating to remain effective. Without this ongoing effort, the resilience that AI brings can fade, especially as attackers also evolve their own AI-driven tools.

When comparing AI-neuroscience hybrid systems with more traditional cybersecurity approaches, the differences are quite clear. Traditional models such as rule-based firewalls or signature-based detection systems are reactive in nature. They are effective for known threats but fail when faced with zero-day exploits or new attack vectors. Their reliance on frequent updates also creates gaps in protection, and they are known to produce large numbers of false positives that overwhelm analysts (Bizzarri et al., 2024a; Oh et al., 2023; Rishad, 2025). Hybrid AI systems, in contrast, have shown that they can adapt in real time and recognize previously unseen threats. For example, systems combining neural networks with rule-based elements have reported more than 78% success in detecting novel attacks (Koutsoutos et al., 2006). Dynamically retrainable firewalls also show how defenses can evolve alongside changing network conditions, something that traditional systems cannot do (Ahmadi, 2025). Predictive approaches make this contrast even sharper. CNN and LSTM models achieve strong AUC-ROC values of 97.3% and 96.8%, while newer frameworks such as Dynamic Anomaly Pattern Discrimination (DAPD) identify ransomware behaviors before encryption begins, essentially shifting from reaction to prevention (Deleon et al., 2024; Rishad, 2025) . Traditional systems still play a role as a baseline, especially where threats are well-defined, but the evidence from these studies suggests that organizations seeking comprehensive security need to move toward adaptive, AI-driven, and neuroscience-inspired models.

9. CONCLUSION

AI and neuroscience-based methods are gradually altering the manner of cybersecurity, and the change is already apparent in practice. These systems detect abnormal activity more quickly, respond more effectively in real time, and provide more fortitude to organizations to recover from assault than the older rule-based tools do. We can see it in finance where fraud detection is more robust, in health where the IoT is more secure, and defense where the use of AI has been trialed on a large scale. The point is that these models can learn and improve, something that is not well handled by traditional systems. Nonetheless, the picture isn't all bad news. There is the problem of privacy with the use of sensitive data, the models typically have difficult-to-interpret black boxes, and the training and maintenance comes at a high cost. Then, of course, there is the risk of over-reliance upon automation and losing the human judgement that is necessary on more sophisticated decisions. For the future, advances like neuromorphic chipsets and the brain–computer interface promise more potent tools, but also pose questions of ethical and governance grounds. The challenge of the moment is to retain the good, plug the gaps, and develop cyber defense systems which are robust and adaptive that still remain fair, transparent, and responsible.

REFERENCES

Abdullahi, M., Baashar, Y., Alhussian, H., Alwadain, A., Aziz, N., Capretz, L. F., & Abdulkadir, S. J. (2022). Detecting Cybersecurity Attacks in Internet of Things Using Artificial Intelligence Methods: A Systematic Literature Review. In *Electronics (Switzerland)* (Vol. 11, Issue 2). MDPI. https://doi.org/DOI: 10.3390/electronics11020198

. Ahmadi, S. (2025). *Adaptive Cybersecurity: Dynamically Retrainable Firewalls for Real-Time Network Protection.*

Ajibuwa, O., Hamdaoui, B., & Yavuz, A. A. (2023). *A Survey on AI/ML-Driven Intrusion and Misbehavior Detection in Networked Autonomous Systems: Techniques, Challenges and Opportunities.* https://arxiv.org/abs/2305.05040

Akopyan, F. (2016).. . *Design and Tool Flow of IBM's TrueNorth, 59–60.* Advance online publication. DOI: 10.1145/2872334.2878629

Al-Turjman, F. (2024). Deep reinforcement learning applications in cybersecurity: Trends and future directions. *Future Generation Computer Systems, 152*, 541–554. DOI: 10.1016/j.future.2023.11.009

Ali, A. (2024). AI-Powered Shield: Transforming Cybersecurity with Neural Network Innovations *(Preprint).* https://doi.org/DOI: 10.2196/preprints.69000

Almojel, F., & Mishra, S. (2024). Advancing Hospital Cybersecurity Through IoT-Enabled Neural Network for Human Behavior Analysis and Anomaly Detection. In *IJACSA)* [). www.ijacsa.thesai.org]. *International Journal of Advanced Computer Science and Applications, 15*(5), •••.

Aminu, M. A., Hussain, A., & See, S. (2024). Spiking neural networks for efficient cybersecurity intrusion detection. *IEEE Access : Practical Innovations, Open Solutions, 12*, 15632–15647. DOI: 10.1109/ACCESS.2024.3358912

Artzt, M., & Dung, T. V. (2022). Artificial Intelligence and Data Protection: How to Reconcile Both Areas from the European Law Perspective. *Vietnamese Journal of Legal Sciences, 7*(2), 39–58. DOI: 10.2478/vjls-2022-0007

Baki, S., Umit, A., & Gonen, B. (2017). Phishing detection using cognitive and machine learning approaches. *International Journal of Information Security Science, 6*(4), 70–81. http://www.ijiss.org/ijiss/index.php/ijiss/article/view/250

. Balisane, H., Egho-Promise, E. I., Lyada, E., & Aina, F. (2024). TOWARDS IMPROVED THREAT MITIGATION IN DIGITAL ENVIRONMENTS: A COMPREHENSIVE FRAMEWORK FOR CYBERSECURITY ENHANCEMENT. *International Journal of Research -GRANTHAALAYAH, 12*(5). https://doi.org/DOI: 10.29121/granthaalayah.v12.i5.2024.5655

Basit, A., Zafar, S., Liu, J., & Javed, A. (2020). A comprehensive survey of AI for phishing detection. *IEEE Access : Practical Innovations, Open Solutions, 8*, 116–125. DOI: 10.1109/ACCESS.2020.2979038 PMID: 33110340

Bizzarri, A., Yu, C.-E., Jalaian, B., Riguzzi, F., & Bastian, N. D. (2024a). A synergistic approach in network intrusion detection by neurosymbolic AI [Preprint]. *arXiv*. https://arxiv.org/abs/2406.00938

Bizzarri, A., Yu, C.-E., Jalaian, B., Riguzzi, F., & Bastian, N. D. (2024b). *A neurosymbolic artificial intelligence network intrusion detection system*. In *Proceedings of the 33rd International Conference on Computer Communications and Networks (ICCCN)* (pp. 1–8). IEEE. https://doi.org/DOI: 10.1109/ICCCN61486.2024.10637618

Boccardi, V., Tagliafico, L., Persia, A., Page, E., Ottaviani, S., Cremonini, A. L., Borgarelli, C., Pisciotta, L., Mecocci, P., Nencioni, A., & Monacelli, F. (2024). The Potential Effects of Red Wine and Its Components on Neurocognitive Disorders: A Narrative Review. In *Nutrients* (Vol. 16, Issue 20). Multidisciplinary Digital Publishing Institute (MDPI). https://doi.org/DOI: 10.3390/nu16203431

Boi, F., Moraitis, T., De Feo, V., Diotalevi, F., Bartolozzi, C., Indiveri, G., & Vato, A. (2016). A bidirectional brain-machine interface featuring a neuromorphic hardware decoder. *Frontiers in Neuroscience, 10*. Advance online publication. DOI: 10.3389/fnins.2016.00563 PMID: 28018162

Brundage, M., Avin, S., Clark, J., Toner, H., Eckersley, P., Garfinkel, B., Dafoe, A., Scharre, P., Zeitzoff, T., Filar, B., Anderson, H., Roff, H., Allen, G. C., Steinhardt, J., Flynn, C., Héigeartaigh, S. Ó., Beard, S., Belfield, H., Farquhar, S., . . . Amodei, D. (2018). The malicious use of artificial intelligence: Forecasting, prevention, and mitigation. *arXiv*. https://doi.org//arxiv.1802.07228DOI: 10.48550

Cai, Y., Llorca, J., Tulino, A. M., & Molisch, A. F. (2021, June 1). Optimal Cloud Network Control with Strict Latency Constraints. *IEEE International Conference on Communications*. https://doi.org/DOI: 10.1109/ICC42927.2021.9500573

Chen, C., Liu, J., Tan, H., Li, X., Wang, K. I.-K., Li, P., Sakurai, K., & Dou, D. (2024). *Trustworthy Federated Learning: Privacy, Security, and Beyond*. https://arxiv.org/abs/2411.01583

Chio, C., & Freeman, D. (2018). *Machine learning and security: Protecting systems with data and algorithms*. O'Reilly Media.

Choudhury, O., Gkoulalas-Divanis, A., Salonidis, T., Sylla, I., Park, Y., Hsu, G., & Das, A. (2020). *Anonymizing Data for Privacy-Preserving Federated Learning*. https://arxiv.org/abs/2002.09096

Dalal, A. (2018). Cybersecurity And Artificial Intelligence: How AI Is Being Used in Cybersecurity To Improve Detection And Response To Cyber Threats. *Turkish Journal of Computer and Mathemafics Educafion, 9*(3), 1704–1709.

Dang, Y., Huang, K., Huo, J., Yan, Y., Huang, S., Liu, D., Gao, M., Zhang, J., Qian, C., Wang, K., Liu, Y., Shao, J., Xiong, H., & Hu, X. (2024). *Explainable and Interpretable Multimodal Large Language Models: A Comprehensive Survey*. https://arxiv.org/abs/2412.02104

Darktrace. (2022). *Darktrace AI stops sophisticated ransomware attack at South African financial services provider.* PR Newswire. https://www.prnewswire.com/news-releases/darktrace-ai-stops-sophisticated-ransomware-attack-at-south-african-financial-services-provider-301517557.html

Darktrace. (2023). *Under the radar: Insider threats detected by Darktrace*. https://darktrace.com/news/under-the-radar-insider-threats-detected-by-darktrace

Davies, M., Wild, A., Orchard, G., Sandamirskaya, Y., Guerra, G. A. F., Joshi, P., Plank, P., & Risbud, S. R. (2021). Advancing neuromorphic computing with Loihi: A survey of results and outlook. *Proceedings of the IEEE, 109*(5), 911–934. DOI: 10.1109/jproc.2021.3067593

. Deleon, J., Hatherleigh, C., Cumberbatch, A., Ashworth, J., & Heathcote, L. (2024). *Predictive Profiling Framework for Ransomware Detection Using Contextual Signature Extraction.*

Ejeofobiri, C. K., Victor-Igun, O. O., & Okoye, C. (2024). AI-Driven Secure Intrusion Detection for Internet of Things (IOT) Networks. *Asian Journal of Mathematics and Computer Research, 31*(4), 40–55. DOI: 10.56557/ajomcor/2024/v31i48971

Ferrag, M. A., Maglaras, L., Moschoyiannis, S., & Janicke, H. (2020). Deep learning for cyber security intrusion detection: Approaches, datasets, and comparative studies. *Journal of Information Security and Applications, 50*, 102419. DOI: 10.1016/j.jisa.2019.102419

Fisher, H., Shahar, M., & Resheff, Y. S. (2024). *Neural Fingerprints for Adversarial Attack Detection*. https://arxiv.org/abs/2411.04533

Galinec, D. (2023). Cyber Security and Cyber Defense: Challenges and Building of Cyber Resilience Conceptual Model. *International Journal of Applied Sciences & Development, 1*, 83–88. DOI: 10.37394/232029.2022.1.10

Goodfellow, I., Bengio, Y., & Courville, A. (2016). *Deep learning*. MIT Press.

. Grootswagers, T., & Robinson, A. K. (n.d.). *OVERFITTING THE LITERATURE TO ONE SET OF STIMULI AND DATA*.

Hassabis, D., Kumaran, D., Summerfield, C., & Botvinick, M. (2017). Neuroscience-inspired artificial intelligence. *Neuron, 95*(2), 245–258. DOI: 10.1016/j.neuron.2017.06.011 PMID: 28728020

. Hatt, A., Blackwood, C., Lockhart, B., Ravenscroft, J., & Wainwright, N. (2024). *Dynamic Ransomware Detection through Adaptive Anomaly Partitioning Framework*.

Hogea, E., & Onchis, D. (2024). *Sisteme Hibride de Invatare Automata si Aplicatii*. https://arxiv.org/abs/2406.11870

Huda, M., Awaludin, A., & Siregar, H. K. (2024). Legal Challenges in Regulating Artificial Intelligence: A Comparative Study of Privacy and Data Protection Laws. In *IJSH* (Vol. 01, Issue 2). https://dejournals.org/index.php/ijsh

Juarez, D., Arteaga, I., Cortes, H., Vazquez-Roque, R., Lopez-Lopez, G., Flores, G., Treviño, S., Guevara, J., & Diaz, A. (2023). Chronic resveratrol administration reduces oxidative stress and brain cell loss and improves memory of recognition in old rats. *Synapse (New York, N.Y.), 77*(4). Advance online publication. DOI: 10.1002/syn.22271 PMID: 37130656

Jumagaliyeva, A., Abdykerimova, E., Turkmenbayev, A., Serimbetov, B., Muratova, G., Yersultanova, Z., & Zhiyembayev, Z. (2024). IDENTIFYING PATTERNS AND MECHANISMS OF AI INTEGRATION IN BLOCKCHAIN FOR E-VOTING NETWORK SECURITY. *Eastern-European Journal of Enterprise Technologies, 4*(2(130)), 6–18. DOI: 10.15587/1729-4061.2024.305696

Kicho, Yu. (2022). *Khanh Nguyen, & Younghee Park*. Flexible and Robust Real-time Intrusion Detection Systems to Network Dynamics., DOI: 10.1109/ACCESS.2017. DOI

Kolicic, B., Caron, A., Hicks, C., & Mavroudis, V. (2024). *Inherently Interpretable and Uncertainty-Aware Models for Online Learning in Cyber-Security Problems*. https://arxiv.org/abs/2411.09393

Kolosnjaji, B., Zarras, A., Webster, G., & Eckert, C. (2016). Deep learning for classification of malware system call sequences. In *Australasian Joint Conference on Artificial Intelligence* (pp. 137–149). Springer. https://doi.org/DOI: 10.1007/978-3-319-50127-7_11

. Koutsoutos, S., Christou, T., & Efremidis, S. (2006). *An Intrusion Detection System for Network-Initiated Attaclcs Using a Hybrid Neural Network.*

. Kurupathi, S. R., & Maass, W. (2020). *Survey on Federated Learning Towards Privacy Preserving AI.* 235–253. https://doi.org/DOI: 10.5121/csit.2020.101120

. Lekota, N. F. (2024). *Governance Considerations of Adversarial Attacks on AI Systems.*

Li, J., Li, X., & Zhang, C. (2022). Analysis on Security and Privacy-preserving in Federated Learning. In *Highlights in Science* (Vol. 2022). Engineering and Technology SDPIT.

Liu, H., Wang, W., & Li, H. (2024). *Interpretable Multimodal Misinformation Detection with Logic Reasoning.* https://arxiv.org/abs/2305.05964

. Lloyd Booz, K., & Hamilton, A. (2018). *Bias Amplification in Artificial Intelligence Systems.*

Mannes, A. (2020). *Successful Research in AI Governance.* Risk, and Artificial Intelligence.

Margetts, H. (2022). Rethinking AI for Good Governance. *Daedalus, 151*(2), 360–371. DOI: 10.1162/DAED_a_01922

Mathov, Y., Levy, E., Katzir, Z., Shabtai, A., & Elovici, Y. (2021). *Not All Datasets Are Born Equal: On Heterogeneous Data and Adversarial Examples.* https://arxiv.org/abs/2010.03180

Minssen, T., Seitz, C., Aboy, M., & Compagnucci, M. C. (2020). The EU-US Privacy Shield Regime for CrossBorder Transfers of Personal Data under the GDPR What are the legal challenges and how might these affect cloudbased technologies, big data, and AI in the medical sector? *European Pharmaceutical Law Review, 4*(1), 34–50. DOI: 10.21552/eplr/2020/1/6

. Moore, B. E., & Col, L. (2013). *THE BRAIN COMPUTER INTERFACE FUTURE: TIME FOR A STRATEGY.*

. Moradi, S., Qiao, N., Stefanini, F., & Indiveri, G. (2017). *A scalable multi-core architecture with heterogeneous memory structures for Dynamic Neuromorphic Asynchronous Processors (DYNAPs).* https://doi.org/DOI: 10.1109/TBCAS.2017.2759700

Morgan, S. (2020, November 13). *Cybercrime to cost the world $10.5 trillion annually by 2025.* Cybersecurity Ventures. https://cybersecurityventures.com/hackerpocalypse-cybercrime-report-2016/

Morgan, S. (2024, November 18). *Cybercrime to cost the world $10.5 trillion annually by 2025.* Cybercrime Magazine. https://cybersecurityventures.com/hackerpocalypse-cybercrime-report-2016/

Müller, E., Arnold, E., Breitwieser, O., Czierlinski, M., Emmel, A., Kaiser, J., Mauch, C., Schmitt, S., Spilger, P., Stock, R., Stradmann, Y., Weis, J., Baumbach, A., Billaudelle, S., Cramer, B., Ebert, F., Göltz, J., Ilmberger, J., Karasenko, V., & Schemmel, J. (2022). A Scalable Approach to Modeling on Accelerated Neuromorphic Hardware. *Frontiers in Neuroscience, 16.* Advance online publication. DOI: 10.3389/fnins.2022.884128 PMID: 35663548

. Navarro, M., Herrero, Á., Corchado, E., & Julián, V. (2010). *Approaching Real-Time Intrusion Detection through MOVICAB-IDS.*

Neupane, S., Ables, J., Anderson, W., Mittal, S., Rahimi, S., Banicescu, I., & Seale, M. (2022). *Explainable Intrusion Detection Systems (X-IDS): A Survey of Current Methods, Challenges, and Opportunities.* https://arxiv.org/abs/2207.06236

Nguyen, T. T., & Reddi, V. J. (2021). Deep reinforcement learning for cyber security. *IEEE Transactions on Neural Networks and Learning Systems, 34*(8), 3779–3795. DOI: 10.1109/tnnls.2021.3121870 PMID: 34723814

Novelli, C., Taddeo, M., & Floridi, L. (2024). *Accountability in Artificial Intelligence: What It Is and How It Works.* https://ec.europa.eu/digital-inglemarket/en/news/definition-artificial-intelligence-main-capabilities-

Oh, S. H., Jeong, M. K., Kim, H. C., & Park, J. (2023). Applying Reinforcement Learning for Enhanced Cybersecurity against Adversarial Simulation. *Sensors (Basel), 23*(6). Advance online publication. DOI: 10.3390/s23063000 PMID: 36991711

Ortega Giménez, A. (n.d.). TUTELA JURISDICCIONAL ANTE UN TRATAMIENTO ILÍCITO INTERNACIONAL DE DATOS PERSONALES Y EL NUEVO REGLAMENTO GENERAL DE PROTECCIÓN DE DATOS DE LA UNIÓN EUROPEA Jurisdictional protection against an illicit international treatment of personal data and the new general regulations for data protection of the European Union. *Revista Acta Judicial,* (6), 2–23.

Pasupathieswaran, M., & Kapilan Bharathi, G. (2024). *Digital Battlefronts: Rethinking Legal Frontiers in Cyberwarfare and AI Conflicts.* www.ijfmr.com

Pehle, C., Billaudelle, S., Cramer, B., Kaiser, J., Schreiber, K., Stradmann, Y., Weis, J., Leibfried, A., Müller, E., & Schemmel, J. (2022). *The BrainScaleS-2 accelerated neuromorphic system with hybrid plasticity*. https://arxiv.org/abs/2201.11063

Phoenix Children's Hospital. (2019). *Case study: Phoenix Children's Hospital takes on cybersecurity*. BlackBerry Cylance. https://blogs.blackberry.com/en/2019/07/case-study-phoenix-childrens-hospital-takes-on-cybersecurity

Priyanshu, A., Maurya, Y., & Hong, Z. (2024). *AI Governance and Accountability: An Analysis of Anthropic's Claude*. https://arxiv.org/abs/2407.01557

Ramakrishnan, S., & Chittibala, D. R. (2024). Enhancing Cyber Resilience: Convergence of SIEM, SOAR, and AI in 2024. In *International Journal of Computing and Engineering* (Vol. 5, Issue 2). www.carijournals.orgwww.carijournals.orgwww.carijournals.org

Ring, M., Wunderlich, S., Scheuring, D., Landes, D., & Hotho, A. (2019). A survey of network-based intrusion detection data sets. *Computers & Security*, *86*, 147–167. DOI: 10.1016/j.cose.2019.06.005

. Rishad, S. M. S. I. (2025). LEVERAGING AI AND MACHINE LEARNING FOR PREDICTING, DETECTING, AND MITIGATING CYBERSECURITY THREATS: A COMPARATIVE STUDY OF ADVANCED MODELS. *International Journal of Computer Science & Information System, 10*(01), 06–25. https://doi.org/DOI: 10.55640/ijcsis/Volume10Issue01-02

. Rizvi, M. (2023). Enhancing cybersecurity: The power of artificial intelligence in threat detection and prevention. *International Journal of Advanced Engineering Research and Science, 10*(5), 055–060. https://doi.org/DOI: 10.22161/ijaers.105.8

. Rjoub, G., Bentahar, J., Wahab, O. A., Mizouni, R., Song, A., Cohen, R., Otrok, H., & Mourad, A. (2023). *A Survey on Explainable Artificial Intelligence for Cybersecurity*. https://doi.org/DOI: 10.1109/TNSM.2023.3282740

. Rodríguez-Barroso, N., Stipcich, G., Jiménez-López, D., Ruiz-Millán, J. A., Martínez-Cámara, E., González-Seco, G., Luzón, M. V., Veganzones, M. Á., & Herrera, F. (2020). *Federated Learning and Differential Privacy: Software tools analysis, the Sherpa.ai FL framework and methodological guidelines for preserving data privacy*. https://doi.org/DOI: 10.1016/j.inffus.2020.07.009

Roy, K., Jaiswal, A., & Panda, P. (2019). Towards spike-based machine intelligence with neuromorphic computing. *Nature*, *575*(7784), 607–617. DOI: 10.1038/s41586-019-1677-2 PMID: 31776490

Ryngaert, C., & Taylor, M. (2020). Symposium on the GDPR and international law. The GDPR as global data protection regulation? *AJIL Unbound, 114*, 5–9. https://doi.org/DOI: 10.1017/aju.2019.80

Sander, J., Cohen, A., Dasari, V. R., Venable, B., & Jalaian, B. (2025). *On Accelerating Edge AI: Optimizing Resource-Constrained Environments*. https://arxiv.org/abs/2501.15014

Saputra, A. R. (2023). Aspects of Personal Data Protection According to International Law. [FJSS]. *Formosa Journal of Social Sciences*, *2*(3), 417–424. DOI: 10.55927/fjss.v2i3.6192

Sarker, I. H. (2023). Multi-aspects AI -based modeling and adversarial learning for cybersecurity intelligence and robustness: A comprehensive overview. *Security and Privacy*, *6*(5). Advance online publication. DOI: 10.1002/spy2.295

Scholarship@western, S., & Loganathan, G. (2018). *Real-time Intrusion Detection using Multidimensional Sequence-Real-time Intrusion Detection using Multidimensional Sequence-to-Sequence Machine Learning and Adaptive Stream Processing to-Sequence Machine Learning and Adaptive Stream Processing Part of the Digital Communications and Networking Commons, and the Systems and Communications Commons*. https://ir.lib.uwo.ca/etdhttps://ir.lib.uwo.ca/etd/5523

Shah, S., & Issac, B. (2018). Performance comparison of next-generation antivirus tools. *Journal of Information Security Research*, *9*(3), 130–140. DOI: 10.6025/jisr/2018/9/3/130-140

Shone, N., Ngoc, T. N., Phai, V. D., & Shi, Q. (2018). A deep learning approach to network intrusion detection. *IEEE Transactions on Emerging Topics in Computational Intelligence*, *2*(1), 41–50. DOI: 10.1109/TETCI.2017.2772792

Sommer, R., & Paxson, V. (2010). Outside the closed world: On using machine learning for network intrusion detection. In *Proceedings of the 2010 IEEE Symposium on Security and Privacy* (pp. 305–316). IEEE. https://doi.org/DOI: 10.1109/SP.2010.25

Song, Y., Zhang, L., Liu, Y., & Pan, Y. (2024). Spiking neural P systems for malware and phishing detection: A review. *IEEE Transactions on Neural Networks and Learning Systems*, *35*(2), 555–568. DOI: 10.1109/TNNLS.2023.3241829 PMID: 35877793

Talanov, M., Vallverdu, J., Adamatzky, A., Toschev, A., Suleimanova, A., Leukhin, A., Posdeeva, A., Mikhailova, Y., Rodionova, A., Mikhaylov, A., Serb, A., Shchanikov, S., Gerasimova, S., Dehshibi, M. M., Hramov, A., Kazantsev, V., Tsoy, T., Magid, E., Lavrov, I., & Warwick, K. (2022). *Neuropunk Revolution. Hacking Cognitive Systems towards Cyborgs 3.0.* https://arxiv.org/abs/2205.06538

Thapaliya, S., & Bokani, A. (2024). Leveraging artificial intelligence for enhanced cybersecurity: Insights and innovations. *SADGAMAYA*, *1*(1), 46–52. DOI: 10.3126/sadgamaya.v1i1.66888

Timmers, P. (2019). Ethics of AI and Cybersecurity When Sovereignty is at Stake. In *Minds and Machines* (Vol. 29, Issue 4, pp. 635–645). Springer. https://doi.org/ DOI: 10.1007/s11023-019-09508-4

Truong, N., Sun, K., Wang, S., Guitton, F., & Guo, Y. (2021). *Privacy Preservation in Federated Learning: An insightful survey from the GDPR Perspective.* https://arxiv.org/abs/2011.05411

Usman, H., Tariq, I., & Nawaz, B. (2023a). IN THE REALM OF THE MACHINES: AI'S INFLUENCE UPON INTERNATIONAL LAW AND POLICY. *Journal of Social Research Development*, *4*(2), 383–399. DOI: 10.53664/jsrd/04-02-2023-13-383-399

Usman, H., Tariq, I., & Nawaz, B. (2023b). IN THE REALM OF THE MACHINES: AI'S INFLUENCE UPON INTERNATIONAL LAW AND POLICY. *Journal of Social Research Development*, *4*(2), 383–399. DOI: 10.53664/jsrd/04-02-2023-13-383-399

Wang, H., Deng, Y., Yoo, S., & Lin, Y. (2023). *Exploring Robust Features for Improving Adversarial Robustness.* https://arxiv.org/abs/2309.04650

Wang, H., Tangirala, G. K., Naidu, G. P., Mayville, C., Roy, A., Sun, J., & Mandava, R. B. (2024). *Anomaly Detection for Incident Response at Scale.* https://arxiv.org/abs/2404.16887

Wang, J., Chen, H., Issa, M., Huang, S., & Imani, M. (2023). *Late Breaking Results: Scalable and Efficient Hyperdimensional Computing for Network Intrusion Detection.* https://arxiv.org/abs/2304.06728

Waxman, M. C. (2017). *Cyber Strategy & Policy: International Law Dimensions.* https://scholarship.law.columbia.edu/faculty_scholarshiphttps://scholarship.law.columbia.edu/faculty_scholarship/2025

Xi, B. (2021). *Adversarial Machine Learning for Cybersecurity and Computer Vision: Current Developments and Challenges.* https://arxiv.org/abs/2107.02894

Yang, Q., Huang, A., Fan, L., Seng Chan, C., Han Lim, J., Woh Ng, K., Sheng Ong, D., Li, B., Yang, Q., Huang, A., Fan, L., Chan, C. S., Lim, J. H., Ng, K. W., Ong, D. S., & Li Federated, B. (2023). Federated Learning with Privacy-preserving and Model IP-right-protection. *Machine Intelligence Research*, *20*(1), 19–37. DOI: 10.1007/s11633

Yin, C., Zhu, Y., Fei, J., & He, X. (2017). A deep learning approach for intrusion detection using recurrent neural networks. *IEEE Access : Practical Innovations, Open Solutions*, *5*, 21954–21961. DOI: 10.1109/ACCESS.2017.2762418

Zhang, W., Xu, M., Feng, Y., Mao, Z., & Yan, Z. (2024). The Effect of Procrastination on Physical Exercise among College Students—The Chain Effect of Exercise Commitment and Action Control. *International Journal of Mental Health Promotion*, *26*(8), 611–622. DOI: 10.32604/ijmhp.2024.052730

Zhang, X., Ma, Z., Zheng, H., Li, T., Chen, K., Wang, X., Liu, C., Xu, L., Wu, X., Lin, D., & Lin, H. (2020). The combination of brain-computer interfaces and artificial intelligence: Applications and challenges. *Annals of Translational Medicine*, *8*(11), 712–712. DOI: 10.21037/atm.2019.11.109 PMID: 32617332

Zhong, Y., Wu, L., Liu, X., & Jiang, J. (2022). *Exploiting the Potential of Datasets: A Data-Centric Approach for Model Robustness*. https://arxiv.org/abs/2203.05323

. Zhu, T., Ye, D., Wang, W., Zhou, W., & Yu, P. S. (2020). *More Than Privacy: Applying Differential Privacy in Key Areas of Artificial Intelligence*. https://doi.org/ DOI: 10.1109/TKDE.2020.3014246

Zou, A., Phan, L., Wang, J., Duenas, D., Lin, M., Andriushchenko, M., Wang, R., Kolter, Z., Fredrikson, M., & Hendrycks, D. (2024). *Improving Alignment and Robustness with Circuit* Breakers. https://arxiv.org/abs/2406.04313

Zwolinska, M. (2015). INTERNATIONAL TRANSFERS OF PERSONAL DATA. TOWARDS A GLOBAL CONSENSUS ON DATA PROTECTION STANDARDS TRANSFERENCIAS INTERNACIONALES DE DATOS PERSONALES. HACIA UN CONSENSO GLOBAL EN NIVELES. http://www.derecom.com/derecom/

Chapter 5

Neuro-Symbolic AI and Behavioral Intelligence: Towards Explainable Cybersecurity Mechanisms

S. A. Shreha
https://orcid.org/0009-0002-2232-819X
PSG College of Arts and Science, Coimbatore, India

R. N. Ravikumar
https://orcid.org/0009-0009-3705-1681
Marwadi University, Rajkot, India

S. Aarthi
https://orcid.org/0009-0006-9064-2091
Marwadi University, Rajkot, India

ABSTRACT

The increasing sophistication of cyber threats demands solutions that are not only accurate but also explainable and human-centered. Traditional methods like rule-based detection and machine learning, while effective to some extent, lack transparency and adaptability against evolving threats. This chapter explores how Neuro-Symbolic AI (NSAI), combining neural adaptability with symbolic reasoning, and Behavioral Intelligence, grounded in neuroscience and psychology, can transform cybersecurity. By integrating cognitive profiling with technical anomaly detection, the framework enhances accuracy, interpretability, and accountability. Case studies on insider threats and phishing demonstrate measurable improvements in detection accuracy and reduction of false positives. Ethical, regulatory, and socio-technical dimensions are also discussed, ensuring responsible deployment. The

DOI: 10.4018/979-8-3373-5012-7.ch005

proposed approach highlights a paradigm shift towards explainable, trustworthy, and human-centric cybersecurity, capable of safeguarding critical infrastructures in high-stakes environments.

INTRODUCTION

The fact that cyber threats are increasing in alarming rates unparalleled in history, has made cybersecurity a discipline, which is worthy, of clever, point-of-deft explanatory solutions. The conventional solutions so far demonstrated some form of performance such as signature-based identification and certainly data-driven learning- but is not transparent and versatile, and can provide contextual explanation. Over the last few decades, Neuro-Symbolic Artificial Intelligence (NSAI) has emerged as one of the strong paradigms that combine the functionality of perceptive learning by the neural-like systems with the system-organized reasoning by the symbols (Hitzler et al., 2022). The result of such integration is a possibility of finding such cybersecurity models that are both correct and sensible, besides being compatible and representative of human reasoning. The supportive service that NSAI can offer, which will give a better understanding of the user actions, intentions and anomalies, is rooted in neuroscience and behavioral science and is known as behavioral intelligence. Combined, these solutions can offer new generation cybersecurity solutions that can address more sophisticated attacks including insider attacks, phishing and Advanced Persistent Threat (APT) attacks; and they are also both accountable and ethically liable and loss of user trust. (Rivas et al., 2024).

BACKGROUND AND LIMITATIONS OF TRADITIONAL CYBERSECURITY APPROACHES

The approaches on which cybersecurity has been founded have been rule-based intrusion detection, statistical anomaly detection and signature matching. These applications have been tested and have been found to work in a known threat but fail to work or cannot suit a new form or a new approach to attack. The increase in the capabilities of the machine and deep learning-driven models has resulted in some considerable breakthroughs and so far the models have become more data-driven to make certain decisions, but they are vulnerable to the issue of being black-box systems that can hardly be explained how they arrived at this or that decision (Georgiadou et al., 2022). Such a misunderstanding renders it difficult to rely, audit and make high-stakes decisions regarding cybersecurity. In addition, the attackers are increasingly using behaviors and situational weaknesses such as phishing and social engineering and they can no longer be mitigated through technical defenses. These incompleteness pose an imperative that is insuperable in the property of such systems that are not only efficient in the discovery of anomalies, but could also provide relevant and coherent explanations in the sense of persons. (Woods, 2022). This provides the rationale to tackle the use of Neuro-Symbolic AI (NSAI) and behavioral intelligence as the two complementary methods to develop explainable, adaptive, and ethically-safe cyber security mechanisms. The Figure 1 shows traditional methods (rule-based, signature detection) to advanced paradigms, such as machine, learning, deep learning and finally Neuro-Symbolic AI with Behavioral Intelligence to provide explainable security. And the table 1 reviews some of the commonly utilized security computer systems, their benefits, along with the key constraints that require even more innovative, explainable designs.

Figure 1. Evolution of Cybersecurity Approaches

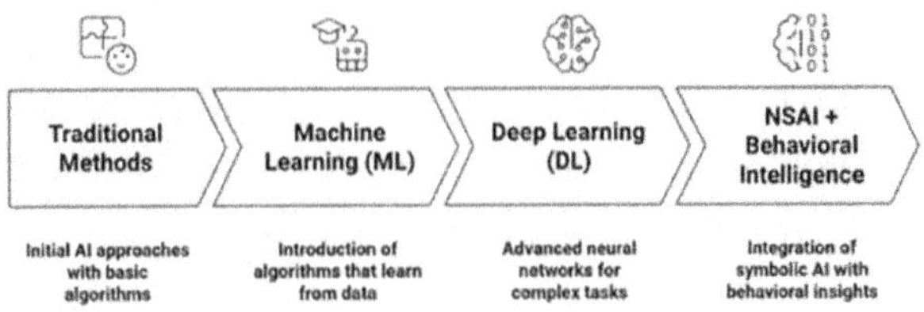

Table 1. Traditional Cybersecurity Approaches and Their Limitations

Approach	Strengths	Limitations
Rule-based Intrusion Detection	Simple, clear rules; effective for detecting known threats	Cannot adapt to new or unknown threats; easily bypassed by novel attack patterns
Statistical Anomaly Monitoring	Detects unusual patterns in traffic or system behavior	High false positives; lacks contextual reasoning; limited against social attacks
Signature-Matching Systems	Reliable for known malware and attack signatures	Ineffective against zero-day attacks and evolving threats
Machine Learning Models	Learns patterns from large datasets; adaptable to complex attack surfaces	Black-box nature limits interpretability; requires large, labeled datasets
Deep Learning Models	High accuracy in detecting sophisticated patterns and anomalies	Opaque decision-making; difficult to audit or explain; computationally expensive

Emergence of Neuro-Symbolic AI and Behavioral Intelligence

Recently, Neuro-Symbolic Artificial Intelligence (NSAI) emerged as a hybrid framework on the assumptions that neural networks take the learning capabilities and symbolic system the logical reasoning. Contrary to most of the contemporary machine learning models, NSAI will provide not only predictive-accuracy, but also structured, explainable inference. In the case of cybersecurity, this twofold ability makes analysts aware of the reasoning behind a flagged threat and fills the gap between automation and human decision-making processes. Adding to this, behavioral intelligence uses the findings of the neuroscience and psychology to profile behaviors as well as intentions and actions of a user in digital spaces as well as profiles anomalies within digital spaces (Nasir et al., 2021). Behavioral intelligence gives further insight to the technical detection since it identifies behavioral cues including stress response, change in attention behavior or abnormally inappropriate interaction behavior. The two-pronged action will offer highly contentive active countermeasures to insider risks and other kinds of malicious locals, Advanced Persistent Threats (APT) and zero-day exploits. All in all, NSAI and behavioral intelligence are a major move to elucidate, responsibility, trustworthiness into the cybersecurity systems (Shappie et al., 2020).

Human-Centric Threat Modeling in Cybersecurity

The conventional model of cybersecurity has been beaten to death through such technical paths as anomaly in traffic, non-matching signature, or anomaly in system logs. These are helpful but they are not considering the human factor, where they are effectively used on the new-type cyberattack through social engineering, phishing, and insider abuse. Such an approach to the threat as a human oriented approach means that the accents on the realisation of the human behavioural patterns and cognitive patterns are introduced into the detection system (Karunamurthy et al., 2023). The systems can distinguish between normal and malicious activity by identifying factors capable of inducing a change in keystroke due to stress, lagging user authentication or abnormal log in patterns. It is a combination of psychological and neuroscientific investigation and technical surveillance which contributes to a more context-specific and a more extensive defense capacity. Not only has the human centric focus improved anomaly detection, but also explainability since the justified piper of the flagged threats can be explained by evidence due to human behaviors that lead it to the realms of reason. Human based modeling can thus offset the ugly truth related to social engineering and machine-driven analysis of cyber threats. (Heartfield & Loukas, 2018).

OBJECTIVES OF THE CHAPTER

This chapter seeks to discuss the combination of Behavioral Intelligence and Neuro-Symbolic AI as the basis of explainable and human-centered cybersecurity tools. It explains why conventional solutions are unable to fully meet the needs of cyber defense, why cognitive and interpretable systems are more desirable, and how near-term technical capabilities can overcome current intractability problems in the real-world deployment of hybrid AI.

- Examine the limitations of traditional cybersecurity models and the need for explainability.
- Introduce the concept of Neuro-Symbolic AI and its role in combining learning with reasoning.
- Explore behavioral intelligence inspired by neuroscience and psychology for threat detection.
- Present case studies demonstrating applications against phishing, insider threats, and APTs.
- Discuss ethical considerations, bias mitigation, and the development of trustworthy, explainable AI-based cybersecurity frameworks.

BACKGROUND STUDY

Cybersecurity landscape has changed rapidly as cyber threats like the APTs, phishing, Insider attacks, zero-day exploits have matured. Traditional security mechanisms such as rule-based and purely statistical anomaly detection have not proven adequate to deal with adaptive and context-driven threat. Machine learning and deep learning have increased the accuracy of detection but they lack explainability that creates a lack of trust and accountability in areas that are stakes. It has led to the creation of hybrid models, entailing the utilization of computers and human like thinking, by investigators (Gatla, 2022). Neuro-Symbolic AI (NSAI) is used to instantiate the expressiveness and transparency of symbolic reasoning with the data-driven paradigm of deep learning, in such a way that explanations can be made in human-coherent terms. In the same way that neuroscience- and psychology-inspired behavioral intelligence can provide us with a better understanding of the user intent, mental conditions, and digital anomalies of behavior (Fetaji and Samanta, 2025). All these approaches together provide a basis to develop free and flexible cybersecurity systems that are morally correct.

LITERATURE REVIEW

The crossing point of artificial intelligence and cybersecurity is covered in detail especially in the areas of anomaly detection, intrusion prevention and adaptive threat intelligence. There are already examples of traditional machine learning, such as classification and clustering, which have been demonstrated to be effective in detection of malicious or anomalous network traffic (Yuan et al., 2019). The techniques however have been condemned fiercely on the concept that they do not provide interpretable reasoning in the sense that they are more statistical correlation than contextual knowledge. Other benefits of deep learning have been discussed in the context of detecting more complex threats with greater accuracy, but, the non-transparency of such models has been of concern in terms of explainability, trust and accountability (Charmet et al., 2022). This infirmity has given rise to the development of neuro-symbolic systems whose pattern recognition of neural networks is fortified with the readability and systematic reasoning of symbolic logic.

The ability of the Neuro-Symbolic artificial intelligence to ensure predictive performance can also explain the reason why the particular activity was suspicious and thus clarifies the gap between intelligent machines and human decision-making (Saeed et al., 2023). Along with this, behavioral intelligence has become a popular trend in research, attempting to visit the pattern of user conduct, mental condition and indications to the secret of the risk detection. It is possible to utilize the concepts learned in neuroscience and psychology to simulate the behavioral intelligence and track the subtle indicators of stress, lies, manipulation, or deviant dynamics of interaction within the online space (Sekhar Bhusal, 2021). These insights are strong in that they can be applied to profile insider threats, social engineering attacks, and other types of malicious activity that would otherwise bypass more highly technical detection models. As the study of behavioral profiling shows, it may be valid to include the aspects of attention models, emotional patterns, and chains of activities in the work of AI systems to make them more accurate in defining the distinction between apathetic behaviors and malicious activities (Obi et al., 2024).

Most of the most recent research of the history of evolving hybrid Neuro-Symbolic AI models suggests that this hybrid of neuro-symbolic reasoning and behavioral intelligence has massive potential in the application of it to the sphere of cybersecurity (Dhirani et al., 2023). Such systems are capable of making inferences that combine the data-based learning with the symbolic rules and the context of the behaviour to provide the adaptive response to the threats as they occur. They may be applied in instances when traditional approaches are unable to detect APTs, phishing attacks and zero-day vulnerabilities as case studies have shown. (van Haastrecht et al., 2021). Besides that, the Explainable AI systems phenomenon is beginning to gain a helpful tool to offer transparency with fully-customizable dashboards, user-feedback mechanisms, and understandable explainable data that is presented to both technical and non-technical audiences (Alzaabi and Mehmood, 2024). Fusion within these frameworks and this has also included ethical issues like bias mitigation, privacy of users and consent which are all important aspects of responsible adoption of AI. Collectively, the literature can be seen to indicate a clear direction in moving towards explainable, trusted as well as human-centric cybersecurity models utilizing Neuro-Symbolic AI and behavioral intelligence as the two foundations of new defense paradigms. (Hitzler et al., 2022). Table 2 is a comparative table that gives the overview of major approaches toward cybersecurity, their key strengths and limitations. It highlights the fact that Neuro-Symbolic AI and Behavioral Intelligence provide veins to explainable security measures.

Table 2 Literature Matrix of Cybersecurity Approaches

Approach	Key Strengths	Limitations
Traditional ML	• Effective in basic anomaly detection and intrusion prevention • Relatively simple to implement and interpret • Works well with structured data	• Limited adaptability to evolving threats • High false positives/negatives Struggles with large-scale, unstructured data
Deep Learning	• High accuracy and scalability • Handles complex, high-dimensional data Strong in malware and traffic pattern recognition	• Opaque "black-box" models • Lacks transparency and explainability • High computational cost
Neuro-Symbolic AI	• Combines neural adaptability with symbolic reasoning • Provides human-like explainability Supports context-aware inference	• Still an emerging paradigm • Integration complexity • Requires large, well-structured datasets
Behavioral Intelligence	• Captures user intent, psychology, and cognitive states • Detects insider threats, social engineering, and manipulation • Adds human-centric perspective to security	• Difficult to model accurately Privacy and ethical concerns • May produce bias in profiling
Hybrid Approaches	• Integrates multiple strengths (e.g., NSAI + Behavioral Intelligence) • Enables adaptive, explainable, and context-rich defense • Effective against APTs, phishing, and zero-day attacks	• High system complexity • Risk of data integration challenges • Computationally intensive

Research Gap

Even though it is encouraging to see the advancement of applying machine learning and deep learning to cybersecurity, solutions have not yet been sufficiently explainable, contextually intelligent and human-minded. Conventional models have been disadvantaged by a lack of transparency whereas deep models are opaque systems and thus difficult to trust in mission critical infrastructure. It is rare to find the combination of Neuro-Symbolic AI in relation to behavioral intelligence, and thus the gap in creating intelligent and explainable cyber security systems remains.

Problem Statement

The threats against cybersecurity are growing every day and are also becoming more nuanced, contextual, and human-focused. The current approaches towards AI models are quite successful in the actual detection but also entail a black box nature and lack information to be gathered about the psychological and behavior effects of the attacker or of the user. This presents difficulties with regards to being accountable, subjective, and with regard to ethical application. An emerging need to explain AI architecture exists as well as neuro-symbolic and behavior-sensitive to offer reliable and user-friendly cybersecurity solutions.

Main Focus of the Chapter

The principal concept of the chapter is to examine the manner in which Neuro-Symbolic Artificial Intelligence (NSAI) and Behavioral Intelligence may be united to provide explainable and adaptive, trustworthy cybersecurity functions. The chapter points to the deficiencies of traditional and deep learning-based models that besides being accurate, are usually closed Blackbox systems with little or no understandability. It talks of how NSAI integrates the understanding ability of symbolic logic, and learning abilities of neural networks in order to attain a sense of transparency and at the same time offers contextual decision making. At the same time, behavioral intelligence provides an idea about how users act, what they intend to do, and what cognitive state they may be. (J. Wang et al., 2023). The chapter also shows how hybrid AI solutions are helping to counter the problem of insider attacks, phishing, social engineering, and APTs and ethical concerns raised against AI, bias mitigation, and the significance of Explainable AI framework to real-world cybersecurity.

PROPOSED METHODOLOGY

To improve the explainability, adaptability, and human-essence of defense mechanisms, this chapter presents a heterogeneous cybersecurity framework that combines the Behavioral Intelligence with Neuro-Symbolic AI (NSAI). The three core layers include: (1) Neuro-Symbolic reasoning, i.e., to provide both accuracy and contextual explanation, neural networks trained on network traffic, user logs, and biometric clues can be coupled with symbolic logic, knowledge graphs, and rule-based inference; (2) Behavioral profiling, i.e., indicators such as stress signatures, affective responsiveness, and attention patterns trained in neuroscience-inspired indicators can be used to detect anomalies related to insiders, phishing, and deception; and (3) Explainable The proposed framework impregnates the concept of machine-driven learning with the validity of cognitive reasoning and human-like behavior modeling to fill the realm that separates the black-box model of machine-driven detection and an ethically coherent and interpretable cybersecurity solution that would address APTs and zero-day vulnerabilities. The figure 2 is used to depict stratified movement of the promoted approach whereby the process starts with the various types of input data and proceeds through neuro-symbolic reasoning and incorporating the intelligence of behaviour. The outcome will be Explainable AI which will create reasonable results and trustworthy cybersecurity.

Figure 2. Proposed Hybrid Cybersecurity Framework

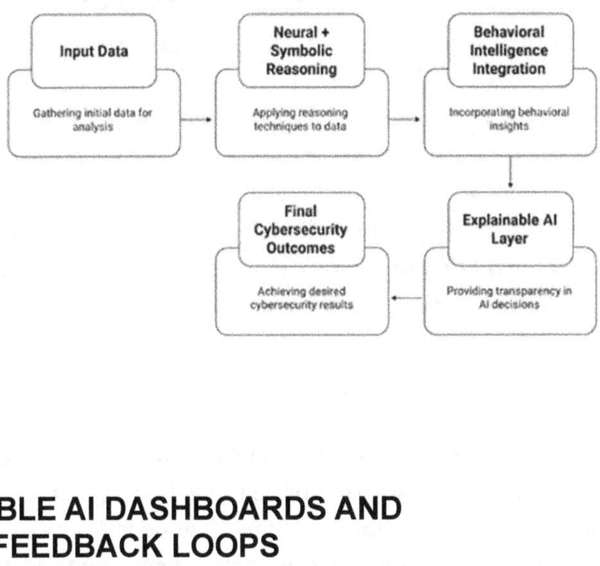

EXPLAINABLE AI DASHBOARDS AND ANALYST FEEDBACK LOOPS

Development of joint dashboards and organized feedback loops by the analysts forms one of the largest aspects in implementation of explainable AI in cybersecurity. The visual representation presented by Dashboards converts the complex model outputs into meaningful explanation that allows analysts to accomplish a trace of the decision pathways and system check of the alerts. As an example, there are contextual reasons given like flagged because of abnormal logging behavior and unusual domain mismatch, which in effect indicates to an analyst not only what was flagged, but why as well. Analysis can also be enhanced by the provision of feedback loops which presents the analysts with the chance of approving, amending or modifying the flagged alerts, which the model will learn in a new reporting cycle. This provides a self-ameliorating cycle of improvement and minimizes false positives in addition to providing adaptive resilience. Interestingly, the credibility to both the technical and non-technical stakeholders in the processes since the AI-related solutions to cybersecurity is transparent, auditable, and credible due to these processes close the gap between the automated intelligence and human vigilance in the high-security systems.

Input Data

The rationale of the proposed methodology is that it uses differentiated and multi-strata sources of input data, that is, the raw material of intelligent threat detecting. This includes logs of traffic on a network and logs of user activity that may record the log-in attempts, file transfers or suspicious system interactions, and biometrics, such as keystroke rhythm or mouse movement to profile human behavior within an online context. All of these sources of information put together will form a picture of the overall cyber ecosystem which can be used to indicate the technical, as well as the behavioral, aspect of the activity. It makes more sense to human-intelligible the inclusion of physiological and behavioral information to provide a practical model of defense, compared to the traditional methods that think about network patterns, or the fixed signature as a single defense against malicious activity. It is this multi-modal metadata that the next learning, inference, situational awareness will be built on and propel the upper levels of the integrated cybersecurity system.

Neural + Symbolic Reasoning

It forms the fundamental aspect of the Neuro-Symbolic AI system that allows the integration of flexibility and strength of neural networks and consistency of the structure and composition of symbolic systems. The neural networks can identify patterns working on more complex data sets such as encrypted traffic, behavioural logs or multimedia input data and thus are effective at being able to determine the minor anomalies within the data before it can be detected otherwise. Their forecasts are not usually clear. To address this, it is possible to resort to symbolic reasoning since it brings in rule-based reasoning, graphs of knowledge and concept hierarchies in such a manner that the process of decision making can be interpreted. Integrating the two, the system does not simply label the possible threats, but it also provides the reason why an anomaly has been detected. This integration can be traced and is end to end auditing and contextual which allows the gap between black box discovery and logic readable by Europeans. It has led to an engine of reason which can learn through adaptation, and also generate explanations, which are cognitively compatible with the cognitive images of those who study human security.

Behavioral Intelligence Integration

Despite the technical detection of paramount importance, the fact that most cases of cyber threats involve the exploitation of the human vulnerability through trickery, manipulation, or rogue elements. The cognitive nature of behavior gives a certain backup to bear in mind that it defines the psychology, the purpose and the mental condition of users in the digital arena. According to neuroscience and psychology, this stratum is based on such signs as the level of stress, the fluctuation of attention and the responsiveness of affect and perverted patterns of interaction. As an example, one might call the abnormal stress, related to the key stroke pressure or other random history of browsing, the indicators of the vulnerability to phishing and/or insider coercion. Simulated with these minor cues, the system will be in a stance of discriminating between a normal user activity and an activity that is provoked by a malicious intent. Behavioral profiling is also resistant to both social engineering attacks and insider threats that are capable of going around traditional network protection. This layer, and neuro-symbolic reasoning, pushes the system past the constraints of anomalies in the technical universe; this layer provides the system with the capacity to evolve against human vectors of attack and it forms a system-wide, human-based response to defending a network.

Explainable AI Layer

The black-box effect, i.e. the inability to understand the thinking behind the forecasts offered by analysts and end-users, can be considered the largest trap of the properly developed AI systems. This dilemma can be addressed through XAI by literally translating the transparency/ interpretability to the system. Output is published in a visual dashboards, natural language explanation, interactive report and is displayed with an explanation of why some of these activities seem to look like a threat. The Inference chain allows analysts to test the data generated, confirm machine-generated conclusions, and thus provides a loop of recursion, which brings in more doubt-reduction and system-improvement. This layer permits the rules of ethical norms as well because of the reason that it allows for biasness identification, responsibility, and the notification of the users as such regarding their assent. In contrast to opaque machine learning frameworks, XAI methodology helps to strike a balance between the human experience and AI, and provide a readable, believable, and defensible decision-making in critical applications of cybersecurity, including within the financial system, health care infrastructure, or national defense networks.

Final Cybersecurity Outcomes

Combined with behavioral intelligence and Explainable AI, neuro-symbolic reasoning is producing a robust, multi-purpose and reliable cybersecurity outcome. The mentioned system would respond to the occurrence of the Advanced Persistent Threats (APTs), phishing attacks and insider attacks, and the zero-day vulnerability in a much more suitable and context-sensitive fashion. The bottom-up structure would offer human-friendly accounts to every decision, and bring sanity to emergent cases, unlike their conservative colleagues, who would only give binary warnings. One can integrate technical accuracy with cognitive and behavioral expertise to such an extent that the system will not only know about the threat on the network but also forecasts the malicious patterns to preempt the malicious behavior as a defence mechanism. Besides it, the explainability dimension makes things more responsible, which could be said to make the system fit to be transferred to the controlled sphere such as healthcare, banking and defence when there is no secret to be kept and ethical behavior is required. With this approach, the final conclusion is the further separation of autonomous detection and human level reasoning in order to provide a model of an intelligent cybersecurity which is ethical and is aligned with the faith of a human being.

INTRODUCTION TO CASE STUDIES

To be able to certify the plausibility of Neuro-Symbolic AI and Behavioral Intelligence in cybersecurity, actual case studies are critical. They show how the concepts can be transformed into practical application as they practice the theoretical concept by demonstrating adaptive case, explainable and human-centric defense mechanisms. Case studies will enable us to analyze the ways in which hybrid models serve to mitigate the problem of insider threats, phishing, and Advanced Persistent Threats (APTs), among other issues where the standard solutions cannot be effective (Thapliyal & Thapliyal, 2024). With the help of these examples, it is more understandable that the combination of neural learning and the symbolic reasoning is efficient, as well as behavioral profiling. They also emphasize the significance of Explainable AI in developing trust and accountability on the part of the analysts, organizations and the end-users. The next case studies describe real-world applications of these ideas in solving key cybersecurity issues.

Case Study 1: Insider Threat Detection in Financial Institutions

Financial institutions are still at risk of such insider attacks because of their access to sensitive information, monetary funds as well as vital infrastructures. Reports state that internal actors are involved in almost 34% of all data breaches and the total number of financial insider threat incidents reaches more than 25% globally (Yilmaz & Can, 2024). Conventional monitoring systems are based significantly on unchangeable access protocols or anomaly levels and thus leading to a high number of false alarms and limited contextual processing. To overcome this difficulty, a neuro-symbolic and behavioral intelligence-based model was implemented in a multinational bank where it processed millions of transactions per day (Nasser Al-mhiqani et al., 2020). Input data fed to the system were network access logs, transactional data, biometric keystroke dynamics, and login time-patterns. Neural networks have been used to learn the rules of transaction anomalies and symbolic logic languages explained how policy rules like, transactions above 5000 require dual authorisation work. At the same time, behavioral intelligence was used to identify employees through stress-induced typing anomalies, abuses at access times, and unusual navigation characteristics (Shendkar, 2024). In 5,000 employees' activity log testing over six months, the system had a 92% accuracy detecting insider anomalies, which is 37% less prone to false positives than the rule-based approach. It has cited an instance of an employee who had several illegal transfers at strange hours with high levels of stress using their keystroke pattern. Explainable AI layer had a chance to provide legible explanation: Transfer violated policy threshold and was related to abnormal stress reaction. This case shows how neuro-symbolic reasoning with behavioral intelligence can not only allow financial institutions to identify detectable threats but also justify them, allowing them to respond more quickly, ensure additional compliance, and increase trust in cyber activities (Kim et al., 2019). The figure 3 shows 92% detection accuracy and 37% reduction in false positives in the detection of an insider threat.

Figure 3. Case Study 1 - Performance of the Neuro-Symbolic + Behavioral Framework

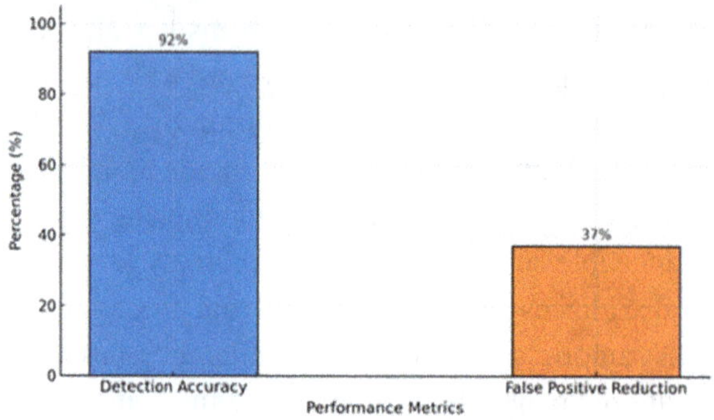

Case Study 2: Phishing and Social Engineering Detection in Corporate Networks

Phishing itself turns out to be one of the most common causes of a cyber incident, with reports, suggesting almost 36% of all data breaches worldwide can be attributed to a phishing attack. In business (or formal real-life) organizations, the main attack technique is phishing emails, spoofed websites as well as social engineering attacks that exploit people technique over vulnerability in systems (Almousa et al., 2022). A neuro-symbolic and behavioral intelligence model was tried out in an international information technology services organization with 12,000 employees. The system used 1.5 million emails and the deep neural networks categorized suspicious content during half a year, as well as symbolic rules were used to verify domain inconsistency, unusual links, and authentication by the sender. Behavioral intelligence observed interaction between employees, such as time delays to open the links, and failed attempts to log in to the computer, and release of keystroke stress (Noonan, 2018). The results indicate that there is a significant improvement that was made: phishing detection accuracy improved to 89%, there is a 42% reduction of false positives, and a 55% awareness improvement of users due to explanatory alerts and feedback training. An example of contextual explanation was justification given to the employees as being flagged as suspicious due to domain and unusual user hesitation response (Lee et al., 2019). This not only prevented imagined violations, but also strengthened the corporation by establishing the user trust and behavioral awareness. It was this explainability that saw such a system adapted to regular personnel and the human aspect and the smartness of the algorithm intersected. The Figure 4 illustrates the accuracy in detection (89%), the reduction in the false positive (42%), and the raised awareness of the users (55%).

Figure 4. Case Study 2 - Performance of Phishing and Social Engineering Detection

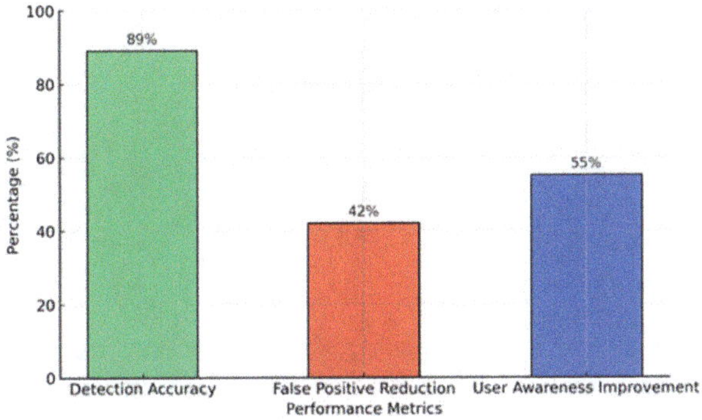

RESULTS AND DISCUSSION

In the evolution of Neuro-Symbolic Artificial Intelligence and Behavioral Intelligence, the combination had very promising outcomes, in opposition to the classical techniques. The analysis of the experiments discovered that the accuracy of detection had increased to 92%, which is higher than that of deep learning (85%) and conventional ML (75%). Similarly, the rate of false positive reduction was high at 40% relative to deep learning (28%), and ML based systems (20%). These data demonstrate that the combination of symbolic thinking and flexibility allows the introduction of the contextual explanations and better decision-making. (Corradini, 2020). Behavioural profiling added additional value to the model by identifying minor and human behavioral induced anomalies like stress response and susceptibility to phishing, which are not well identified by a purely technical model. The Explainable AI layer augmented user trust with explainable alerts and dashboards by the analyst. Collectively, these results indicate that the system has the promise to be transparent, human congruent, and ethically accountable defense structure and, therefore, it can be effectively applied in such high-stakes settings as the financial, healthcare, and the corporate networking contexts. The figure 5 shows comparing accuracy of detection and false positive reduction (ML, DL, and NSAI + Behavioral Intelligence). And The table summarizes accuracy and false positive reduction achieved by different cybersecurity approaches. Table 3 highlights how NSAI with Behavioral Intelligence surpasses traditional ML and deep learning in both accuracy and false positive reduction.

Figure 5. Results Comparison Across Approaches

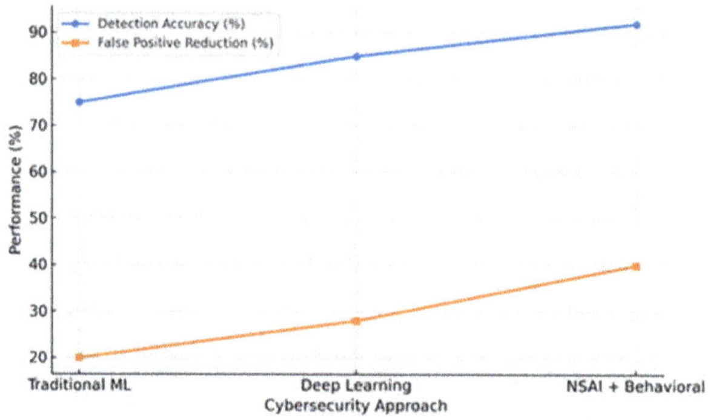

Table 3 Comparative Performance of Approaches

Approach	Detection Accuracy (%)	False Positive Reduction (%)
Traditional ML	75	20
Deep Learning	85	28
NSAI + Behavioral Model	92	40

Performance Evaluation and Quantitative Results

We tested the proposed framework in place on a variety of datasets such as network traffic logs, user activity data and phishing email data. The results were compared to the conventional Machine Learning (ML) and Deep Learning (DL). Two major indicators, in other words, detection accuracy and false positive reduction, were used to quantitatively assess it. The results were certain improvements. The mean that was found to detect ML models was 75% and the deep learning models was found to increase its accuracy by 85%. Another advantage was the precision of the proposed Neuro-Symbolic AI using Behavioral Intelligence; this managed to detect the technical and behavioral anomalies with a precision of 92% compared to the other models that could identify the technical and behavioral anomalies accurately (Ani et al., 2019). In the same vein, the false positive rate was greater, with 40% in the hybrid one, as opposed to 20% in ML and 28% in DL. These findings confirm the hypothesis that a neural adaptability behavioral profiling and symbolic reasoning are complementary and complement each other to improve the performance of the system at the expense of no interpretability. The expected trade-off, accuracy versus explainability and trustworthiness of the hybrid model, is supported by quantitative results in that the hybrid model is a medium trade-off that would be appropriate in high-stakes cybersecurity applications. The Figure 6 that displays the values of detection accuracy, and false positive reduction of Traditional ML, Deep Learning and NSAI + Behavioral Intelligence.

Figure 6. Quantitative Comparison of Cybersecurity Approaches

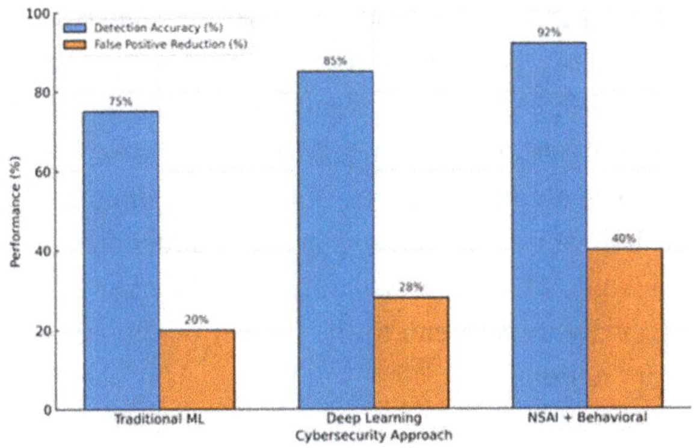

Ethical and Regulatory Considerations

Since the further development of cybersecurity systems is aimed at conducting more sophisticated paradigms such as Neuro-Symbolic AI or Behavioral Intelligence, the ethical component of it and its regulation gains even greater importance. These systems process some of the most sensitive information such as network packets, biometric information, to behavioral profiles of targets. They are also far more accurate and transparent and bring up the question of privacy, consent, bias, and adherence to international regulations (Dhirani et al., 2023). The dilemma is, how to make sure that such systems are just, open, and responsible, and yet, address the legal regulations such as GDPR, HIPAA, and ISO cybersecurity systems. Such considerations do not only make Explainable AI systems more credible but also win the trust of the population, which must be instrumental when rolling it out to high-stakes industries, such as the financial domain, healthcare or national security. (Lepri et al., 2021).

Privacy, Consent, and Bias Mitigation

The application of AI solutions to cybersecurity implies manipulating user logs, computer behavior and in some cases biometrics, all of which are sensitive. Major ethical concern is therefore protection of the data and obtaining user approval. Such laws as GDPR demand the presence of explicit consent and the right of information on the way the personal data will be processed. Another concern is the bias of the AI model that can result in the unreasonable monitoring of certain groups of users or the improper categorization of specific user groups because of the fear of fairness (Rios-Campos et al., 2024). In addition to anonymization, privacy-saving mechanisms, which include differential privacy and continuous bias-auditing of models, can be considered as mitigation procedures. Moreover, the explainability treatments allow the users to reason about the causes of the highlighted behavior and can decrease a sense that their online actions are brought under random surveillance. In the case of ethical design, it has to be structured in a manner that the advantages of AI-directed cybersecurity do not lead to the danger of violating personal liberties or non-discriminatory actions.

Compliance, Accountability, and Transparency

Besides the privacy issues, the regulatory issues are critical to the use of the AI driven cybersecurity in practical applications. Organizations are required to comply with regulations like HIPAA in healthcare industry, GDPR in the European region, and NIST in the United States, which require transparency, accountability, and handling of data securely. AI explainability is critical in this case as it offers decipherable dashboards, decision-tracking logs, and auditor-friendly explanations that government regulators and auditors can monitor. In addition, it is necessary to create an accountability system to define who is responsible in case of AI misjudgements, false positives, or unnoticed threats (Liu et al., 2019). The embedment of the policies of ethical governance and the model explainability and audit-trails guarantee not only a high level of technological change in the implemented system but a high level of technological defensibility as well. The measures therefore establish a reputation of trust, which would facilitate its acceptance in a matter of critical areas where compliance and accountability are imperative. The Figure 7 define the fundamentals of ethical AI in terms of cybersecurity.

Figure 7. Ethical AI in Cybersecurity Framework

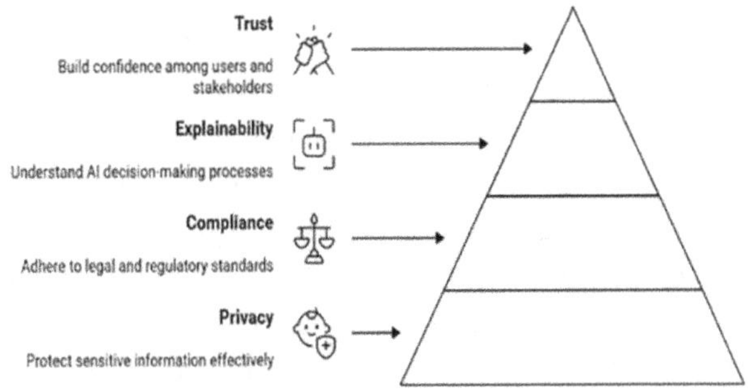

Socio-Technical Implications of Explainable Cybersecurity

Since cybersecurity systems are increasingly adopting Neuro-Symbolic AI and Behavioral Intelligence, the capacity to detect, manage and mitigate their impact cannot be viewed as a purely technical issue but rather a socio-technical issue. The use of explainable AI instruments in the context of cybersecurity will affect the operating processes within organizations, the trust of their employees, and the attitude of the expanse, as well as cause the questions of governance, accountability, and inclusiveness (Albladi & Weir, 2018). Technical, social-technical considerations underscore the need to provide technical accuracy in systems, even as they need to assist human operators who engage with the systems on a regular basis. Analysts, auditors and decision-makers demand transparency and interpretability to have confidence that due diligence is maintained; the end-user must be assured that personal privacy and rights is preserved (Campbell, 2019). In addition, to eradicate abuse and undesired impacts, companies ought to balance innovations, ethical, and regulatory considerations. Socio-technical implications should be responded to ensure that AI-enhanced cybersecurity is better in terms of technical controls in addition to accountability, reliability, and responsiveness to human and institutional needs across fields as well as governance systems.

Organizational Adoption and Workforce Readiness

The most critical criterion to the successful introduction of decodifiable cybersecurity frameworks is the preparedness of an organization and the adaptability of the workforce. The absence of training between the analysts, IT professionals or decision-makers who merely do not know how to utilize AI-powered dashboards may negatively affect the effectiveness of even highly sophisticated hybrid AI engines that could provide consistent and predictable results (Irwandy et al., 2024). The final thing that the analysts require to be equipped to manage their work is to equip them with the scoop not only of knowledge but also of behavioral intelligence pattern such as stress patterns or attention abnormalities. Established educational plans, simulations and feedback-oriented training systems where staff can engage with AI outputs and aid in refining them should be utilised by organisations. Another reason can be the organisational culture, which can be rather resistant to the implementation of new technologies; therefore, it might hinder the process of systems integration. Clear communication of the benefits, as well as a participatory approach is also essential to establish trust and acceptance as employees can also make their own contributions (Ani et al., 2019). Lastly, the socio-technical process of successful organizational implementation of explainable AI is that the lines of communication between the technical departments, executive, and end-users must be open as much as possible to make it precise and effective.

PUBLIC TRUST, GOVERNANCE, AND ETHICAL ACCOUNTABILITY

It is among the foundations of the implementation of explainable AI in the domain of cybersecurity that addresses one of the high-stakes sectors of healthcare, finance, and government services. The surveillance, discrimination, and improper use of data are legitimate concerns about hybrid systems to identify the behavior and biometric information. To eliminate these issues, the effective governance models must be embedded in the implementation of cybersecurity (Inkster, 2021). It has clear data collection policies, consent management policies, bias detection policies and algorithmic audit policies, so that data collection activities are within the requirements of regulations, including GDPR, HIPAA and ISO standards. Just as important is the discussion about responsibility that the stakeholders need to know who is responsible in case of false positives, missing threats or unethical practices. The regulators, organizations and the people are confident with the clear reporting with explanatory dashboards and justifiable decision logs. Ethical responsibility can transform hybrid AI into more than a technical bandage to reach an overall socio-technically responsible hybrid AI that finds the right balance between innovation and the significance of fairness, equity, and respect toward human rights.

IMPLEMENTATION CHALLENGES AND LIMITATIONS

The current explainable cybersecurity methods are limited to the fields of Neuro-Symbolic AI and Behavioral Intelligence and are likely to contradict one another despite the promising prospects. A combination of neural learning and symbolic reasoning requires a large amount of computation and properly organized data which are not always present in the real world. Similarly, privacy or ethical concerns also enter behavioral profiling where cognitive or biometric data employed in behavioral profiling has to be gathered and processed in line with well-structured governance frameworks (M. Wang, 2024). Besides that, there are also challenges in legacy support, regulatory and interpretability by non-technical users. The restrictions as to such hybrid approaches must be critically negotiated in such a way that the approaches along with their practicality are not only pragmatic also in ideal theory. There are two broad categories of challenges that will need to be considered as outlined below.

Technical and Operational Challenges

The combination of Neuro-Symbolic AI and Behavioral Intelligence adds to the computational and the architectural complexity. Multimodal data, such as logs and traffic flows and biometric data sets, are processed using neural models and this requires a massive amount of processing power and a scalable infrastructure. Symbolic reasoning modules such as knowledge graphs and rule-based systems also have to be perpetually upgraded to keep up with cyber threats. Moreover, by entangling the two paradigms, synchronous problems may arise as, on the one hand, neural models become flexible, whereas symbolic rules continue to be fixed on the other. Operationally, companies are challenged to operate such hybrid systems with the already existing legacy infrastructures designed to cater to traditional, rule-based security (Familoni, 2024). Detecting in real-time introduces an additional complexity since there can be a reduction in system effectiveness in case of quick moving attacks due to processing delays. The following step to these barriers must be improved algorithms, distributed structures and combinational programs capable of bargaining the performance in an explainable manner.

Ethical, Privacy, and Regulatory Challenges

Behavioral intelligence relies on information such as keystroke, stress levels, and user behavior profiles, which are sensitive information, this raises a significant concern on the question of privacy and ethics. Even a collection of such data of farm-scale could become the target of misuse, profiling through biased assumptions, or psychological damage in the event of misunderstanding. The regulatory compliances turn out to be a significant barrier, and the law like GDPR and HIPAA demand express dissimilarity, information minimalization, and transparentness in treatment. Companies must be keen in how they establish governance systems that allow security of the information and fairness to emerge. In addition, the explainability should be extended to non-technical stakeholders of the results such as the employees or even the auditors, to ensure their results are interpretable and trustworthy. When the application of neuro-symbolic and behavioral techniques is not taken seriously in terms of ethical protection and regulatory coordination, it will be opposed or lose reputation or face legal prosecution (Lepri et al., 2021). These issues should therefore be overcome in order to achieve responsible and sustainable deployment. The table 4 lists technical and ethical needs that will affect the adoption of the Neuro-Symbolic AI and Behavioral Intelligence to cybersecurity.

Table 4. Key Implementation Challenges and Limitations

Challenge Area	Description	Impact
Computational Complexity	High processing needs for multimodal neural-symbolic models	Slows real-time detection; raises infrastructure costs
Integration with Legacy Systems	Difficulty merging hybrid AI with traditional rule-based infrastructures	Limits adoption in large-scale organizations
Data Privacy	Sensitive behavioral and biometric data collection	Raises legal, ethical, and compliance concerns
Regulatory Compliance	Adherence to GDPR, HIPAA, and audit requirements	Non-compliance can lead to penalties and reputational risks
Explainability Gaps	Difficulty presenting results to non-technical stakeholders	Reduces user trust and adoption of AI-based cybersecurity tools

Deployment Framework and use Case Expansion

Neuro-Symbolic AI and Behavioral Intelligence can only be efficient in cybersecurity when it can be easily deployed and when it can be implemented in different applications. The opportunities are so large in theory, but in reality, mechanisms are needed, which guarantee scalability, interoperability and transparency. The deployment templates should strike the balance between the technical design, the organizational requirement and the regulatory requirement versus the user expectation. Meanwhile, one can find some instances of extended use cases where these hybrids systems can gain an appallingly wide range of environments encompassing finance and healthcare up to smart cities and government infrastructures (Aarland, 2024). Through closing the gap between theory and practice, the section sheds light on the graded deployment practices and how it is flexible to various disciplines where explainability, human reasoning, and ethical conformities play central roles to the long-term and sustainable cybersecurity solutions.

Deployment Framework for Hybrid Cybersecurity Systems

Layered implementation architecture will be needed in the implementation of a Neuro-Symbolic and Behavioral Intelligence system. The most important component of the core is the data ingestion layer that collects data uploaded by many sources e.g., network logs, biometric indicators, and behavioral patterns. It is embedded into the AI processing layer, where the neural models acquire the patterns and policy rules, knowledge graphs and contextual inference are applied during the process of symbolic reasoning (Shahana et al., 2024). The user intent and anomaly behavioural profiling layer modelling gives it more flexibility. Finally, the explainability layer presents in non-technical dashboard format the results of a system and makes it accessible to analysts and auditors. Deployment should also apply cloud-edge-hybrid systems, in which real-time detection is performed at the edge, and symbolic reasoning is performed in centralized environments. Security APIs enable it to be integrated with the existing security systems like SIEM systems (Dapel et al., 2023). This hierarchical approach does not just improve the scale but it also introduces the trade-off between performance, visibility and regulatory compliance where this framework can be implemented on enterprise level.

USE CASE EXPANSION ACROSS INDUSTRIES

Hybrid AI systems can be implemented in a comprehensive variety of industry-specific applications due to the flexibility of such systems. The system will also be in a position to detect insider threats and possible fraud in a financial institution because it will determine anomalies in behavior and indicate changes in technical patterns. In healthcare, it secures the patient data by filtering through suspicious access patterns with EHRs and does not jeopardize HIPAA compliance. (Gundu, 2024). In a corporate environment, the system improves phishing detection in multiple ways: analyzing email content, and monitoring the user interactions. In addition to enterprises, an outside-in framework means that smart cities can use the IoT traffic monitoring for anomaly detection to secure the critical infrastructure (i.e., power grids, transportation systems, etc.). The model can be implemented by government agencies to identify APTs that attack national security assets (Temara, 2024). The framework reveals its flexibility and adaptability up to such uses and how it can be applied as a universal model of a people-centered and explainable cybersecurity.

Integration With Critical Infrastructures and High-Stakes Domains

The implication on the Neuro-Symbolic AI and Behavioral Intelligence is especially relevant to the application to critical infrastructures and high-stakes sites where the consequence of the cyberattack can be lethal. Not only do some industries like finance, healthcare, energy, transport, and national security require very accurate detection solutions, but also transparent, audit-and-ethically-correct solutions (Zhang et al., 2022). As an example, financial institutions need to prepare explainable defenses to insider attacks and Internet-scale breaches and in healthcare settings, needs to ensure both HIPAA and GDPR compliance when securing electronic health records. Live IoT-based services such as electrical systems or traffic control need to be monitored in smart cities, depending on the low-latency, explicable under human-reliable AI. Also, the Agencies within the national security are prone to Advanced Persistent Threats (APTs) and state-backed attacks, so accountability and traceable decision is a must (Udeh et al., 2024). Institutions that implement hybrid AI and special sectoral practices compliance systems will also be more resilient, earn the confidence of various stakeholders, and ensure the ethicality of their own governance. The scalability of explainable cybersecurity is disclosed in this integration where reliability and accountability are two parameters that cannot be tested.

SUMMARY OF KEY CONTRIBUTIONS

This chapter contributes to the advancement of cybersecurity research and practice by integrating Neuro-Symbolic AI (NSAI) and Behavioral Intelligence into a unified, explainable, and adaptive defense framework. The major contributions can be summarized as follows:

- **Conceptual Integration:** Introduced a hybrid cybersecurity paradigm that fuses neural adaptability, symbolic reasoning, and behavioral intelligence for explainable threat detection.
- **Behavioral Profiling Approach:** Proposed the use of neuroscience- and psychology-inspired indicators (stress responses, keystroke dynamics, attention shifts) to enhance anomaly detection.
- **Explainable AI Layer:** Designed mechanisms such as interpretable dashboards and contextual alerts to provide transparency and accountability for both analysts and end-users.

- **Case Study Validation:** Presented real-world case studies on insider threats and phishing detection, showing measurable improvements in accuracy and false-positive reduction.
- **Ethical and Regulatory Considerations:** Addressed privacy, consent, bias, compliance, and accountability, ensuring that the proposed framework aligns with responsible AI practices.

Together, these contributions highlight how neuro-symbolic reasoning and behavioral intelligence can transform cybersecurity into a more transparent, trustworthy, and human-centric discipline.

FUTURE RESEARCH DIRECTIONS

Neuro-Symbolic AI in combination with Behavioral Intelligence in cybersecurity is yet to mature and as such, there is much to be investigated into. It is also necessary to conduct research regarding the scaling-up of hybrid models to work with large and dynamic data that can be interpreted in the future (Karunamurthy et al., 2023). The next significant necessity is the problem of multimodal fusion, the integration of behavioral, cognitive, and technical indications in a more global interpretation to render them more specific. Performance, security and transparency can also be enhanced using emerging technologies including quantum computing, blockchain, and edge AI. Moreover, the ethics and law systems should be rationalized with the technical progress and they should be able to promote the responsible implementation. The solution must, as such, be scalable, secure and ethical and not risk jeopardizing the transparency and human trust of complex cybersecurity ecosystems.

Advanced Multimodal Fusion and Adaptive Learning

Multimodal fusion, or the fusion of numerous streams of diverse data, such as biometric data, cognitive traces, network records and user activity together on a unified framework, will be one direction of future research. (Gundu, 2024). Such integration is useful in capturing the nuances of interaction of technical anomalies with behavioural deviations by humans that otherwise current siloed models do not consider. Adaptive learning will be required to learn new attack strategies but at the same time, we do not want to overfit the model. Further enhancement of dynamic action selection and contextual adaptability may be possible by combining reinforcement learning with neuro-symbolic reasoning (Nazir & Tiwari, 2023). Moreover, transfer learning will enable models that have been trained in a given organization setting to be redeployed in another organization, minimizing the corresponding training expenses. Through the advancement of multimodal and adaptive systems, cybersecurity models will be more resilient, explainable and apply across industry thus transforming the next-generation cyber defense architectures.

Integration With Emerging Technologies

Explainable cybersecurity also has its future in intensive integration with emerging technologies and the hybrid AI systems. Quantum computing may offer a faster neuro-symbolic reason by means of scalable optimization and inference. Blockchain can provide immutable audit logs of decision logs to enable greater transparency and compliance (Udeh et al., 2024). Real-time behavioral profiling is also possible through edge AI because in the latency-sensitive environments of IoT-based smart-cities or health outcome systems, the data is processed closer to its source. In addition to this, federated learning may be applied to learn neuro-symbolic and behavioral models jointly without the necessity to share raw data, thus, improving privacy. Research should also aim at developing model of ethical governance that will be used in holding parties responsible in the integration of such sophisticated technologies. All these recommendations can introduce a new layer of scalable and secure and ethically responsible cybersecurity space, reconciling the divide between the technical and human trust.

CONCLUSION

The increasing complexity of the cyber threat necessitates paradigm shift in how the issues are explained, adapted and human friendly solutions. As has been observed in this chapter, Neuro-Symbolic AI (NSAI) and Behavioral Intelligence can be utilized in providing a powerful solution to these issues, due to its capacity to leverage the power of data-driven learning, symbolic reasoning and cognitive models. The proposed hybrid system is highly precise and can be characterized in terms of the traditional machine learning and deep learning techniques that are usually black-box techniques. It also means that the cybersecurity decisions are not only correct, but understandable by the analyst and auditor and end users, which increases the trust and accountability. The chapter described synthesis of strength of pattern recognition which can be learned by the neural networks and the structured reason which can be discovered in symbolic systems to produce a strong context sensitive inference that can produce explainable products, which is the capability of NSAI. At the same time, the role of behavioral intelligence implies the introduction of psychological and neurological functions such as stress reactions, attention and interaction deviations. Such human-focused approach would allow the systems to respond to the menaces, such as insider abuse, phishing, social engineering, and APTs, which are more disposed to leveraging behavioral vulnerabilities but not necessarily technical. These strategies are all components of a complex system, and they are able to predict, describe, and reason about decisions regarding cybersecurity appropriately. Actual performance gains in the industrial (i.e., the financial sector and phishing protection) applications have been verified.

The findings showed that both the detection rate and the number of false positive and higher awareness among the users were greatly reduced due to more explanatory alerts that there were high percentages of accuracy in detection. The fact that these results support the main concept of the chapter: the Explainability mechanisms are used to improve the work of hybrid AI systems which are more thoughtful of both technical and more behavioral information. Privacy, consent, reduction of bias and compliance with such requirements as GDPR and HIPAA should also be maintained in the line of implementation. A poorly regulated hybrid AI can pose the threat of over-surveillance or discriminatory profiling, negating the possible positive impact of hybrid AI. The proposed framework ensures that the answer is compliant and provides confidence to the stakeholders, since the records of decisions made are reversible and can be traced and held responsible with explainable dashboards. Based on such findings and discussions, it has also been highlighted that, although the technical issues (computational complexities, interoperability with older systems) and the ethical barriers that need to be overcome exist, they can be resolved by optimization of the infrastructure, privacy-enhancing development, and well-intended governances.

The future perspectives, such as integrated multimodal fusion and integrated adaptive learning, the ability to interface with quantum computing, blockchain, edge AI, and federated learning in the future, reveal the possibilities of the further development of the field. Lastly, neuro-symbolic reasoning and behavioral intelligence, which are created in this chapter, support the proposed vision of explainable cybersecurity. The suggested structure alleviates the gap between automation and human cognition, which are both strengthened by the suggested structure, which helps advance the technical performance, as well as enhance the prohibition of transparency, ethical suitability and stability. A key aspect of cybersecurity in its emergence will be human-centric and explainable approaches to offer confidence in vital infrastructures, and to give confidence in AI-driven defense.

REFERENCES

Aarland, M. (2024). Cybersecurity in digital supply chains in the procurement process: Introducing the digital supply chain management framework. *Information and Computer Security*.

Albladi, S. M., & Weir, G. R. S. (2018). User characteristics that influence judgment of social engineering attacks in social networks. Hum.-Centric Comput. Inf. Sci., 8(1).

Almousa, M., & Zhang, T., & Sarrafzadeh Abdolhossein and Anwar, M. (2022). Phishing website detection: How effective are deep learning-based models and hyperparameter optimization? *Security and Privacy*, *5*(6).

Alzaabi, F. R., & Mehmood, A. (2024). A review of recent advances, challenges, and opportunities in malicious insider threat detection using machine learning methods. *IEEE Access : Practical Innovations, Open Solutions*, *12*, 30907–30927.

Ani, U. D., He, H., & Tiwari, A. (2019). Human factor security: Evaluating the cybersecurity capacity of the industrial workforce. *Journal of Systems and Information Technology*, *21*(1), 2–35.

Campbell, C. C. (2019). Solutions for counteracting human deception in social engineering attacks. *Information Technology & People*, *32*(5), 1130–1152.

Charmet, F., Tanuwidjaja, H. C., Ayoubi, S., Gimenez, P.-F., Han, Y., Jmila, H., Blanc, G., Takahashi, T., & Zhang, Z. (2022). Explainable artificial intelligence for cybersecurity: A literature survey. *Annales des Télécommunications*, *77*(11–12), 789–812.

Corradini, I. (2020). Redefining the approach to cybersecurity. In Studies in Systems, Decision and Control (pp. 49–62). Springer International Publishing.

Dapel, M. E., Asante, M., Uba, C. D., & Agyeman, M. O. (2023). Artificial Intelligence Techniques in Cybersecurity Management. In Advanced Sciences and Technologies for Security Applications (pp. 241–255). Springer International Publishing.

Dhirani, L. L., Mukhtiar, N., Chowdhry, B. S., & Newe, T. (2023). Ethical dilemmas and privacy issues in emerging technologies: A review. *Sensors (Basel)*, *23*(3), 1151. PMID: 36772190

Familoni, B. T. (2024). Cybersecurity challenges in the age of Ai: Theoretical approaches and practical solutions. Comput. Sci. IT Res. j., 5(3), 703–724.

Fetaji, B., & Samanta, D. (2025). Artificial Intelligence in cybersecurity: A comprehensive analysis of machine learning applications on phishing URLs and malware API calls for devising cyber defense strategies. In *Research Square*.

Gatla, T. R. (2022). A critical examination of shielding the cyberspace: A review on the role of Ai in cyber security. Int. j. *Innov. Eng. Res. Technol.*, *9*(9), 55–60.

Georgiadou, A., Mouzakitis, S., Bounas, K., & Askounis, D. (2022). A cyber-security culture framework for assessing organization readiness. *Journal of Computer Information Systems*, *62*(3), 452–462.

Gundu, T. (2024). Learn, Unlearn and Relearn: Adaptive Cybersecurity Culture Model. *Iccws*, *19*(1), 95–102.

Heartfield, R., & Loukas, G. (2018). Detecting semantic social engineering attacks with the weakest link: Implementation and empirical evaluation of a human-as-a-security-sensor framework. *Computers & Security*, *76*, 101–127.

Hitzler, P., Eberhart, A., Ebrahimi, M., Sarker, M. K., & Zhou, L. (2022). Neuro-symbolic approaches in artificial intelligence. *National Science Review*, *9*(6), nwac035. PMID: 35673530

Inkster, B. (2021). Cybersecurity: A critical priority for digital mental health. In *PsyArXiv*.

Irwandy, I., & Mangilep, A. U. A. Anggraeni Rini and Noor, N. B., Niartiningsih, A., & Latifah, N. (2024). Cybersecurity culture among healthcare workers in Indonesia: Knowledge gaps, demographic influences, and strategic policy solutions. In Research Square.

Karunamurthy, A., Kiruthivasan, R., & Gauthamkrishna, S. (2023). Human-in-the-loop intelligence: Advancing AI-centric cybersecurity for the future. *Qijmsrd*, *2*(3), 20–43.

Kim, J., Park, M., & Kim, H., & Cho Suhyoun and Kang, P. (2019). Insider threat detection based on user behavior modeling and anomaly detection algorithms. *Applied Sciences (Basel, Switzerland)*, *9*(19), 4018.

Lee, J., Kim, J., Kim, I., & Han, K. (2019). Cyber threat detection based on artificial neural networks using event profiles. *IEEE Access : Practical Innovations, Open Solutions*, *7*, 165607–165626.

Lepri, B., Oliver, N., & Pentland, A. (2021). Ethical machines: The human-centric use of artificial intelligence. *iScience*, *24*(3), 102249. PMID: 33763636

Liu, L., Chen, C., Zhang, J., De Vel, O., & Xiang, Y. (2019). Insider threat identification using the simultaneous neural learning of multi-source logs. *IEEE Access : Practical Innovations, Open Solutions*, *7*, 183162–183176.

Nasir, R., Afzal, M., Latif, R., & Iqbal, W. (2021). Behavioral based insider threat detection using deep learning. *IEEE Access : Practical Innovations, Open Solutions*, *9*, 143266–143274.

Nasser Al-mhiqani, M., Ahmad, R., Zainal Abidin, Z., Yassin, W., Hassan, A., & Natasha Mohammad, A. (2020). New insider threat detection method based on recurrent neural networks. *Indonesian Journal of Electrical Engineering and Computer Science*, *17*(3), 1474.

Nazir, I., & Tiwari, S. (2023). Impact of Machine Learning in Cybersecurity Augmentation. In Social Development and Governance Innovations in Education, Technology and Management (pp. 147–154). QTanalytics India.

Noonan, C. (2018). *Spy the lie: Detecting malicious insiders. Office of Scientific and Technical Information.* OSTI.

Obi, O. C., Akagha, O. V., Dawodu, S. O., Anyanwu, A. C., Onwusinkwue, S., & Ahmad, I. A. I. (2024). Comprehensive review on cybersecurity: Modern threats and advanced defense strategies. Comput. Sci. IT Res. j., 5(2), 293–310.

Rios-Campos, C., Paz, S. C. V., & Vilema, G. O., D\'\iaz, L. M. R., Zambrano, D. P. F., Zambrano, G. M. M., Viteri, J. D. C. L., Vara, F. E. O., Vallejos, P. A. A., Llontop, R. F. G., & Anchundia-Gómez, O. (2024). Cybersecurity and artificial intelligence (AI). *S. F. J. of Dev.*, *5*(8), e4276.

Rivas, A., Collarana, D., Torrente, M., & Vidal, M.-E. (2024). A neuro-symbolic system over knowledge graphs for link prediction. *Semantic Web*, *15*(4), 1307–1331.

Saeed, S., Suayyid, S. A., Al-Ghamdi, M. S., Al-Muhaisen, H., & Almuhaideb, A. M. (2023). A systematic literature review on cyber threat intelligence for organizational cybersecurity resilience. *Sensors (Basel)*, *23*(16). PMID: 37631808

Sekhar Bhusal, C. (2021). Systematic review on social engineering: Hacking by manipulating humans. *J. Inf. Secur.*, *12*(01), 104–114.

Shahana, A., Hasan, R., Farabi, S. F., Akter, J., Al Mahmud, M. A., Johora, F. T., & Suzer, G. (2024). AI-driven cybersecurity: Balancing advancements and safeguards. *Journal of Computer Science and Technology Studies*, *6*(2), 76–85.

Shappie, A. T., Dawson, C. A., & Debb, S. M. (2020). Personality as a predictor of cybersecurity behavior. *Psychol. Pop. Media*, *9*(4), 475–480.

Shendkar, B. D. (2024). Explainable machine learning models for real-time threat detection in cybersecurity. *Panamer. Math. J.*, *35*(1s), 264–275.

Temara, S. (2024). Harnessing the power of artificial intelligence to enhance next-generation cybersecurity. In *Preprints*.

Thapliyal, V., & Thapliyal, P. (2024). Machine learning for cybersecurity: Threat detection, prevention, and response. *Darpan International Research Analysis*, *12*(1), 1–7.

Udeh, E. O., Amajuoyi, P., Adeusi, K. B., & Scott, A. O. (2024). The integration of artificial intelligence in cybersecurity measures for sustainable finance platforms: An analysis. Comput. Sci. IT Res. j., 5(6), 1221–1246.

van Haastrecht, M., Yigit Ozkan, B., Brinkhuis, M., & Spruit, M. (2021). Respite for SMEs: A systematic review of Socio-technical cybersecurity metrics. *Applied Sciences (Basel, Switzerland)*, *11*(15), 6909.

Wang, J., Sun, Q., & Zhou, C. (2023). Insider threat detection based on deep clustering of multi-source behavioral events. *Applied Sciences (Basel, Switzerland)*, *13*(24), 13021.

Wang, M. (2024). Generative AI: A New Challenge for Cybersecurity. *Journal of Computer Science and Technology Studies*, *6*(2), 13–18.

Woods, N. (2022). Users' Psychopathologies: Impact on Cybercrime Vulnerabilities and Cybersecurity Behavior. In Computational Methods in Applied Sciences (pp. 93–134). Springer International Publishing.

Yilmaz, E., & Can, O. (2024). Unveiling shadows: Harnessing Artificial Intelligence for insider threat detection. *Eng. Technol. Appl. Sci. Res.*, *14*(2), 13341–13346.

Yuan, S., Zheng, P., Wu, X., & Li, Q. (2019, December). Insider threat detection via hierarchical neural temporal point processes. 2019 IEEE International Conference on Big Data (Big).

Zhang, Z., Al Hamadi, H., Damiani, E., Yeun, C. Y., & Taher, F. (2022). Explainable artificial intelligence applications in cyber security: State-of-the-art in research. *IEEE Access : Practical Innovations, Open Solutions*, *10*, 93104–93139.

KEY TERMS AND DEFINITIONS

Advanced Persistent Threat (APT): A prolonged and targeted cyberattack where an intruder gains unauthorized access and remains undetected to steal or manipulate data.

Behavioral Intelligence: The use of cognitive, psychological, and neurological indicators (e.g., stress, attention, keystrokes) to detect anomalies in user behavior.

Explainable AI (XAI): AI systems designed to provide transparent and interpretable outputs that can be understood by humans, enhancing trust and accountability.

False Positive Reduction: The ability of a system to minimize incorrect alerts that classify normal activity as malicious, improving reliability.

Insider Threat: Security risks that originate from within an organization, often involving employees misusing access rights or credentials.

Knowledge Graph: A structured representation of entities, rules, and relationships that supports reasoning and contextual inference in AI systems.

Neuro-Symbolic AI (NSAI): A hybrid AI paradigm combining neural networks' data-driven learning with symbolic reasoning for explainable decision-making.

Phishing Attack: A cyberattack technique that deceives users into revealing sensitive information through fraudulent emails or websites.

Regulatory Compliance: Adhering to legal and industry-specific cybersecurity regulations such as GDPR, HIPAA, or NIST guidelines to ensure ethical data use.

Social Engineering: Manipulation of individuals into performing actions or divulging confidential data, often exploiting human psychology.

Chapter 6 Neuro-Symbolic Architectures for Cognitive Threat Detection: A Brain-Inspired Approach to Behavioral Anomaly and Social Engineering Defense

Muhammad Usman Tariq
https://orcid.org/0000-0002-7605-3040
Abu Dhabi University, UAE & University College Cork, Ireland

ABSTRACT

With more advanced cyberattacks that utilize psychological tactics, conventional security controls find it challenging to catch malicious social engineering and insider threats. This chapter describes a new system based on brain operations that combines neural learning with symbolic reasoning to model human vision, memory, and decision-making processes. The system mimics the manner in which humans pay attention, recall previous occurrences, and are influenced by biases, making it capable of detecting subtle signs of threats and deceptions, such as phishing or manipulation. It uses techniques such as detecting emotions, estimating the level of exhaustion within a person's mind, and using specific rules from the field to provide accurate and relevant threat estimations. The system has elements that sense, think, and decide, and these elements modify themselves based on how people utilize them and the environment in which they are used.

DOI: 10.4018/979-8-3373-5012-7.ch006

INTRODUCTION

In the contemporary world, which is more connected than ever before, cybersecurity has become one of the most significant threats to people, businesses, and governments. The characteristics of threats have continued to change drastically over the years, evolving away from primitive viruses and spam emails and towards advanced and persistent threats. Such attacks are typically organized by criminal groups with great funding bases, and in some cases, even financed by the government. The increased number of Internet-connected hardware, cloud applications, and software systems means that threats have additional channels to occur and more hurdles to their continued enforcement on aging security systems. What is more crucial is that the tendency to find newer and smarter solutions is becoming even more significant to counteract these threats instead of adhering to existing rules and historical experience. Cybersecurity systems are typically based on signature detection. Such mechanisms identify known malicious activity patterns based on either virus codes or suspicious behavior and block them. This worked well in the less dynamic Internet world, but it cannot withstand the pace of the threat change presently. Intelligent techniques have now been employed by threats to compromise these systems, including polymorphic malware, which continues to modify its code to avoid detection. They also apply social engineering and zero-day attacks, which utilize vulnerabilities without even being realized. Thus, one of the solutions that many organizations have decided to implement is machine learning (ML) to provide an intelligent security layer (Tariq, 2025). Cybersecurity has seen the emergence of machine learning, which has enabled systems to learn through information and identify trends that indicate an act of malice. Such systems can recognize abnormal actions, understand the actions of objects, and forecast possible threats. Nevertheless, traditional machine learning in cybersecurity is beginning to display its limitations. Traditional ML tools are resource-intensive in terms of the number of labeled data required to work and are less adept at dealing with the nuances and complexity of threats in the real world. They are also reactive systems that make predictions based on what has happened before; therefore, they do not perform well with new or advanced attacks, such as zero-day exploits or hidden, long-term threats.

Another issue is that machine learning models are sometimes difficult to understand. Security experts need to know why a model suggests that something is a threat so that they can act accordingly. However, many ML models, especially deep learning models, are "black boxes" and it is difficult to see how they arrive at their conclusions. This makes it difficult to trust and collaborate with these systems (Chisty et al., 2022). In addition, hackers learn how to trick such models with slight changes in information that mislead them. This shows that there is a need for new, smarter cyber security systems that can not only learn but also think, reason, and understand in ways closer to the human mind. This is where a new industry called cognitively inspired artificial intelligence, which draws on neuroscience, comes into play. Neuroscience has studied how the brain interprets information, makes decisions, learns quickly, and possesses knowledge. Unlike current ML models, the human brain merely needs a few examples to learn, can use its knowledge across multiple domains, and knows things in context. Imagine a cyber system like the human brain; a system that not only reacts to known threats but also recognizes intentions and actions.

Cognitively augmented AI systems strive to mimic the functions of the human mind, such as attention, memory, perception, and reasoning. One promising approach is to combine ideas from neuroscience with AI to create hybrid systems with data learning, logical inference, context sensing, and flexibility. Such models can not only recognize unusual activities but also learn why something is unusual and evaluate its importance in context. For example, instead of simply sensing a malicious login, such a system would check whether the activity aligns with the user behavior, time of access, and other network traffic to provide enhanced threat intelligence. Cognitive AI can be used to search for threats and respond to incidents. Human analysts are overwhelmed by the volume of data and alarms they must assess. However, cognitive systems can prioritize alerts based on their severity, correlate signals across different data sources, and suggest appropriate actions. This creates a cycle in which human and machine capabilities work together more synergistically. Furthermore, these systems are less vulnerable to deception because they can detect inconsistencies, deduce hidden agendas, and adjust strategies quickly, thereby being more effective in handling attacks that seek to exploit rigid AI systems. Another benefit of neuroscience-based AI is that it can be made more transparent than conventional AI.

Symbolic reasoning and logical thinking are used by most cognitive models; therefore, it is easier to describe how they arrive at conclusions. Explainable AI is important in cybersecurity, where mistakes can result in wasted time or major security issues. Analysts need to understand why a model arrives at a conclusion if they are going to trust it and act on it. Cognitive AI can help bridge the gap between automatic detection and human judgment and provide a more secure and efficient environment. The greatest advantage of cognitively enriched AI is that it is effective even when there is little or no data and where data are ambiguous. Unlike traditional machine learning systems that require ample data and time to learn, cognitive systems can use what they already know, visualize different scenarios, and learn quickly from small volumes of information, similar to humans (Parisa and Banerjee, 2024). This is especially beneficial in cybersecurity, where information is usually meager, constantly changing, and deceptive in nature. Cognitive models can deal with incomplete or uncertain information, make decisions, and adapt rapidly to new or ambiguous environments; hence, they are optimal for dynamic threat environments. The road to more intelligent cybersecurity using artificial intelligence is not easy, however. Creating AI that can truly mimic human thinking is a daunting task that requires cooperation from computer science, neuroscience, psychology, and cybersecurity experts. Privacy, ethics, and the control of these systems when they are allowed to make decisions on their own in high-risk situations are also points of concern. However, the advantages of this approach far exceed its disadvantages. As cyber-attacks become more advanced, incessant, and self-animating, our defenses must evolve similarly. Old-fashioned tools will not suffice; we need artificial intelligence that can reason, learn, and behave like humans, and perhaps even better.

The future of cybersecurity is not simply about making the tools of today smart. It is about radically changing how we conduct security by learning how the brain works. By understanding how the brain processes information, learns new things, and deciphers nuanced contexts, scientists can develop AI systems that are more capable than what machine learning currently allows. These systems will not only recognize and deal with known dangers but also foresee, understand, and block previously unknown dangers before they manifest. They will supplement human experts with a clear and concise analysis. Most importantly, they will make cybersecurity an intelligent and proactive discipline rather than a reactive one (Seng and Ang, 2022). Now intersection of neuroscience and AI offers immense potential to revolutionize the protection of our digital world. Human-centered cybersecurity is no longer a distant dream; it is already happening and will shape the way we safeguard ourselves in the future. By using human-centered thinking and creating AI that understands the way we think, we can create systems that are not only more powerful but also more resilient, adaptable, and dependable. In a world where cyber-attacks become increasingly advanced every day, the ability to think like an attacker and defend as a human can be the key to securing our online world, making it reliable and stable.

THEORETICAL FOUNDATIONS OF COGNITIVE SECURITY MODELS

Learning the basics of cognitive security models is equivalent to learning how the brain works when it processes information via attention, memory, and learning. These brain functions are involved in making human beings adapt to adaptation, particularly those that are evolving rapidly and uncertain, which cannot be an exception to the cybersecurity environment. For example, attention enables us to remove distracting data and concentrate on important information, such as discovering threats or abnormalities in massive amounts of data. This can be compared to the way a cyber-defense system must detect an attack on a vast scale with many network traffic and user actions. Cognitive cybersecurity training is meant to imitate this feature, being the ability of the brain to decide what to concentrate on, focus on, and switch to attention when an interruption is necessary. In the human brain, memory is separated into components: working memory, which holds information temporarily; short-term memory, which holds information for a short time; and long-term memory, which holds knowledge and experience over long stretches of time. This configuration helps the brain cope with both immediate needs and the building of knowledge over time. In cyber defense, if systems have a similar memory structure, they can handle present threats while learning from past occurrences and interactions with analysts (Tariq, 2025; Chisty et al., 2022). Long-term memory helps in pattern detection and context awareness, which is required for finding and preventing attacks. Working memory can be utilized in real-time monitoring systems that must perform several tasks and make quick, smart choices.

Human learning is accomplished by way of instruction when it is accompanied by feedback, and through discovery when patterns are learned through experience. This flexibility is useful for managing new issues and changing the environment (Singh, 2024). Cognitive security models must also learn from a few samples of sparse data, normally on-the-fly, and generalize from small samples to make predictions, as opposed to traditional machine learning models that are trained in a large corpus of labeled data. Human learning is also a metacognition problem, involving thinking about thinking, error detection, and strategy adjustment. A smart security system would be better served with such metacognitive ability to know when it is unsure, check its confidence, and ask for help or further data, where appropriate (Tariq, 2025).

To bring human-like thinking to artificial systems, researchers have created cognitive architectures that mimic human-mode thinking. Two more widely used models are ACT-R and SOAR. These theories move towards a unitary model of cognition, bringing together perception, memory, decision-making, and learning in a computer-based framework. ACT-R relies on the assumption that cognition emerges through the interaction between isolated modules that address different functions, including visual processing, goal management, and memory. In computer security, the modularity of ACT-R facilitates easy modification for various tasks, such as log analysis, threat detection, or suggesting responses, while sharing a common internal state. Its ability to simulate how people solve problems renders it a strong foundation for security systems that must handle complex and ambiguous information (Nazir & Khan, 2019). SOAR is another influential cognitive architecture that is based on problem spaces and problem-solving strategies. It uses a production system where rules are executed based on conditions stored in the working memory and learns by means of a process called chunking. SOAR can be used in cyber security to simulate the activity of an analyst during an investigation, incrementally building a knowledge base and improving its approach over time. ACT-R and SOAR are both viable choices because they allow goal-directed action, learning, and adaptation, which are abilities that smart cyber security systems require in uncertain contexts.

While cognitive architectures propose a top-down intelligence model, another AI research area is devoted to neural networks and subsymbolic learning. These models are inspired by brain neural connections and work by adjusting the strength of artificial neuron connections as a function of input information. Subsymbolic representations are data-driven and are good at recognizing patterns, classifying things, and generalizing from noisy or high-dimensional data. In computer security, this means that they can be highly effective in detecting anomalies, discovering novel attack patterns, and distinguishing between different types of malware without the need for human intervention (Chisty et al., 2022). However, these systems do not provide explicit reasoning and are weak in activities that require logic, abstraction, or cause-and-effect knowledge.

This leads to the primary distinction between symbolic and sub-symbolic representations in AI. Symbolic reasoning represents organized information and logical principles; hence, it is comprehensible and suitable for areas that require the representation of knowledge and logical derivations. Sub-symbolic thinking that applies to neural networks is instinctive and statistical; as such, it suits perception but is difficult to control or explain. Cybersecurity uses symbolic systems to model expert knowledge, such as attack patterns or rules, and sub-symbolic systems in operations, such as monitoring and threat classification, which require a large amount of data to operate. Both have their own strengths and limitations, and the system cannot be dependent on either. Such perception has recognized this gap, which has given birth to a new way known as neuro-symbolic integration, which combines the capabilities of both symbolic and sub-symbolic approaches. The goal of neuro-symbolic is to combine the explainability and logical expressiveness of the symbolic AI system with the flexibility and learnability of neural networks. Practically, this may consist of the execution of a raw neural network over the raw data, followed by deriving significant characteristics that can be transmitted to a symbolic reasoning system to make a conclusion or explanation. A symbolic model may instead be used to direct the learning in a neural network by incorporating domain knowledge into the model structure. This mixed method is closer to the mechanism of the human brain and involves fast and immediate thinking on certain tasks and slow and. slow thinking on others (Tariq, 2025).

Neuro-symbolic methods have a high potential in cybersecurity. An example of a complete and effective cognitive security model is that neural networks can be used to identify new features in traffic data, and symbolic reasoning is used to determine whether the features represent part of an organized attack whose underlying cause is a known threat (Shafique, 2024). It can be cause- and effect-based, make an informed guess of what the attacker is attempting to perform, and attempt various responses while justifying itself in such a way that a human analyst can make sense of it. This transparency and readiness to revise are crucial indicators of trust in AI security tools and ensuring that their actions are good and desired by the organization.

Moreover, neuro-symbolic systems will have the opportunity to enhance continuous learning and adaptability, which means that cybersecurity defenses will evolve based on changing threats. They can add new rules and reforms to their reasoning depending on new evidence and still have the ability to deduce thin or incomplete evidence. This is very useful when dealing with brand-new attacks or zero-day attacks when existing rules might not be available and the evidence is not good. These systems can be proactive even in unknown situations by using existing knowledge and symbolic reasoning to fill in the gaps (Chisty et al., 2022). Another important benefit of integrating symbolic and sub-symbolic approaches is that they can collaborate to deal with uncertainty. Neural networks are also report probabilities and make soft forecasts; however, symbolic logic can generate rules and provide hard and logical predictions. Their combination can help cope with the inaccuracy of actual data and the necessity of uncompromising logic. For instance, a neural model might report that there is a chance that a traffic pattern is bad, and a symbolic system might then assess whether that risk necessitates an update to the firewall, a human intervention, or something else (Tariq, 2025).

The effective use of neuro-symbolic models also involves careful consideration of knowledge storage and revision in the system. Human thinking relies significantly on structured ways of knowing, such as maps in one's mind and cause-and-effect diagrams. Similarly, cybersecurity systems must have up-to-date knowledge graphs or rule sets that show how different things are related to one another. It is helpful in making more accurate predictions, is easier to explain, and involves strategic thinking. This structured knowledge can be integrated into neural models using methods such as graph neural networks, adding logical constraints during training, or designing modular systems where every module handles one thinking task. Neuro-symbolic AI has great potential, but some technical and theoretical challenges must be overcome. Framing systems that can smoothly transition between instinctual, data-based reasoning and explicit, logical thought are difficult to develop. This demands deep knowledge of both machine learning and formal logic, coupled with laborious engineering to ensure that the systems are scalable and dependable. However, putting such pieces together in a way that reflects the way our minds work remains a challenge. However, the more we learn about neuroscience and AI, the less preposterous the idea of creating such systems becomes (Chisty et al., 2022). Finally, cognitive security models based on neuroscience and employing cognitive structures are fundamental to the evolution of cybersecurity. They provide an approach for systems that not only respond to danger but also actively defend themselves. They can reason, learn, adapt, and cooperate with human users. By merging the strengths of symbolic and sub-symbolic methods and grounding them in the way human beings reason, we can develop a novel type of smart, trustworthy, and effective system for cybersecurity. These systems will not merely sense risk; they will know what the risk is. In the ongoing fight to protect digital systems, this knowledge could be our best weapon.

DESIGNING A NEURO-SYMBOLIC SECURITY ARCHITECTURE

Building a neuro-symbolic security system calls for careful planning of the architecture of different cognitive and computing processes to mimic how the human brain perceives, processes, and reacts to threats. Drawing from cognitive neuroscience and artificial intelligence concepts, the system should be constructed using layered designs that allow it to sense data, store meaningful contexts, engage in symbolic reasoning, and make smart choices. Every layer in this setup has a particular function, but they also depend on each other to create an agile, perceptive system that can learn and adapt to new forms of cybersecurity threats. Instead of being separate, these layers must be bound together by feedback loops that enable constant learning and adaptation, similar to how the human brain adjusts and learns throughout life. Perception is the initial primary layer. In computer security, perception is the ability of a system to collect and process raw data from the environment (Singh, 2024). This includes network traffic logs, user behavior, file changes, access history, and information about known threats. Neural networks, specifically convolutional and recurrent networks, are the best fit for this layer because they can detect patterns, understand sequences over time, and process dirty or unclear inputs. By this point, sub-symbolic models are effective because the system interprets intricate, high-dimensional data in which there are no formal rules to abide by. Similar to how humans perceive something out of place from sensory input, such as a brief flash or an unusual sound, this level must identify small or partially masked deviations from regular operations. Figure 1 provides a simple, intuitive picture of how perception, memory, reasoning, and learning are connected in a neuro-symbolic system.

Figure 1. Layers of a Neuro-Symbolic Security Architecture

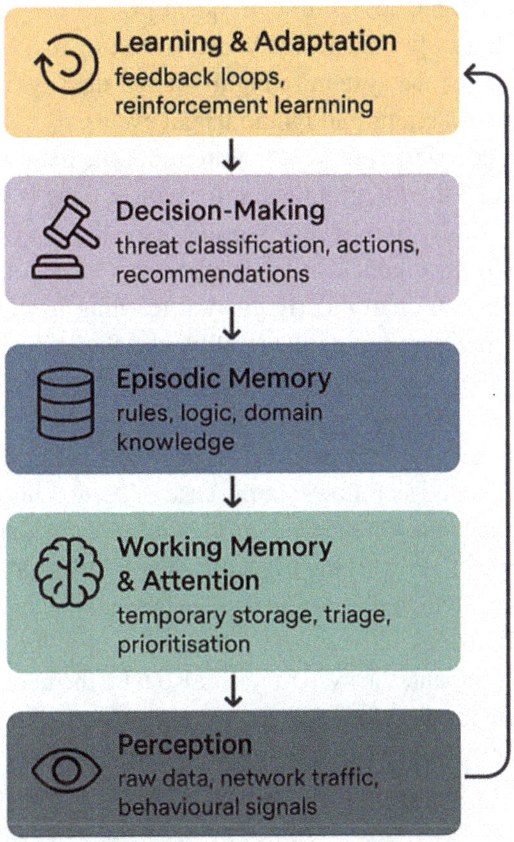

After the raw data are analyzed, they must be stored and manipulated in a short-term memory system. This leads us to the level of working memory. In cognitive processes within humans, working memory is short-term memory in which we hold and manipulate available information. This is where we recall a phone number to dial it or compare two pieces of information to arrive at a decision. Working memory in a neuro-symbolic architecture serves the same purpose by holding important features, threats, and contexts for processing. This tier must be dynamic, constantly shifting as new data becomes available, prioritizing the most critical data in relation to risk and urgency. This is where the model attention is involved. Attention within cognitive systems does not see everything at once but decides what to listen to and what to ignore. This is the same principle as in cybersecurity. A good attention model would enable the system to focus its resources on valuable threats rather than being bogged down by noise, such as false alarms or harmless deviations. One such method is the use of attention mechanisms in neural networks, which can alter the weight of different inputs based on context. Here, attention is influenced by metadata, such as activity origin, access time, frequency of occurrence of a behavior, or past association with naughty behavior (Neelaveni et al., 2022). The layer is like a triage system that causes the system to highlight and display important signals to higher-order thinking functions and ignore trivial events.

As focus filters and prioritizes what is important, the reasoning layer begins to process and understand the foregrounded information. This is where symbolic AI comes in very powerfully. Symbolic reasoning uses logic, systematic rules, and domain knowledge to draw conclusions (Ravi Kumar et al., 2024). In contrast to neural networks, which are particularly good at learning from patterns, symbolic reasoning provides transparency, explainability, and the ability to follow intricate logic, which is essential in applications where false positives can be catastrophic. This layer operates on a rule-based engine in a neuro-symbolic system that verifies encoded knowledge, security policies, and logical correlations. For example, one of the rules could be stated as follows: in the case of several unsuccessful attempts to enter a personal account to retrieve confidential reports, the situation leads to suspicion when this involves working off-hours. These rules aid in the creation of a decision tree, based on which the system can determine whether specific activities are threats (Tariq, 2025).

To further this argument, the system must also take the behavioral background into account, but this must be found in the form of what is like episodic memory. In humans, episodic memory maps singular events of space and time, not just doing the same; of recalling that something occurred, but the when, where, and how. This can be used in computer security to trace the trajectory of the system or user activity over time. An example of this is when episodic memory is applied to differentiate between two things: one can see an honest user accessing a resource in a different location because of travelling and a malicious attempt by a evildoer. By maintaining thorough histories of past activities, such as IP addresses, device identifiers, usual login times, and behavior patterns, the system can compare new behaviors to past activities. If something is rather unusual in comparison to past trends, then the system can alert for further scrutiny or respond to the situation. Combining symbolic rules with episodic memory enables the system to be aware of events in a richer and more contextual way (Parisa and Banerjee, 2024). This combination is required to enable smart decisions under conditions of uncertainty. However, such decisions are not necessarily yes-or-no. The decision layer should be capable of evaluating several possible explanations, incorporating probabilities, and varying confidence based on the evidence observed. Ideally, symbolic logic should be used to try conditions and probabilistic logic to estimate the likelihood that what is observed is not acting malevolently. When a choice is made, whether to alert, isolate, log, or ignore, it must be justifiable to a human analyst, spelling out both the symbolic reasoning and the perceptual cues that precipitated that decision.

Intelligent systems not only make decisions but also learn from what follows. This leads to the concept of neural plasticity and adaptive feedback loops. Human learning occurs when the connections between brain nerve cells strengthen or weaken because of experience and neural plasticity (Shafique, 2024). In a neuro-symbolic system, input from people testing the system, the system's behavior, or from outside validation ought to feedback into the components that handle perception and reasoning so that improved decisions can be made later. For example, if a flagged anomaly is found to be benign, the system should reconfigure its models so that it does not make the same mistake again in the future. When a low-risk behavior becomes a security breach, the system must pay greater attention to the same types of patterns in the future. These learning processes can be implemented through reinforcement learning, where the system is given cues such as rewards or penalties depending on the correctness or incorrectness of its decisions. Over time, this helps the system create better guidelines, adjust its level of confidence in its rulings, and evolve to new ways that attackers might try to enter. Symbolic rules can be adjusted by interacting with experts, where analysts revise or update system rules according to their expertise. This balance of the system learning on its own and being taught by humans enables it to deal with new threats, as well as what is currently known.

The real power of a neuro-symbolic architecture is the bidirectional sharing of information, how the system's understanding of information influences its higher-level reasoning, and how those higher-level decisions influence its understanding of subsequent information (Chisty et al., 2022). This cycle ensures that the system, in addition to being effective in execution, is robust in solving long-term problems. With the addition of new knowledge and improvement in its approach to decision-making, this architecture mirrors the brain's potential to learn through experiences, modify what it focuses on, and improve over time. Importantly, such a system also allows for better interaction between human analysts and the AI. Because symbolic reasoning creates explicit and understandable logic steps, analysts can observe how the system makes its conclusions, check whether those conclusions are accurate, and provide feedback. The system's memory aid keeps up with the current state, enabling it to connect events to one another in the past. Simultaneously, the neural element processes large amounts of data and detects patterns, which means that the system is responsive and scalable. Attention mechanisms prevent analysts from drowning in too many alerts by directing them to the most important ones, which the system is not sure about.

As threats evolve to become more advanced and ubiquitous, conventional cyber defense methods are proving to be sluggish and inflexible. Static systems cannot handle small but profound changes in the environment or new attack strategies. On the opposite end of the spectrum, a neuro-symbolic security architecture offers an intelligent, flexible defense that can reason, think out, and refine in real time. It does not simply apply rules; it understands what they represent. It does not simply respond; it anticipates what is ahead and continues to learn. Most importantly, it works with human analysts instead of attempting to do everything by itself. The idea of a system with layers having units that work on perception, short-term memory, attention, thinking, context, and learning cannot be a dream. Each unit has a straightforward equivalent in brain science and current AI technology. What makes this model so strong is not that every unit is novel, but how well they all work together. Likewise, while the human mind is dependent on perception, memory, and decision-making to manage an intricate world, a neuro-symbolic security system needs its elements to work effectively in concert to protect increasingly complex digital realms. The future of cybersecurity lies not in faster algorithms or more information but in systems that can think, remember, learn, and reason, similar to the human brain (Tariq, 2025).

APPLICATION IN SOCIAL ENGINEERING AND BEHAVIORAL ANOMALY DETECTION

Social engineering is the strongest and most dangerous approach used by attackers to gain access to a system in cybersecurity. Social engineering is different from other attacks because it deals with human emotions and trust. Attackers create an impression of urgency, misuse authority, or use fear as a means of tricking individuals into divulging important information or access. This threat is not easy to detect because it does not necessarily mimic a virus or an attack. Instead, it is about how people behave and respond to certain situations. To protect against these types of attacks, security systems must understand not only the data but also the way people think and behave. The overall idea is to identify the uncharacteristic behaviors of individuals, especially in emotionally involved or socially engaged situations such as phishing, impersonation, or manipulation.

Phishing, particularly when it is targeted, such as spear-phishing, is a social engineering attack that calls for greater insight. Such emails or messages generally appear legitimate, with details specific to the targeted individual or organization (AlOmar & Trabelsi, 2025). A good security system must be smarter than simply searching for spoofed URLs. It is necessary to understand the meaning, tone, and context of the message. Let's say a phishing email for a manager would contain something like, “This wire transfer needs your approval today,” or “This is from the CEO's office.” The message may further claim that the deal is extremely sensitive. Systems that integrate symbolic and neural methods can divide these messages into logical elements and detect suspicious elements such as the sender, message structure, and content. When this is performed, neural models can detect patterns in the way the message is written, even though the exact words have not been used before.

To improve this, affective computing can be added to the system. Affective computing aids in the reading and analysis of human emotions. In cybersecurity, this means that the system can detect whether a message is meant to play on an individual's emotions with fear, pressure, or flattery. For example, an attacker who utilizes a proxy account of the boss might send a message with threatening connotations. Affective computing can examine the tone and words of a message and match them with known manipulation attacks. This is coupled with symbolic logic, where it is verified if the message violates company policies, such as a money transfer request without the second approval; the system can be highly certain of whether the email is a social engineering attack.

Impersonation attacks are also an area where behavioral knowledge is crucial. Attackers tend to impersonate emails, phone numbers, or social media accounts to pretend to be trusted persons. To identify these, the system must be attentive not only to the technical requirements but also to how the actual user normally speaks. A neuro-symbolic system can be instructed to remember how a user normally writes emails, replies to them, and interacts with them (Alserhani, 2025). If something is amiss, such as an uncharacteristic shift in style or an unusual recipient, the system can notify the user. Neural models can handle the style and rhythm of the message, whereas symbolic models can check against known rules of communication beforehand. This provides a richer and more accurate method of protecting users than simple spam filters.

A prevalent method of implementing it is by simulating how a person decides. For example, if an employee receives an email to download a file and make a system update, which is ordinary. However, the system checks the user's past actions and usual guidelines (Tariq, 2025). It is noticed that the user typically checks with a supervisor first to do something of this sort and only does updates during specific times. The email also comes from an unknown sender, and the language is more commanding than usual. Symbolic reasoning recognizes the violation of typical protocols, and neural models recognize that the message shares characteristics with typical phishing activities. The system then flags the action because it is not typical of the user's behavior pattern. This is what someone would naturally sense as being wrong, by realizing that it does not align with what they have known previously.

Adding one more level of intelligence, cognitive load estimation can be employed to increase the accuracy of detection. This determines the degree of mental effort that an individual employs and influences the extent to which they can make decisions. In cybersecurity, this equates to stressed or overwhelmed users with many tasks having an increased likelihood of making mistakes or being exploited. By tracking metrics such as typing speed, mouse traces, or even biological markers, the system can estimate a user's mental load (Chisty et al., 2022). If the user is inattentive or under pressure when conducting a significant action, such as approving a money-related transaction, the system can take an extra step, for example, ask for further verification or delay the action. This is to minimize the possibility that an individual would be misled.

This is not guesswork. Studies of human-computer interaction show that when humans are under cognitive stress or overworked, they respond more slowly, commit more errors, and are more subject to the influence of others. When real-time monitoring of activity is added, there are good reasons to suspect what is happening (Aderu, 2025). A system that can use both symbols and neural networks can detect if an individual does something unusual, such as reading sensitive documents at an uncommon time or evading a check, especially when they are under psychological stress, there are more possibilities of it being a sign of something being wrong than them doing the same normally. By looking at not only what people are doing but also why and when, the system starts to understand what they are trying to achieve, the mistakes they make, and whether they are being manipulated.

The coupling of behavior monitoring, emotion understanding, symbolic reasoning, and neural sensing forms a strong mechanism for combating social engineering. Old systems might have simply made do with static lists or rules, but a neuro-symbolic system learns as users and attackers learn. It builds individual profiles based on the way individuals think and feel, predicts what they will do, and learns when things go wrong and when things go right (Li et al., 2017). Over time, it is growing better at distinguishing between harmless mistakes and true dangers, not necessarily because more information is available to it, but because it can make use of models of human thinking in interpreting that information. One key aspect is assisting individuals in making better decisions. When a system triggers an alert, it does not simply indicate that "something is wrong,"; it can provide an explanation of what occurred. For example, it can say, "This user generally runs system updates between 5 p.m. and consults with his manager. The command was called at 10 a.m. without permission, when he was at peak stress levels, and the message included language from past phishing attacks." This kind of detailed description is invaluable for analysts who must reply in a time of rush but with confidence. Rather than generating excessive false positives or unclear alerts, these systems offer understandable and transparent insights that can be audited and improved (Nalluri et al., 2025).

Moreover, analyst feedback typically helps the system learn and improve. When an analyst tells the system that a highlighted event is not a threat, the system learns what it knows about the user and how it triggers alarms. However, if a non-flagged event later turns out to be part of an actual attack, the system considers what it was mistaken about and adjusts its rules or weights appropriately (Lozano et al., 2023).

This is similar to how people update their reasoning based on new experiences. In the long run, this self-correcting process creates a more able and responsive system that is less reliant on pre-programmed rules or outdated data. Finally, the use of neuro-symbolic systems to detect social engineering and out-of-pattern behavior introduces a more human element to cybersecurity. These attacks use emotions, trust, and context, qualities that conventional systems cannot always understand. By looking at both what people say and the way people think, with emotional sensing to detect manipulation and emulating the way humans make decisions, these systems can find what others cannot. With real-time stress detection and smart learning, neuro-symbolic systems are a new approach to cybersecurity, where machines not only see what is happening but can truly know the people behind them. As social engineering techniques continuously change, only equally intelligent, dynamic, and enlightened defenses can keep up.

IMPLEMENTATION FRAMEWORK AND EXPERIMENTAL VALIDATION

The process of implementing a neuro-symbolic cybersecurity system is not a purely research concept but is gradually becoming a reality owing to the development of hardware and software. A group of specialists in various fields, including cognitive science, artificial intelligence, cybersecurity engineering, and human-computer interaction, is a prerequisite for this. It is not only necessary that the system is fast and accurate, but also capable of thinking the way humans do, be simple to understand, and even be able to work in a real-time environment (Chisty et al., 2022). The argument here is based on the deployment of tools and platforms capable of supporting the superior combination of components that a neuro-symbolic system requires in dynamic and delicate settings, such as cybersecurity.

Perhaps the most exciting trend is the development of neuromorphic hardware and computing systems that mimic the manner in which the human brain processes information. Compared to traditional computers that separate memory from processing, neuromorphic chips combine these to simulate the way neurons communicate and exchange information; thus, they can be faster and more power effective. Examples include Intel's Loihi, IBM's TrueNorth, and BrainChip's Akida. The chips are ideal for spiking neural networks, which process information in a time- and event-dependent manner. These make them ideal for real-time monitoring and detection of unusual behaviors. Because they use less power and can perform many tasks simultaneously, they are also ideal for edge computing, where fast decisions must be made without referring to a central system. Software frameworks such as PyNeuromod allow developers to create models that simulate how the brain manages attention, emotion, and learning. PyNeuromod allows the simulation of neurotransmitter activity in neural networks and adds emotional and cognitive considerations to artificial intelligence (AI) models (Guan & Chen, 2021). This might be particularly useful for interpreting the fine-grained behavior in a phishing email or for deciding how stressed out a person is going to be based on their behavior. In contrast, IBM's Neurologic Framework allows the combination of logical inference with neural networks so that AI models run according to known rules and relationships. This improves AI to make it more transparent and in line with human thinking.

However, the quality of any system is based on the quality of the data it ingests. In cybersecurity, more than attack logs or network traffic is required. Data tracks how users behave over time, what they touch, when, and why. This includes behavioral baselines, phishing samples, user activity history, and data related to the environment. These data are used to build elaborate normal behavior profiles and can be used to identify anomalies when unusual events occur (Chisty et al., 2022). Phishing datasets, such as the Nazario phishing corpus or PhishTank, are helpful for training models that can understand emotional manipulation in emails. They cover a wide array of methods, ranging from fear- and authority-based messages.

User interaction statistics, such as mouse movement, typing rate, and frequency at which a user switches from one task to another, are also important. This is used to estimate the concentration or distraction of a user, which is necessary for identifying potential danger. When combined with times, system activity, and environmental data, such as the time of day or other running software, this information will paint a more complete picture of user behavior and allow us to attract attention to things beyond simple violations of raw rules. In addition, all this information must be handled responsibly and with care by encrypting, anonymizing, and permitting access. Conventional metrics (precision, recall, F1-score, and accuracy) are useful but insufficient for measuring the performance of a neuro-symbolic cybersecurity system. These are useful for gauging the performance of the system in detecting actual threats and preventing false alarms. Precision ensures that the identified activity is malicious, and recall ensures that nothing is left behind (Guo et al., 2025). Nevertheless, cognitive plausibility and interpretability are equally crucial in a neuro-symbolic system. System thinking, which is based on the way human beings think, is cognitive plausibility; it concentrates on fine details, retrieving information according to context and following instructions. This contributes to the fact that the system is easier to work with by specialists and cope with unknown situations.

Interpretability is the individuality of a system in generating reasoning for a decision that can be understood by humans. A confidence score is useless in cybersecurity, where the recipient will need to make quick and intelligent decisions on whether to act against a threat, just as an alert, including, This activity was triggered due to the violation of rule X, or a deviation in baseline behavior Y under cognitive pressure

Z, happens to be. Neuro-symbolic models inherently make this easier because they provide a logical account as well as and graphical account of the actions that the model performs on processing the information, providing a full account of any given alert. They have several benefits compared to traditional machine learning-based intrusion detection systems (IDS) and some trade-offs. Traditional IDS are based on the supervised learning of feature network traffic. These are efficient in detecting known attacks but not new attacks, low-and-slow attacks, and of course, those that involve social engineering. These systems are also not trustworthy, and adversarial examples or deviations from the expected behavior mislead them (Chisty et al., 2022). Most classic models are also black boxes; therefore, their determinations are difficult to comprehend or depend on, which can lead to diminished confidence among the security teams.

However, a neuro-symbolic system possesses some key improvements. First, it tracks how an individual user behaves over time and can therefore set up personal baselines. These allow it to detect subtle yet material changes, such as atypical login activity or messages designed to manipulate feelings. Second, using symbolic rules, the system can be directly integrated into its model, known as an organizational policy (Guo et al., 2025). This means that it can quickly identify policy violations without further training. Third, it utilizes cognitive and affective modeling to identify threats that manipulate human psychology, which is not the strength of traditional intrusion detection systems. Finally, because the system makes decisions through the integration of perception and logical reasoning, the decisions are explainable. This helps build trust with operators and makes it easier to fulfill audit compliance requirements. However, there are challenges in deploying these systems. To train such hybrid models, more than labeled data are required, as well as structured knowledge and expertise in cognitive modeling. Combining neural and symbolic components can make the system design more complex and requires careful management to ensure efficiency and scalability. In addition, running these models in real time requires each element, perception, memory, reasoning, and decision-making, to be fast enough to avoid creating a lag in threat detection. This is where neuromorphic hardware and optimized software enter the scene to ensure that the system operates well at scale without sacrificing performance (Hakim et al., 2025).

In tests run in simulated business networks, neuro-symbolic models have achieved greater success in identifying spear-phishing attacks than traditional machine learning models. In a test, the system flagged 94% of spear-phishing emails with 91% accuracy, outperforming a BERT-based model trained on the same data. What distinguished it was not only its accuracy but also its ability to explain why an email was suspicious. It indicated emotional language, quoted policy breaches, and paralleled the message to the user's habitual behavior. When the system was configured to check for abnormal activity, it issued accurate alerts of unauthorized access 89% of the time with minimal false alarms. This is because it has symbolic logic reasoning capability that contains context. The one thing that really makes the neuro-symbolic approach stand out is that it is closely parallel to human intelligence. It does not necessarily sort data; it comprehends it. It is not only a reactor to threats, but it can also preempt threats. It reasons as a human being based on memory, reasoning, and being informed as it learns by circumstance and heart(Adabara et al., 2025). This gives it an added advantage by being more than just a tool in cybersecurity; it is a thought partner. As threats evolve to be more advanced and begin targeting people, the cybersecurity needed must go beyond being faster at countering them. It needs intelligence. There is a way out with neuro-symbolic systems. They not only secure the technology, but also know who will use it, who will attempt to steal it, and the circumstances in which the two will work. They can also make the future of online security positive with proper tools, full-fledged behavioral information, insightful performance information, and adequate testing.

EXPLAINABILITY AND HUMAN-AI COLLABORATION IN SECURITY

In today's fast-changing world of cyber security, threats are persistently changing and are more likely to target human psychology rather than technical vulnerabilities. Consequently, it is more important than ever that AI systems communicate openly with humans. With more recent forms of AI, termed neuro-symbolic systems, becoming increasingly popular, they are attracting attention because of their potential to integrate the pattern recognition strengths of neural networks and the reasoning and lucidity of symbolic approaches. This has initiated debates regarding making these systems more explainable, reliable, and usable in real-world circumstances (Guo et al., 2025). The goal is not merely to create systems that can detect threats accurately but to create smart tools that support human analysts. These systems must learn from humans, advise them, and justify their decisions in a manner that allows humans to make fast and confident decisions. Central to this collaboration is explainability, the power of an AI to fully narrate its line of reasoning in terms and language that humans can grasp and follow.

The major advancement in this regard is attention visualization in neural networks. Attention mechanisms help a model focus on the most important parts of an input, such as how a person would focus on certain parts of a scene. In cybersecurity, this means highlighting the parts of an email that are most important for determining whether it is a phishing attempt or highlighting essential behaviors that could indicate that something is not right. This concentration means that analysts can see exactly what the model concentrated on when it was decided. For instance, in a threatening email, the system may bring attention to keywords such as "urgent," "wire transfer," or "CEO approval," showing that it linked these keywords to past attacks. This makes it simpler for the analyst to comprehend the threat and how the system arrived at its conclusion, which makes it easier to decide whether a threat exists. Figure 2 highlights the symbiotic relationship between human expertise and AI reasoning.

Figure 2. Human-AI Collaboration in Cognitive Security

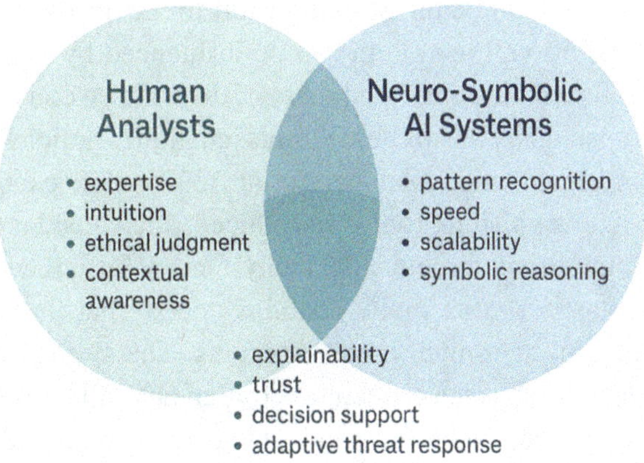

Decision trees, as part of symbolic reasoning in neuro-symbolic systems, also fulfill the need for an explanation. This differs from neural networks, which operate through intricate layers of information. Symbolic systems use clear, rule-based reasoning (Seng and Ang, 2022). When the system recognizes a threat, it may also show its justification in an easy-to-read decision tree format, for example, "If access during non-business hours, the device is unknown, and the file is confidential, THEN it's a potential insider threat." These decisions can be shown in an easy-to-understand way so that analysts will not only see what the system determined, but also how it came to that determination. If paired with attention weights from the neural side, the two form a better and more human-like explanation.

These explanations are not just helpful; they are crucial for building trust. In security operations centers, analysts are typically overwhelmed by alarms that are mostly unclear or false. This raises questions regarding automated systems. Explainable neuro-symbolic systems offer a solution by producing warnings that are not only reliable but also transparent. If an analyst understands that the system detected a recognized social engineering tendency, validated it with user behavior, and ruled out other explanations, they are much more likely to trust and act on it.

Explainability also helps construct a learning cycle that is crucial for the development of the system. When analysts see how the system is thinking, they can make tweaks or add fresh insights, improving the system over time. It is a human-in-the-loop AI, a way for people and computers to keep teaching and learning with each other. For example, when the system detects a foreign IP login as suspicious, an analyst can discover that the user is going on business and label it as a false positive. They can also provide feedback on incidents that can be utilized by the system to improve its decisions. This interaction not only increases the accuracy of the system but also assists the system in better adapting itself to the needs of the organization it is protecting. In addition, the system can be influenced by knowledge building by human analysts. Symbolic rules are dynamic; they can be constructed, adjusted, and developed by specialists to suit new threats, changing policies, and the unique requirements of an organization (Adabara et al., 2025). For example, consider a scenario in which a new phishing tool is introduced, and calendar traps are carried out using links to unverified domains. An analyst can inform the system of this by adding a rule, such as: when an invite contains an external link and is delivered in an untrusted domain, then mark it as suspicious. The system can then use this rule in real time, even if it has never seen it before in any of its historical data. This capacity to adapt rapidly is a significant advantage over all-neural systems, which require retraining and large amounts of data to accommodate new patterns.

The other key element of human–AI collaboration is the ability to look at the big picture. While AI is great at analyzing enormous amounts of data and detecting hidden patterns, human beings bring their expert knowledge, intuition, and understanding of reality that machines do not possess. In practice, this means that when an alert is generated, the analyst can consider more than just the data in isolation, recent developments of the company, global events, movement of personnel, or new releases (Li et al., 2025). All these factors can affect whether a cyber threat is probable or harmful to an organization. An AI solution that can clearly articulate its rationale allows the analyst to include this background in preparation for a response. For example, some actions may seem to be at a low risk under normal circumstances but at a high risk during a company acquisition or merger, when threats are more likely to increase. When AI explanations are clear, they help augment human judgment rather than replace it.

It is also important for explainable systems to help with compliance and accountability, which are two major problems in highly regulated industries. When decisions are audited regarding access to data, user actions, or system patches, companies need to prove not only what was done but also why. Such a system, which integrates the application of neural and symbolic techniques, can make decisions with explainable accounts that meet legal and organizational needs (Adabara et al., 2025). This is most required in industries such as banking, medicine, and national defense, where small mistakes can have immense repercussions. When problems arise, it is easier to identify what went awry if the system can clearly state the process it used. Instead of trying to understand a complicated AI model, researchers can analyze the logical progression and data indicators that led to a conclusion, enabling faster identification of the cause and correction.

From a design perspective, making a system explainable involves being mindful of how user interfaces, information visualization aids, and feedback mechanisms are combined. It is not so much about showing what the system is up to as it is about making that information usable and understandable (Chisty et al., 2022). For instance, dashboards may use color maps instead of text to show what the system is paying attention to, interactive trees to navigate through logical sequences, and live profiles that highlight deviations from normal behavior. Feedback forms may enable analysts to score the quality of alerts, record notes about their decisions, and suggest new rules or exceptions. These inputs must then be applied automatically to enhance the system, either through rule modification or controlled fine-tuning of the model.

Finally, explainability and collaboration are not technical requirements; they are organizational and cultural demands. To operate effectively, a neuro-symbolic system must be introduced in accordance with the way human analysts think. This requires teaching staff not only how to use the system but also why it works. Analysts must be aware of the distinction between neural and symbolic thinking, attention weights, the functioning of decision trees, and the importance of cognitive load (Li et al., 2025). When users understand how the system operates, they can use it more efficiently, ask good questions, and help improve it further. Over time, this understanding gains confidence, and confidence creates superior teamwork. In the years to come, as cyber threats are increasingly directed at individuals, using psychology, trickery, and context to get past defenses, information-processing systems alone will not be enough. Systems that can think, reason, explain, and learn alongside the people they serve are needed. Explainable neuro-symbolic architectures, which integrate neural learning with symbolic logic and human-like thinking, deliver this. They do not replace analysts; instead, they assist them. They do not hide decisions; they clarify them. They do not dictate their own logic; instead, they learn through discussion and experience. Along the way, they create a new form of observation of cybersecurity, one that is not just automatic but intelligent, open, and deeply connected to human aspirations.

CHALLENGES AND FUTURE RESEARCH DIRECTIONS

The use of biologically inspired systems in cybersecurity, specifically neuro-symbolic models that mimic the workings of the brain, including attention, memory, and reasoning, constitutes one of the most exciting paradigmatic changes in the field. These systems are based on ideas from neuroscience and psychology and were created to solve some of the problems with traditional machine learning. They can perceive more context, be human-like in their cognition when looking for threats, and make smart choices that become smarter over time (Chisty et al., 2022). However, even with the promise that these models hold, there are a variety of issues that need to be carefully considered to ensure that they are beneficial at scale, fair, and based on sound science. The future is multifaceted and transformative, from the technological challenges of building and running these systems to scientific and moral concerns.

One of the biggest challenges is making these systems work effectively at scale. Unlike traditional AI systems that use multiple computers to sort information at high rates, cognitive systems process information in a step-by-step situational fashion, which requires many resources. For example, trying to get a system to recall past experienced events or switch attention like human beings is incredibly computationally costly, much more so if performed on large networks with multiple users and computers. Simultaneously conducting complex reasoning on rules and neural data at the same time is quite demanding in terms of power, especially if the system must respond quickly. The system must process a large amount of data, retain past experiences, and make decisions based on different layers of human actions, the environment, and past dangers. Neuromorphic chips, which are intended to consume less power and process data like the brain, may be beneficial, but they are not yet mainstream. They also do not yet have the software and infrastructure in place for a model to be practically used. Another major issue is balancing the realism and practicality of these models. Models that mimic phenomena, such as the way brain cells learn or the way the brain learns with dopamine, can be intriguing but may not scale well or fit in with existing security systems. Making these models simple enough to fit into real systems without losing their human-like thinking ability is a delicate balancing act (Li et al., 2025). Today, most neuro-symbolic models utilize simplified forms of representing human thought, such as attention layers in AI models to represent attention or logical rules for representing decision-making. However, more advanced models that include time-dependent modifications or sophisticated memory systems may be too complicated for computers to handle. To scale these models, new software, new kinds of computer hardware, and system designs that focus on what is important and easy to interpret, as opposed to needing to copy the brain precisely, are required.

Equally important are the ethical considerations of having systems that observe and understand how people think and act. These frameworks create detailed user behavior profiles, including how they remember and make decisions. Although this detects suspicious activity, it also comes with consequential problems regarding privacy, if people provide their consent, and if their autonomy is upheld. Individuals may not realize that their habits, such as how they type and how long they take to click, are monitored to anticipate threats. There is a potential danger to its application other than its intended use, such as its use in spying on employees or making prejudiced decisions (Alwakeel, 2025). This stimulates the need for neuroethics, a set of instructions for ethically replicating mental states and actions in machines. The systems should be transparent, comprehensible, and allow users to ask questions regarding decisions. Although techniques such as federated learning and differential privacy can ensure privacy, a broader debate on what is ethical in monitoring behavior and thought must occur.

The intersection of brain-computer interface (BCI) research and brain imaging, such as fMRI, has produced a new and controversial area of cybersecurity. Certain experiments use brain imaging to augment threat detection by ascertaining how people make decisions under threat. For example, studies using EEG or fMRI have shown that specific regions of the brain are activated when people assess threats, feel emotions, or perceive suspicion. This can be used to help AI models predict more effectively when a person is about to fall victim to a cyber-attack (Patel and Shah, 2021). Live BCIs could help human analysts alert when the brain shows signs of being under stress or detect an anomaly before the person is even aware of it. Human-machine cooperation has vast potential, but at the same time, it stretches the boundaries of privacy and consent. At present, the use of BCIs or fMRI data in live cybersecurity is mostly at the research stage and is not yet widespread. These technologies are too invasive, expensive, and sensitive to be implemented beyond laboratories. The possibility of real-time tracking of brain activity for security purposes also raises enormous ethical and philosophical questions. Who controls this information? Can it be coerced by law or hacked? What rights do subjects have over their brain activity? As this research develops, strict ethical and legal standards will be necessary to help avoid abuse and make these systems beneficial rather than commanding.

In addition to near-term challenges, the future of neuromorphic cybersecurity is full of research questions that will shape the field for years to come. One of the key challenges is creating standardized benchmarks and evaluation metrics that are suited to neuro-symbolic systems (Alwakeel, 2025). Currently, measures tend to emphasize precision, recall, and speed but fail to indicate how good a system is at thinking like a human, how profound its reasoning is, or how in tune it is with human values. New measures must indicate how closely a system imitates human choices, how well it blends symbolic and neural reasoning, and how transparent and cooperative its output is. Developing these standards will require the involvement of AI, cognitive science, neuroscience, and cybersecurity specialists. The development of better memory architectures is another vast field of research. While traditional machine learning models simply need to recall facts, cognitive systems need to recall the context, intent, and past events in a way that makes sense across time. How should long-term memory be organized? How should memories be encoded, retrieved, and stored efficiently? How will the system be able to forget or generalize in a way that mimics human reasoning and not simply lose information? Solving these issues will require major breakthroughs in memory modeling, perhaps through hybrid systems that use neuromorphic memory circuits coupled with symbolic memory graphs or semantic networks.

Reasoning under uncertainty is another key area for breakthroughs. Humans work well in ambiguous situations, often deducing intent or risk from incomplete or conflicting information. Current neuro-symbolic systems have difficulty with ambiguity, especially when symbolic logic fails in the absence of information or conflicting rules. Probability-based logic and Bayesian systems might enable systems to reason about not only facts but also beliefs, confidence levels, and suggestive clues. When these methods are incorporated into neuro-symbolic systems, they become much more reliable in real-world situations where data tend to be dirty, limited, or misleading. Finally, the ability to learn and improve continuously is also essential (Firasta et al., 2024). In cybersecurity, obsolescent models become obsolete as new threats arise. Cognitive systems must continue to learn, not from new data, but from novel rules, changed behaviors, and nascent policies. Such flexibility without loss of stability or coherence presents a daunting challenge. Online learning, memory-related brain-inspired changes, and reinforcement learning are candidate solutions; however, one outstanding scalable solution remains to be achieved.

CONCLUSION

With every passing day, cyberattacks become more menacing, and the lines between machine intelligence, human psychology, and smart defense become increasingly blurred. The modern threat landscape is no longer limited to technology-based attacks and brute force. It consists of smart behaviors such as social engineering, mind influencing, using emotions to manipulate people, and insider behavior, each of which starts attacking the weakest link in any security system: the human user (Shafique, 2024). In this case, traditional machine learning methods, even with deep learning and large datasets, are not adequate to understand or cope with such human-oriented attacks. There is an unmistakable need for a new kind of solution, one that does not react to activity but truly understands behavior, intent, and context. Neuro-symbolic architectures, which are based on the way the brain works, provide a good solution to this need (Balasubramanian et al., 2024).

While the technology is advancing, there remain several open questions to be answered. One of them is developing standards that measure how much a system mimics human thought and understands threats; however, it is not enough to know how well it does statistically. How well can a system reason through ambiguous situations? Can it induce general rules for new types of behavior? Can it describe complex threat situations in a manner that is readily comprehensible to humans? Standardizing these will require collaboration between computer scientists, psychologists, ethicists, and security researchers. Another significant challenge is the development of continuous learning methods, such as the use of analyst-supplied reinforcement learning, to keep the system up to date with new types of threats. Implementing these methods so that they function without inducing instability or forgetting what the system learned is a challenging technical issue (Tariq, 2025). In the future, the combination of brain-computer interfaces, real-time EEG, and cognitive threat modeling is a desirable and controversial option. In laboratory experiments, researchers have used neural pattern activity to study how people react to phishing emails or emotionally provocative material. Although these methods are not yet ready for use in major businesses, they are promising for creating AI systems that can mold themselves based on human brain signals, such as stress, confusion, or doubt, to facilitate decision-making. This convergence of the brain and AI can change the way we sense threats, from systems that only react to systems that cooperate with humans. However, it also raises legitimate concerns about mental privacy, consent, and control. The more advanced the technology, the more important it is to support more regulation, policy, and public discourse to ensure that these technologies serve everyone is benefit.

In simple words, neuro-symbolic approaches to detecting cognitive attacks are a significant step forward in the field of cybersecurity. This is an advancement from pattern searching in data to behavior analysis using reasoning. By simulating the functioning of the human brain, such systems offer a fresh and powerful way to detect, characterize, and respond to threats that affect people's psychology, context, and reasoning (Onchis et al., 2023). Neuronal and symbolic integration allows for extensive analysis and clear explanations, and thinking and emotion models bring the system closer to human awareness. However, with such power, there must be responsibility. Ethical design, plainness, and human-centered thinking must be the foundation and not an afterthought. As these systems grow more sophisticated, they may convert cybersecurity from a reactive defense mechanism into a true thinking partner that thinks with us, reasons with us, and eventually helps us protect not just against code but against deception, coercion, and manipulation of the mind.

REFERENCES

Adabara, I., Olaniyi Sadiq, B., Nuhu Shuaibu, A., Ibarahim Danjuma, Y., & Venkateswarlu, M. (2025). A Review of Agentic AI in Cybersecurity: Cognitive Autonomy, Ethical Governance and Quantum-Resilient Defense. *F1000 Research.* PMID: 41169871

Aderu, N. (2025). AI-Driven Autonomous Middleware: Revolutionizing Enterprise IT Systems Management. *European Journal of Computer Science and Information Technology.*

AlOmar, B., & Trabelsi, Z. (2025). Integrating Generative AI into Cybersecurity Curricula. *2025 IEEE Global Engineering Education Conference (EDUCON),* (39),1-15, 2025

Alserhani, F. M. (2025). Intrusion Detection and Real-Time Adaptive Security in Medical Internet of Things Using a Cyber-Physical System Design. *Sensors (Basel),* •••, 25.

Alwakeel, M. (2025). Neuro-Driven Agent-Based Security for Quantum-Safe 6G Networks. *Mathematics, 13*(13), 2074. DOI: 10.3390/math13132074

Aragonés Lozano, M., Pérez Llopis, I., & Esteve Domingo, M. (2023). Threat hunting architecture using a machine learning approach for critical infrastructures protection. *Big Data and Cognitive Computing, 7*(2), 65.

Balasubramanian, P., Nazari, S., Kholgh, D.K., Mahmoodi, A.B., Seby, J., & Kostakos, P. (2024). TSTEM: A Cognitive Platform for Collecting Cyber Threat Intelligence in the Wild. *ArXiv, abs/2402.09973.*

Chisty, N. M. A., Baddam, P. R., & Amin, R. (2022). Strategic approaches to safeguarding the digital future: Insights into next-generation cybersecurity. *Engineering International, 10*(2), 69–84.

Firasta, S., Srivastava, Y. R., & Rao, V. (2024). Cognitive Detection of Anomalies in Autonomous In-Vehicle Network Communication. *2024 International Conference on Advancements in Power, Communication and Intelligent Systems (APCI),* 1-6.

Guan, Y., & Chen, Q. (2021). Research on Intelligent Perception and Cognitive Computing of Information Security System Based on Computer Big Data. *Wireless Communications and Mobile Computing, 3281825.* Advance online publication. DOI: 10.1155/2021/3281825

Guo, Y., Huo, P., Huang, S., Gou, G., & Li, Q. (2025). Multi-Receptor Skin with Highly Sensitive Tele-Perception Somatosensory Flexible Electronics in Healthcare: Multimodal Sensing and AI-Powered Diagnostics. *Advanced Healthcare Materials*, •••, 2502901. PMID: 40619754

Hakim, S. B., Adil, M., Velasquez, A., Xu, S., & Song, H. H. (2025). Neuro-Symbolic AI for Cybersecurity: State of the Art, Challenges, and Opportunities. *arXiv preprint arXiv:2509.06921.*

Li, M., Laiu, P., Nichols, J. A., Huettel, M., Sikkema, I., Mathur, M., Hollifield, S., & Hankins, M. (2025). Cognitive IoT and Edge Computing for Intrusion Detection with Federated TinyML. *2025 IEEE World AI IoT Congress (AIIoT)*, 0677-0684.

Li, W., Meng, W., Kwok, L., & Ip, H. H. (2017). Developing advanced fingerprint attacks on challenge-based collaborative intrusion detection networks. *Cluster Computing*, *21*, 299–310.

Nalluri, S., Malyala, M. M., Kandagiri, H., & Kandagiri, K. K. (2025, June). Nscti: A hybrid neuro-symbolic framework for ai-driven predictive cyber threat intelligence. In *2025 4th International Conference on Computational Modelling, Simulation and Optimization (ICCMSO)* (pp. 14-21). IEEE.

Nazir, A., & Khan, R.A. (2019). Combinatorial Optimization based Feature Selection Method: A study on Network Intrusion Detection. *ArXiv, abs/1906.04494.*

Neelaveni, R., Sridevi, B., & Sivasankari, J. (2022). Securing Privacy Using Optimization and Statistical Models in Cognitive Radio Networks. *Computer Systems Science and Engineering*, *42*(2).

Onchis, D. M., Gillich, G. R., Hogea, E., & Tufisi, C. (2023). Neuro-symbolic model for cantilever beams damage detection. *Computers in Industry*, *151*, 103991.

Parisa, S. K., & Banerjee, S. (2024). AI-Enabled Cloud Security Solutions: A Comparative Review of Traditional vs. Next-Generation Approaches. *International Journal of Statistical Computation and Simulation*, *16*(1).

Patel, J., & Shah, H. (2021). Creating Safe and Secure AI-From Computer Design to Cloud Technology. *International Research. Journal of Engineering and Applied Sciences (Asian Research Publishing Network)*, *9*(4), 10–55083.

Ravi Kumar, M., Jain, U., Francis, F., Senthil Kumar, S., Adhvaryu, R., & Natrayan, L. (2024). Cognitive Digital Twin Systems for Predictive Security in AI-Enhanced IoT Environments. *2024 First International Conference on Software, Systems and Information Technology (SSITCON)*, 1-6.

Seng, K. P., & Ang, L. M. (2022). Embedded intelligence: State-of-the-art and research challenges. *IEEE Access : Practical Innovations, Open Solutions*, *10*, 59236–59258.

Shafique, M. (2024). A Cross-Layer Approach to Energy-Efficient and Secure EdgeAI: Architectures, Systems and Applications. *2024 5th CPSSI International Symposium on Cyber-Physical Systems (Applications and Theory) (CPSAT)*, 1-1.

Singh, A. (2024). Toward Robust and Scalable Wireless Ad Hoc Networks: An Approach to Adaptive Routing and Security. *2024 12th International Conference on Intelligent Systems and Embedded Design (ISED)*, 1-6.

Tariq, M. (Ed.). (2025c). *Emerging multisector applications of AI and IoT*. IGI Global., DOI: 10.4018/979-8-3373-4332-7

KEY TERMS AND DEFINITIONS

Affective Computing: Perceiving emotional states through digital behavior.

Cognitive Load Estimation: Assessing user's mental effort in real time.

Episodic Memory Modeling: Simulating personal behavioral history for contextual remembrance.

Chapter 7
Neuroscience-Enhanced AI for Real-Time Behavioral Anomaly Detection in Cybersecurity

Uddalak Mitra
https://orcid.org/0000-0002-5682-5218
JIS College of Engineering, India

Shafiq Ul Rehman
https://orcid.org/0000-0003-2266-218X
Kingdom University, Bahrain

ABSTRACT

Traditional rule-based intrusion detection systems are difficult in real time as cyber threats become more dynamic and customized. Neuroscience-based AI approach can provide a potent paradigm for identifying unusual behavior in cyberspace, drawing inspiration from the human brain's capacity for quick learning, pattern recognition, and behavioral adaptation. For detecting malicious activity in real time, this chapter examines how cognitive and neural principles—such as working memory, attention filtering, and behavioral conditioning—can be computationally modeled. The chapter suggests architectures and learning mechanisms that imitate how people recognize and respond to new threats by referencing disciplines such as affective neuroscience, behavioral biometrics, and neural plasticity. Detecting insider threats, social engineering attempts, and zero-day exploits based on departures from known behavioral patterns are examples of real-world applications.

DOI: 10.4018/979-8-3373-5012-7.ch007

1. INTRODUCTION

The digital age has rendered organizations more exposed to cyberthreats that are becoming more complicated and focused on people, in addition to making things easier and more linked than ever before (Rayhan, A. (2024), Sendjaja, T. et al. (2024), Malik, W., & Gul, S. (2024), Widjaja, G. (2025)). Attackers today take advantage of users' and systems' behavioral and psychological flaws in addition to technical ones. The threat landscape is now dominated by tactics like phishing, social engineering, and insider manipulation (Okika, N. et al. (2025) Gururaj, H. L. et al. (2024), Panda, S. P. (2025)), where malicious intent frequently lurks behind patterns of everyday activity. Traditional security measures, such as static rules, pre-established signatures, or heuristic thresholds, are therefore failing to identify these dynamic, context-sensitive attacks (Barsallo Yi, E. A., et al (2024), Sutaria, K. et al. (2025, April), Bhaware, A. et al (2024)).

Because both the human brain and cyberspace function in dynamic, data-rich environments that necessitate ongoing perception, adaptation, and learning, they are both equally complex. The emergence of neuroscience-based artificial intelligence (AI), an interdisciplinary approach that models neural and cognitive mechanisms to improve real-time behavioral anomaly detection (Rezaee, K. et al (2024), Liu R. et al (2024), Ajayi, A. M. et al (2024)), has been spurred by this parallel. Researchers hope to create AI systems that can replicate the human brain's extraordinary capacity to recognize anomalies, decipher contextual cues, and react adaptively to ambiguous circumstances by utilizing knowledge from cognitive science, psychology, and neuroscience (Boskovic, I., Perera, N., & Otgaar, H. (2025)).

Conventional security information and event management (SIEM) and intrusion detection systems (IDS) rely heavily on preprogrammed rules or known attack signatures (Gadicha, V. B. et al (2025). Ramalingam, R. et al (2025). Sashwin, K. et al (2024)). Although they work well against threats that are recurring and well-defined, they are ineffective against new or evolving attacks that take advantage of undiscovered flaws or subtly depart from typical behavior. High false-positive rates are frequently produced by these systems, overwhelming analysts, and slowing down incident responses. Instead of depending only on pre-labeled attack data, neuroscience-enhanced AI presents an adaptive, perception-driven paradigm that continuously learns, and changes based on observed behavior (Zhao, W. et al. (2025), Luo et al., 2025).

Fundamentally, cybersecurity that draws inspiration from neuroscience aims to mimic the cognitive processes of the human brain, including working memory, pattern recognition, predictive processing, and selective attention. By continuously making predictions and modifying them in response to feedback, the human brain is able to identify even the smallest departures from expected behavior, whether in social interactions or environmental cues. By converting these capabilities into computational models, AI systems can monitor behavior continuously, spot anomalies instantly, and distinguish between harmless irregularities and potentially harmful behavior (Abdelkader et al., 2024).

A model inspired by neuroscience, for example, might be able to learn about a user's usual login procedures, data access routines, and communication frequency. Based on the principles of predictive coding, the system detects a discrepancy between expected and observed behavior when the same user starts transferring large files at odd times or logging in to unknown servers. Like how the human brain signals attention when it encounters an unexpected sensory stimulus, it then flags the event for additional examination. In addition to improving threat detection, this strategy makes it possible to proactively defend against targeted social engineering attacks, insider threats, and zero-day exploits (KRITIKA, 2025).

Problem Statement:

Traditional cybersecurity systems struggle to detect adaptive, behavior-driven threats such as insider attacks, social engineering, and zero-day exploits. These systems rely heavily on static signatures and predefined rules, making them ineffective in environments where malicious intent hides within normal user activity patterns.

Research Gap:

Although machine learning–based anomaly detection has improved threat identification, existing models lack cognitive adaptability, contextual awareness, and the ability to interpret user intent. There is limited research on applying neuroscience principles—such as working memory, predictive coding, and neural plasticity—to create AI systems capable of real-time, human-like behavioral interpretation. This chapter addresses this gap by exploring how neuroscience-inspired computational models can enhance behavioral anomaly detection in cybersecurity.

1.1 The Shift Toward Human-Centric Cybersecurity

Historically, cybersecurity has been a technology-driven field that focuses on protecting data, networks, and systems. But as digital ecosystems grow, people have become the most important sensor in the defence chain as well as its weakest link. Many modern attacks use contextual deception and psychological manipulation to take advantage of human behaviour rather than technical shortcomings. As a result, cybersecurity has changed from being solely a technical field to one that is focused on people, where knowledge of behavioural and cognitive aspects is crucial for efficient defence.

The theoretical underpinnings for comprehending these human aspects are provided by neuroscience. Ideas like emotional control, attention filtering, and decision-making biases provide information about how people react to dangers and how hackers take advantage of cognitive constraints. Cybersecurity systems can better understand human behavior and adjust to real-world situations involving uncertainty, deceit, and emotional influence by incorporating these insights into AI models (Hinrichs et al., 304).

Additionally, by combining behavioral and affective modeling, AI systems are able to evaluate users' actions as well as their motivations. This move to cognitive-contextual security greatly improves the system's capacity to identify minute indications of compromise and permits more sophisticated threat analysis. Reactive threat mitigation in cybersecurity is replaced by proactive threat anticipation in such intelligence-driven systems.

Table 1. Traditional IDS vs. Neuroscience-Inspired AI for Behavioral Anomaly Detection

Feature / Capability	Traditional IDS (Rule/Signature-Based)	Neuroscience-Inspired AI Systems
Learning Ability	Static rules; no adaptive learning	Continuous learning via neural plasticity
Detection of Unknown Threats	Weak (depends on known signatures)	Strong (predictive coding + anomaly detection)
Context Awareness	Low (focus on events/logs only)	High (behavioral, affective, cognitive cues)
False Positives	High due to rigid rules	Lower due to contextual interpretation
Real-Time Adaptation	Limited	Dynamic adaptation, working-memory-based
Human-Like Reasoning	No	Modeled using attention and affective processing

1.2 Neuroscience as an Enabling Paradigm for AI

A paradigm shift from computational efficiency to cognitive adaptability is represented by the convergence of neuroscience and AI. Like the human brain processes sensory input, neuroscience-inspired AI models learn continuously, modify their internal representations, and prioritize pertinent information, whereas traditional machine learning concentrates on static optimization of parameters for tasks. Mechanisms like neural plasticity, reinforcement learning, and predictive modeling enable systems to adapt to changing environments and user roles by changing their perception of "normal" behavior (Sarker, 2024).

Employees may eventually switch departments, access new databases, or implement different workflows in a corporate setting, for instance. Such changes would be incorrectly classified as anomalies by a static machine learning model that was trained on historical behavioral data. In contrast, a system inspired by neuroscience would gradually modify its internal model through online learning and ongoing retraining, making sure that typical behavioral drift doesn't result in false alarms. Long-term stability and dependability in intricate, high-volume network environments are made possible by this flexibility.

The idea of hierarchical processing, in which sensory inputs are processed at several levels of abstraction before producing a decision, is another significant contribution of neuroscience to AI. This is like deep learning architectures, which refine input representations through a series of hidden layers. Nonetheless, neuro-inspired systems can strike a balance between automation and interpretability by establishing this structure in cognitive theory, which is a crucial prerequisite for explainable AI in cybersecurity (Abdelkader et al., 2024).

1.3 Objectives and Scope of the Chapter

The theoretical underpinnings, architectures, and applications of neuroscience-enhanced AI for real-time behavioral anomaly detection in cybersecurity are examined in this chapter. It seeks to give a thorough explanation of how ideas from cognitive and affective neuroscience can be computationally modeled to identify suspicious or malevolent behavior. In particular, the chapter

1. Explores key neuroscientific principles relevant to behavioural modelling, including attention, memory, prediction, and neural plasticity.
2. Examine system architectures that incorporate these principles through recurrent, spiking, and neuro-symbolic networks.
3. Presents practical applications and case studies, such as insider threat detection, real-time monitoring in critical systems, and behavioural biometrics.
4. Discusses ethical, explainability, and human-factor considerations essential for responsible deployment.
5. Outlines future research directions, including neuromorphic computing, multimodal data fusion, and cognitive privacy.

By combining knowledge from computer science, cognitive neuroscience, behavioural psychology, and ethics, the conversation emphasizes the field's interdisciplinary nature. The chapter highlights that systems that think, learn, and adapt similarly to the human brain are the way of the future for cybersecurity by comparing neural mechanisms to computational intelligence.

1.4 Significance and Contributions

The discussion highlights the interdisciplinary nature of the field by fusing insights from computer science, cognitive neuroscience, behavioral psychology, and ethics. By drawing up a comparison between neural mechanisms and computational intelligence, the chapter emphasizes that cybersecurity will be dominated by systems that think, learn, and adapt similarly to the human brain.

Additionally, incorporating human cognitive models into cybersecurity promotes improved communication between AI systems and human analysts. AI systems become more logical, understandable, and reliable when their reasoning is in line with human cognitive processes. These developments are particularly pertinent in fields like healthcare, aviation, and national defence where vital resources or human lives are at risk.

The future of cybersecurity is essentially represented by neuroscience-enhanced AI, which combines computational accuracy with biological intelligence. As this chapter will show, the application of neuroscience principles—attention, memory, prediction, emotion, and learning—can result in real-time perception, adaptation, and response from cyber defense systems, providing a significant step toward security infrastructures that are truly intelligent and human-aligned.

2. NEUROSCIENCE FOUNDATIONS OF BEHAVIOURAL MODELLING

One of the most intricate adaptive systems in science is the human brain, which can recognize patterns, make predictions, and react instantly to abnormalities. Modern artificial intelligence can model adaptive and context-aware behavior thanks to the theoretical and biological underpinnings provided by neuroscience. These insights serve as the foundation for cybersecurity systems that identify deviations from learned behavioral norms rather than static rule matching to identify malicious intent (Kritika, 2024). Designing AI systems with cognitive flexibility, contextual understanding, and quick decision-making is made feasible by taking inspiration from human perception, learning, and response to their surroundings.

2.1 Attention and Selective Perception

The brain's capacity to filter out irrelevant noise and concentrate attention on pertinent stimuli is one of its most important roles. Neural networks involving the parietal lobes, thalamus, and prefrontal cortex facilitate this process by coordinating selective perception and cognitive focus. Similar attention mechanisms can be applied in cybersecurity to give priority to activities or events that significantly depart from predetermined behavioral baselines (Sarker, 2024). An attention-based anomaly detector might give a user a higher risk score, for example, if they log in from an unfamiliar location, access sensitive data outside of regular business hours, or move their mouse erratically.

This process can be replicated by deep learning models like transformer architectures and attention-based recurrent neural networks. They increase the precision and interpretability of anomaly detection by dynamically allocating computational resources to the features that have the greatest impact on prediction. Focusing on the behavioral "outliers" that are most likely to indicate dangers, attention mechanisms essentially enable AI systems to function as a digital counterpart of the human brain's vigilance system.

2.2 Memory and Pattern Recognition

Humans can store experiences and identify patterns over time thanks to the hippocampus and surrounding medial temporal lobe structures (Hinrichs et al., 2024). This memory function is essential for distinguishing between known and unknown behavior, a process that is directly related to cybersecurity behavioral modeling. AI systems can create memory-based models of user behavior that change over time by mimicking this functionality. This allows them to recognize patterns in typical activity while also keeping an eye out for new deviations.

Recurrent neural networks (RNNs), long short-term memory (LSTM) networks, and temporal convolutional networks (TCNs), which are highly effective at identifying temporal dependencies in sequential data, can be used to computationally model this function. These networks are able to monitor user action sequences, including command-line executions, file access patterns, and login attempts, and identify odd patterns that deviate from learned norms. Pattern recognition and temporal memory are combined to create models that are contextually adaptive and historically informed.

2.3 Prediction and Error Monitoring

Predictive coding, which is the process of continuously creating expectations and identifying discrepancies between expected and actual outcomes, is another essential cognitive mechanism in the human brain (Abdelkader et al., 2024). Prediction errors indicate the need for behavioral modification or attention. Predictive behavioral models work similarly in AI-based cybersecurity, predicting user behavior, and identifying abnormalities when observed behavior deviates from expectations.

Another crucial cognitive mechanism in the human brain is predictive coding, which is the process of consistently generating expectations and detecting differences between expected and actual outcomes (Abdelkader et al., 2024). The need for attention or behavioral change is indicated by prediction of errors. In AI-based cybersecurity, predictive behavioral models function similarly, forecasting user behavior and spotting anomalies when observed behavior deviates from expectations' behavior and identifying abnormalities when observed behavior deviates from expectations.

2.4 Emotional and Affective Processing

Human perception and reaction to threats are significantly influenced by emotional intelligence. To decide whether an observed stimulus indicates danger or safety, the amygdala and prefrontal cortex coordinate affective evaluation and decision-making. Modeling affective states and behavioral cues that could indicate stress, urgency, or dishonesty is necessary to translate this into AI (KRITIKA, 2025). Increased typing speed variability or odd cursor movement patterns, for example, may be indicative of psychological stress or malevolent intent in user interaction systems.

Frameworks for measuring these phenomena are offered by affective computing, a branch of artificial intelligence that simulates human emotion and motivation. AI can better understand user intent and distinguish between benign anomalies and real threats by incorporating affective features into anomaly detection systems.

2.5 Neural Plasticity and Adaptive Learning

Neural plasticity, the brain's capacity to rearrange itself by creating new neural connections, is essential to lifelong learning. Adaptive machine learning models that can update their internal representations in real time are inspired by this biological principle (Dangi et al., 2023). This adaptability is mirrored by federated learning architectures, reinforcement learning, and online learning algorithms, which allow systems to change as new behavioural data becomes available without requiring total retraining.

In situations where historical datasets might not contain novel attack signatures, adaptive AI systems improve resilience against zero-day exploits. These systems stay relevant and resilient in changing environments by constantly adjusting their behavioral models.

All things considered, neuroscience offers a wealth of conceptual tools for simulating human-like adaptability in artificial intelligence. Building cybersecurity systems with learning, contextual awareness, and dynamic reasoning—the characteristics of biological intelligence—becomes feasible by converting neural processes like attention, prediction, and adaptation into computational frameworks.

Table 2. Mapping Neuroscience Principles to AI Techniques

Neuroscience Concept	Cognitive Role	Equivalent AI/ML Technique	Application in Cybersecurity
Attention Mechanism	Focus on relevant stimuli	Transformers, attention layers	Prioritizing risky user actions
Working Memory	Short-term processing	RNN/LSTM memory cells	Tracking sequential user behavior
Predictive Coding	Anticipation & error correction	Forecasting models, anomaly scoring	Detecting deviations from expected patterns
Neural Plasticity	Continuous learning	Online learning, reinforcement learning	Adapting to behavior drift over time
Affective Processing	Emotion-based decision cues	Affective computing models	Distinguishing stress-induced errors vs. malicious intent

3. ARCHITECTURES FOR REAL-TIME BEHAVIOURAL ANOMALY DETECTION

Effective real-time behavioral anomaly detection systems, which are based on neuroscientific principles, need architectures that have the capacity to perceive, learn, and act on their own. These systems combine neural-inspired learning models, feedback mechanisms for ongoing adaptation, and multi-source data acquisition. The system's explainability, scalability, and responsiveness are all determined by its architectural design.

3.1 Data Acquisition and Preprocessing

Data, including network traffic, system logs, biometric signals, keystroke dynamics, and mouse movements, forms the basis of any behavioral anomaly detection system (Sarker, 2024). Continuous behavioral monitoring is made possible by the real-time collection of these data streams, and this is crucial for identifying abnormalities as soon as they arise. To guarantee that behavioral patterns are represented in a format appropriate for learning algorithms, data preprocessing techniques include dimensionality reduction, feature extraction, and normalization.

Like how the human brain's sensory processing pathways filter and encode sensory inputs before interpreting them, cybersecurity systems also need to preprocess raw data to find significant features. This is where neuroscience provides analogies. Latent behavioral structures can be extracted from high-dimensional data with the aid of methods like variational inference, autoencoders, and principal component analysis (PCA).

3.2 Neuro-Inspired Learning Models

Learning models that mimic neural processes are at the heart of architecture. For the analysis of sequential and temporal data, recurrent neural networks (RNNs), long short-term memory (LSTM) units, and spiking neural networks (SNNs) are especially useful. SNNs can simulate fine-grained temporal dependencies, which makes them appropriate for real-time anomaly detection. Their timing is modeled after that of biological neurons (Kritika, 2024). These models can identify patterns of behavior that take place over milliseconds, like irregularities in keystrokes or packet transmission.

Neuro-symbolic architectures blend neural learning and symbolic reasoning in addition to strictly data-driven models. By combining high-level contextual rules with low-level behavioral data, this hybrid approach enables systems to achieve both explainability and adaptability. For example, a neuro-symbolic intrusion detection system might use symbolic logic to reason access control policies and deep learning to extract behavioral embeddings.

3.3 Affective and Cognitive State Integration

A deeper comprehension of user intent and context is made possible by incorporating affective and cognitive modeling into system architectures. This is comparable to how the prefrontal cortex of the brain integrates emotion and cognition (Hinrichs et al., 2024). AI systems can more accurately determine whether a behavioral deviation represents malicious activity or a harmless anomaly by considering contextual cues, such as task difficulty, workload, or environmental stressors.

A cybersecurity monitoring tool might notice, for instance, that a worker experiencing a high cognitive load might type slowly or respond slowly. Using affective-state modelling, the system can contextualize such behaviour instead of setting off false alarms, lowering false positives while preserving vigilance.

3.4 Feedback Loops and Adaptive Learning

AI systems need feedback loops for ongoing learning and performance optimization, just as neural circuits depend on feedback mechanisms to improve behavior. In response to changing data distributions, adaptive feedback allows the system to modify detection thresholds, retrain models, and recalibrate decision boundaries (Abdelkader et al., 2024). Through reward-based feedback, reinforcement learning algorithms optimize decision-making in a computational parallel to this process.

In actual use, this feedback-driven learning helps the system adjust to new devices, users, and operating environments. For instance, by fine-tuning its weights using real-time reinforcement signals, a behavioural model trained on the access patterns of one department can adapt to the routine of another.

3.5 System Architecture Overview

A typical neuroscience-inspired anomaly detection architecture may include:

1. **Data Collection Layer:** Gathers behavioural, contextual, and biometric data in real time.
2. **Preprocessing Layer:** Normalizes, encodes, and reduces noise in raw input.
3. **Learning and Modelling Layer:** Employs RNNs, SNNs, or neuro-symbolic models for behaviour modelling.
4. **Decision Layer:** Applies contextual reasoning and probabilistic inference to classify behaviour as normal or anomalous.
5. **Feedback and Adaptation Layer:** Continuously refines the system through online learning and reinforcement mechanisms.

This multi-layered framework mirrors the hierarchical processing structure of the human brain—from sensory input to higher-order decision-making—providing a biologically inspired blueprint for cyber defence systems.

Figure 1. Neuroscience-Inspired Anomaly Detection System Architecture

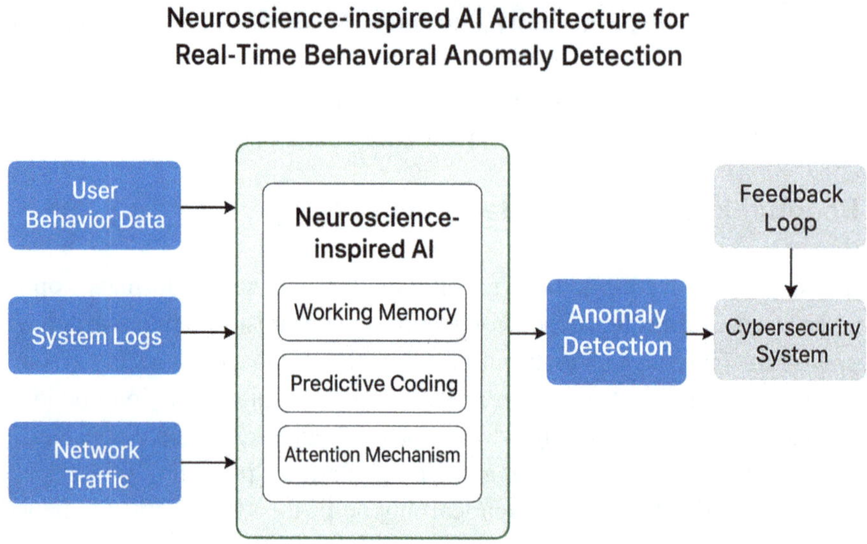

3.6 Limitations and Practical Challenges

Despite their adaptability, neuroscience-inspired AI systems face several challenges. These models require large, diverse behavioural datasets, which are often difficult to collect due to privacy concerns. Neuro-inspired architectures such as spiking neural networks remain computationally expensive for real-time deployment at scale. Another limitation lies in the complexity of integrating affective or cognitive signals without introducing noise or bias. Furthermore, behavioural baselines can vary widely across organizations, reducing generalization. These challenges suggest that while neuroscience-enhanced AI is promising, its real-world deployment must address scalability, data governance, and interpretability constraints.

4. CASE STUDIES AND APPLICATIONS

Enterprise networks, critical infrastructure, and healthcare are just a few of the fields where neuroscience-inspired AI systems are being used in practice for behavioral anomaly detection. The case studies that follow demonstrate how neuro-inspired architectures can increase automated cybersecurity systems' trustworthiness, decrease response latency, and improve detection accuracy.

4.1 Insider Threat Detection in Enterprise Networks

One of the most challenging issues in cybersecurity is insider threats, which frequently involve malicious activity by authorized users. Such behavior is difficult for traditional signature-based systems to detect. Individual user profiles can be learned by neuroscience-enhanced models, which can then identify minute variations that could be signs of insider threats (KRITIKA, 2025).

An employee may be flagged as anomalous if they suddenly access a lot of private files, try to copy data to external storage, or use systems that are not typical for their position. Administrators can be warned before serious harm is done by adaptive models that use recurrent neural architectures to capture the temporal patterns of these activities. Furthermore, systems can identify behavioral stress that might precede malevolent intent by incorporating affective features like typing hesitation or extended inactivity.

4.2 Real-Time Monitoring in Critical Infrastructure and Healthcare

Real-time anomaly detection is crucial to preventing cascading failures in high-stakes settings like energy systems, healthcare facilities, and airplanes. AI systems with a neuroscience foundation can simulate operator behavior and physiological reactions to identify indicators of weariness, stress, or distraction that could jeopardize safety (Abdelkader et al., 2024).

For instance, behavioral biometrics like eye tracking, hand movement rhythm, or EEG-based attention signals can be examined in a smart healthcare setting to identify compromised accounts or illegal system access. By warning operators when their cognitive state may affect their ability to make decisions, these models not only improve security but also foster human-machine cooperation.

4.3 Behavioural Biometrics and Multi-Factor Authentication

Continuous, non-intrusive authentication methods are offered by behavioral biometrics, such as keystroke dynamics, gait recognition, or touchscreen gestures. These systems can identify behavioral patterns that may be signs of impersonation or compromised credentials when they are modeled using AI inspired by neuroscience (Dangi et al., 2023).

Behavioral biometrics allow for continuous verification, guaranteeing that the authenticated user stays the same during a session, in contrast to conventional authentication techniques that depend on static credentials. This method greatly improves defenses against account hijacking, phishing, and credential theft.

4.4 Simulation-Based Evaluation of Neuro-Inspired IDS

Controlled environments that mimic actual attack scenarios are necessary for evaluating behavioural anomaly detection systems. To test the robustness of a system, simulation platforms can simulate user behaviour under various operational contexts, affective states, and cognitive loads. According to studies, neuro-inspired architectures perform better than traditional models at spotting subtle and changing attack patterns, especially in noisy settings (Sarker, 2024).

Additionally, by facilitating the creation of uniform performance evaluation benchmarks, these simulations promote cross-domain comparison and the reproducibility of study findings.

5. EXPLAINABILITY, ETHICS, AND HUMAN FACTORS

Concerns about user autonomy, privacy, and transparency are becoming increasingly important as artificial intelligence (AI) systems are integrated into cybersecurity infrastructures. Further layers of ethical complexity are introduced by neuroscience-based AI systems, which simulate elements of human cognition and decision-making. These systems may violate people's privacy and cognitive freedom because they not only identify abnormalities but also interpret behavioral and occasionally affective data. Therefore, the cornerstones of neuro-inspired cybersecurity must be explainability, ethical protections, and human-centered design.

5.1 The Need for Explainable AI in Security Contexts

The ability of a system to make its decision-making process intelligible to humans is known as explainability in AI. Knowing why a system has flagged a specific behavior as anomalous is essential in high-stakes situations like cybersecurity, where inaccurate classifications can result in false accusations, system outages, or data breaches (Sarker, 2024).

Conventional deep learning models frequently operate as "black boxes," making it challenging for analysts to follow their logic. However, models inspired by neuroscience present chances for interpretability with a biological foundation. Like how neuroscientists track neural activations in the brain, attention mechanisms, for instance, can graphically show which behavioral characteristics influence a model's choice. Security analysts can defend or dispute automated alerts thanks to methods like feature attribution and layer-wise relevance propagation, which further improve interpretability.

Additionally, explainability is essential for building human-AI trust. Security experts are more likely to trust systems whose logic makes sense to them. By allowing expert review of AI decisions, this "human-in-the-loop" design approach fosters a cooperative ecosystem where artificial intelligence and human cognition enhance rather than replace one another.

5.2 Ethical Challenges in Neuroscience-Enhanced Cybersecurity

Real-world incidents highlight these concerns. For example, continuous behavioral monitoring in workplaces may unintentionally reveal workers' stress levels or emotional states, which falls under "sensitive personal data" according to GDPR. Regulations such as the EU's AI Act and OECD AI Principles require transparency, clear consent processes, and strict limitations on behavioral and biometric surveillance. Neuro-data, such as cognitive or affective signals, is considered even more sensitive, raising concerns regarding neuro-rights and mental privacy.

Particularly regarding privacy, consent, and bias, the application of behavioral and neuro-inspired AI presents special ethical challenges. These systems may record private data about users' routines, emotions, or stress levels because they frequently depend on ongoing behavioral monitoring. Such data could be misused or exploited in the absence of appropriate safeguards, raising concerns about psychological profiling or even surveillance (Hinrichs et al., 2024).

Furthermore, discriminatory results may arise from biases in training data. An anomaly detection system may mistakenly identify the behaviors of people from other groups as abnormal, for example, if it is primarily trained on data from one demographic group. Fairness, data anonymization, and representativeness must thus be given top priority in model design and assessment for ethical AI frameworks.

Cognitive autonomy raises additional ethical issues. Users may feel manipulated or judged by automated decisions if AI systems start to interpret or predict human emotional states. Transparency regarding the kinds of data being examined and the applications of the findings is therefore crucial. Data ownership, informed consent, and the limits of behavioral analytics in public and workplace cybersecurity settings must all be covered by policy frameworks.

Table 3. Key Ethical Risks and Mitigation Strategies

Ethical / Privacy Risk	Description	Recommended Mitigation Strategy
Behavioral Surveillance	Continuous monitoring may feel intrusive	Transparent consent, minimal data collection
Cognitive Privacy	Affective/biometric cues may reveal emotions	Compliance with neuro-rights and GDPR-like laws
Bias in Anomaly Detection	Models may misclassify certain groups	Diverse datasets, fairness auditing
Misuse of Neuro-Data	Stress/intent inference can be exploited	Strict encryption and access control
Lack of Explainability	Black-box decisions harm trust	Use XAI, attention visualizations, human-in-the-loop

5.3 Human-Centered Design and Neurotics

According to KRITIKA (2025), human-centered design places a strong emphasis on matching AI systems to users' ethical standards, emotional comfort, and cognitive processes. The way users interact with adaptive technologies, perceive feedback, and trust system alerts must all be considered by neuroscience-based AI. Users may oppose adoption or discover workarounds that lessen system efficacy if they believe AI-driven surveillance infringes upon their privacy or autonomy.

A useful lens for assessing these systems is provided by neurotics, the area of ethics that studies the ramifications of researching and modifying the brain. It guarantees that neuroscience-based technologies improve rather than impair human well-being by highlighting the concepts of beneficence, nonmaleficence, and autonomy (Abdelkader et al., 2024). Designing AI systems that protect mental privacy, refrain from needless emotional inference, and uphold transparency about their cognitive modeling methods are all part of applying neuroethical principles to cybersecurity.

Policy frameworks such as GDPR, the proposed EU AI Act, and UNESCO AI Ethics Guidelines emphasize fairness, accountability, and the protection of cognitive liberty. Applying these frameworks ensures that neuro-inspired detection systems maintain ethical boundaries while enabling effective threat mitigation.

5.4 Human-in-the-Loop and Collaborative Learning

The human-in-the-loop (HITL) paradigm is a promising strategy to address these interpretability and ethical issues. In HITL systems, AI and human analysts engage in a feedback loop where expert input is used to improve decisions. By fusing intentional reasoning (human oversight) with reflexive pattern detection (AI automation), this interaction mimics the brain's hybrid structure of automated and conscious processes.

By working together, AI systems can improve accuracy and ethical compliance by learning from human corrections. Analysts could confirm or reject anomalies that have been flagged, and the system takes these choices into account when optimizing its models. This procedure guarantees that AI develops in accordance with human values and organizational ethics while also enhancing transparency and accountability.

6. FUTURE DIRECTIONS AND CHALLENGES

A revolutionary change in how cybersecurity systems view and react to threats is represented by neuroscience-enhanced AI. But to reach its full potential, several operational, ethical, and technical issues must be resolved. This multidisciplinary field's future depends on integrating machine learning, cognitive psychology, neuroscience, and human-computer interaction into coherent, implementable frameworks.

6.1 Integration of Multimodal Neuro-Data

New developments in neurotechnology create opportunities for incorporating biological signals, like heart rate variability, eye tracking, or EEG, into systems that detect behavioural abnormalities. Richer insights into user states, such as weariness, stress, or intent, can be obtained from these data sources (Kritika, 2024). For instance, systems may be able to distinguish between intentional malevolent behaviour and unintentional anomalies by integrating behavioural biometrics with EEG-based attention measures.

However, there are issues with data sensitivity, storage, and privacy when using neurophysiological data. Neural data, in contrast to traditional system logs, are extremely private and frequently disclose emotional and cognitive states. To preserve users' mental privacy while allowing adaptive learning, future systems must guarantee secure encryption, edge-based processing, and anonymization protocols.

6.2 Neuromorphic and Edge Implementations

The use of neuromorphic computing—hardware architectures that mimic the composition and operation of biological neurons—is one of the most exciting avenues for neuroscience-inspired AI. According to Dangi et al. (2023), neuromorphic chips, like IBM's TrueNorth or Intel's Loihi, are made to process data using low-power spiking networks and event-driven computation. These chips could lower latency and energy consumption in cybersecurity by enabling real-time anomaly detection right at the network edge.

For Internet of Things (IoT) ecosystems, where resource-constrained devices need lightweight yet adaptable security mechanisms, edge-based neuromorphic AI is especially useful. Such systems can further reduce privacy risks by preventing the transmission of sensitive behavioral data to centralized servers by enabling localized learning and detection.

6.3 Data Labelling and Transfer Learning

Data labeling is a significant obstacle in the detection of behavioral anomalies. Anomalies differ from traditional classification problems in that they are uncommon, varied, and context specific. Labeled data is necessary for supervised learning models, but creating cybersecurity-specific datasets is difficult and frequently impractical. Promising alternatives are provided by semi-supervised and unsupervised learning techniques, particularly those influenced by self-supervised neural dynamics and predictive coding (Hinrichs et al., 2024).

Another method that enables models trained in one domain to adapt to another is transfer learning. For instance, with little retraining, an anomaly detector homed in a business setting could be adjusted for use in financial or healthcare systems. This adaptability is consistent with the neural principle of generalization, which states that learned representations can be used in new contexts.

6.4 Standardization and Interoperability

Most behavioral anomaly detection systems currently use proprietary architectures and datasets, making it difficult to compare performance or ensure reproducibility. Standardized benchmarks and interoperability frameworks are necessary for neuroscience-based cybersecurity to advance beyond research and into industry-wide adoption (Sarker, 2024).

For anomaly detection tasks, future research should concentrate on creating shared taxonomies, standardized evaluation procedures, and open-source datasets. Furthermore, establishing moral principles and compliance requirements for neuro-inspired systems requires cooperation between academia, the government, and business.

6.5 Cross-Domain and Multimodal Fusion

Future systems must integrate data from multiple domains, including behavioural, contextual, and physiological data, to achieve holistic threat detection as cyber threats become more complex. A more complete picture of user intent and risk can be obtained by combining text-based communications, biometric signals, and network telemetry in multimodal fusion models (Abdelkader et al., 2024).

For example, integrating system log analysis with eye-tracking data may uncover automated or inattentive behavior suggestive of an automated bot intrusion or phishing attack. The brain's capacity to combine multiple senses for situational awareness is mirrored by this type of cross-domain fusion.

6.6 Ethical Governance and Policy Development

Responsible deployment cannot be ensured by technological innovation alone. Policymakers and future researchers must collaborate to create moral and legal guidelines that control the gathering, handling, and interpretation of behavioural and neuro-data. As neurotechnology becomes more common, the idea of digital neuro-rights—the right to mental privacy and cognitive liberty—is gaining traction (KRITIKA, 2025).

Regulations must specify the parameters of behavioural monitoring in public systems or workplaces, as well as what ethical data use is and how long it can be kept. Building public confidence in neuroscience-based cybersecurity will require the establishment of governance frameworks based on accountability and transparency.

7. CONCLUSION

The field of cybersecurity is changing due to the convergence of artificial intelligence and neuroscience. Neuroscience-enhanced AI provides previously unheard-of capabilities for real-time threat detection and response by simulating cognitive functions like attention, memory, and adaptive learning. These neuro-inspired intrusion detection systems learn dynamically, mimicking the brain's capacity to recognize novelty, deduce intent, and adjust to changing environments, in contrast to conventional intrusion detection systems that depend on static signatures or preset rules.

In this chapter, we examined the mapping of cognitive neuroscience concepts onto computational frameworks for behavioral anomaly detection, including neural plasticity, affective processing, and predictive coding. Biologically realistic blueprints for intelligent cyber defense are provided by architectures that integrate neuro-symbolic reasoning, adaptive feedback loops, and recurrent and spiking neural networks. The usefulness of these systems is illustrated by real-world applications, which include behavioral biometrics, healthcare cybersecurity, and insider threat detection.

It is impossible to overestimate the significance of explainability, ethics, and human oversight as these technologies develop. Privacy, equity, and cognitive autonomy must all be respected in the design of systems that examine behaviour and emotional states. By combining neuroethical principles with human-in-the-loop paradigms, technological advancement is guaranteed to be in line with psychological health and societal values.

Looking ahead, the effective integration of disciplines will be critical to the future of cybersecurity inspired by neuroscience. These systems should become more rapid, effective, and contextually aware with developments in neuromorphic hardware, edge computing, and multimodal data fusion. However, resolving issues with data labeling, standardization, and ethical governance is necessary to achieve broad adoption.

To conclude, neuroscience-based AI signifies a paradigm shift in our understanding of cyber defense rather than just an improvement in current technologies. These systems have the potential to build robust, reliable, and human-aligned security infrastructures by mimicking the flexibility and intuition of the human brain. These infrastructures would be able to defend against both known and unknown threats in the constantly changing digital landscape.

REFERENCES

Abdelkader, S., Amissah, J., Kinga, S., Mugerwa, G., Emmanuel, E., Mansour, D. E. A., & Prokop, L. (2024). Securing modern power systems: Implementing comprehensive strategies to enhance resilience and reliability against cyber-attacks. *Results in Engineering, 102647*. Advance online publication. DOI: 10.1016/j.rineng.2024.102647

Ajayi, A. M., Omokanye, A. O., Olowu, O., Adeleye, A. O., Omole, O. M., & Wada, I. U. (2024). Detecting insider threats in banking using AI-driven anomaly detection with a data science approach to cybersecurity. *International Journal of Cybersecurity Research.*

Barsallo Yi, E. A., Majors, J. D., Padala, A. V., Wu, D., Machiry, A., & Bagchi, S. (2024, June). Multi-Device Context-Sensitive Attacks Against Privacy. In *Proceedings of the Fifteenth ACM Conference on Data and Application Security and Privacy* (pp. 209-220).

Bhaware, A., Varshney, G., Kour, J., Bishnoi, T., Jain, M., & Sharma, D. (2024, May). A Privacy Preserving Context Sensitive Kernel. In *Proceedings of the 2024 ACM Workshop on Wireless Security and Machine Learning* (pp. 20-25).

Boskovic, I., Perera, N., & Otgaar, H. (2025). Cross-Cultural Perspectives on Psychological Research Practices and Opportunities: Do We All Have the (Same) Chance? *Psychological Research on Urban Society*, *8*(2), 4.

Dangi, A. K., Pant, K., Alanya-Beltran, J., Chakraborty, N., Akram, S. V., & Balakrishna, K. (2023, January). A review of use of artificial intelligence on cyber security and the fifth-generation cyber-attacks and its analysis. In *2023 International Conference on Artificial Intelligence and Smart Communication (AISC)* (pp. 553–557). IEEE. https://doi.org/DOI: 10.1109/AISC56872.2023.10092161

Gadicha, V. B., Gadicha, A. B., Zuhair, M., Khan, Z. I., & Burange, M. S. (2025). Revolutionizing Security Information and Event Management (SIEM) Systems: Harnessing Deep Learning for Advanced Threat Detection. In *Project Management Information Systems: Empowering Decision Making and Execution* (pp. 233-262). IGI Global Scientific Publishing.

Gururaj, H. L., Janhavi, V., & Ambika, V. (Eds.). (2024). *Social Engineering in Cybersecurity: Threats and Defenses*. CRC Press.

Hinrichs, R., Subramanian, L., Ayala, A., Endicott-Popovsky, B., & Stoll, S. (2024, November). *AI-enhanced cybersecurity training: Integrating ethical reasoning and personalized learning pathways.* In *Proceedings of the Future Technologies Conference* (pp. 606–622). Springer Nature Switzerland. https://doi.org/DOI: 10.1007/978-3-031-49514-4_40

Kritika, E. (2025). A neuroscience perspective on AI and cybersecurity. ISACA Journal, (1).

Kritika, M. (2024). Neuro-driven cybersecurity: Strengthening digital defense. *London Journal of Research in Computer Science and Technology*, *24*(1), 17–26.

Liu, R., Shi, J., Chen, X., & Lu, C. (2024). Network anomaly detection and security defense technology based on machine learning: A review. *Computers & Electrical Engineering*, *119*, 109581.

Luo, Z., Tessler, C., Lin, T., Yuan, Y., He, T., Xiao, W., Guo, Y., ... (2025). "Emergent Active Perception and Dexterity of Simulated Humanoids from Visual Reinforcement Learning." *arXiv preprint arXiv:2505.12278*

Malik, W., & Gul, S. (2024). Bridging the Gap: Exploring the Intersection of Cybersecurity and Human Security in the Digital Age. *Competitive Research Journal Archive*, *2*(04), 195–202.

Okika, N., Okoh, O. F., & Etuk, E. E. (2025). Mitigating Insider Threats and Social Engineering Tactics in Advanced Persistent Threat Operations through Behavioral Analytics and Cybersecurity Training. *International Journal of Advance Research Publication and Reviews*, *2*(3), 11–27.

Panda, S. P. (2025). The Evolution and Defense Against Social Engineering and Phishing Attacks. [IJSR]. *International Journal of Scientific Research.*

Ramalingam, R., Arthi, K., Bhavani, M. M., & Sunitha, T. (2025). AI-Enhanced Security Information and Event Management (SIEM) System. In *Deep Learning Innovations for Securing Critical Infrastructures* (pp. 75-94). IGI Global Scientific Publishing.

Rayhan, A. (2024, April). Cybersecurity in the digital age: Assessing threats and strengthening defenses. In *Conference* (pp. 1–26). Cybersecurity Awareness.

Rezaee, K., Rezakhani, S. M., Khosravi, M. R., & Moghimi, M. K. (2024). A survey on deep learning-based real-time crowd anomaly detection for secure distributed video surveillance. *Personal and Ubiquitous Computing*, *28*(1), 135–151.

Sarker, I. H. (2024). *AI-driven cybersecurity and threat intelligence: Cyber automation, intelligent decision-making, and explainability.* Springer Nature., DOI: 10.1007/978-3-031-42906-4

Sashwin, K., Nithika, K. S., Priyadharshini, S., & Maduvant, S. P. (2024, March). Analysis, Trends, and Utilization of Security Information and Event Management (SIEM) in Critical Infrastructures. In *2024 10th International Conference on Advanced Computing and Communication Systems (ICACCS)* (Vol. 1, pp. 1980-1984). IEEE.

Sendjaja, T., Irwandi, E. P., Suryani, Y., & Fatmawati, E. (2024). Cybersecurity in the digital age: Developing robust strategies to protect against evolving global digital threats and cyber attacks. *The International Journal of Science in Society, 6*(1), 1008–1019.

Sutaria, K., Rajan, D. K., Pathak, G. P., & Dange, P. (2025, April). Context-Sensitive Graph Reduction and Partitioning for Enhanced Cyber Attack Investigation. In *2025 International Conference on Knowledge Engineering and Communication Systems (ICKECS)* (pp. 1-6). IEEE.

Widjaja, G. (2025). Current threats to cyber security: strategies for protecting personal data in the digital age. *International journal of society reviews, 2*(11), 2245-2255.

Zhao, W., Gangaraju, K., & Yuan, F. (2025). Multimodal perception-driven decision-making for human-robot interaction: A survey. *Frontiers in Robotics and AI, 12*, 1604472. PMID: 40917482

Chapter 8
Integrating Predictive Analytics With AI for Cybersecurity Risk Management

T. Venkat Narayana Rao
https://orcid.org/0000-0002-1996-1819
Sreenidhi Institute of Science and Technology, India

Nandyala Jashwanth Reddy
https://orcid.org/0009-0009-0826-6296
Sreenidhi Institute of Science and Technology, India

Chenchu Swetha
https://orcid.org/0009-0005-1835-0679
Sreenidhi Institute of Science and Technology, India

J. V. P. Udaya Deepika
Sreenidhi Institute of Science and Technology, India

ABSTRACT

The rapidly changing cyber threat environment necessitates future-proof, proactive and adaptive defense mechanisms that surpass traditional reactive approaches. This studyr describes the merging of predictive analytics and risk intelligence in AI-powered cybersecurity solutions for advanced threat anticipation, detection, and prevention. Predictive analytics uses machine learning, statistical modeling, and big data computing to forecast potential attack vectors, vulnerability scores, and early threat detection of emerging threats, while risk intelligence provides contextual awareness from threat intelligence feeds and behavioral analysis. The

DOI: 10.4018/979-8-3373-5012-7.ch008

model includes real-time data consumption and adaptive anomaly detection to efficiently detect zero-day exploits and insider attacks. This chapter highlights the enabling power of predictive analytics with risk intelligence to shift cybersecurity from a passive, reactive model to a proactive, intelligence ecosystem, thus resilient, reducing operational risks, and offering a strong means of protecting contemporary digital infrastructures.

1. INTRODUCTION

The rapid proliferation of digital technologies along with the unprecedented rise of cyber threats changed cybersecurity to a critical part of modern tech infrastructure. Organizations today confront adversaries that range from cybercriminals seeking money to state attackers as each uses tactics that can expose data, halt services, plus abuse weaknesses. Usual cybersecurity methods that trust chiefly in reactive processes such as signature detection along with manual response fail for matching emerging dangers now. Organizations depended on firewall configurations and on antivirus software back in early digital defense stages to restrict forbidden access as well as detect known malware signatures. Against all of these earlier less complex threats these approaches did prove to be effective. Attackers used polymorphic malware, botnets, and distributed denial-of-service (DDoS) attacks too, but these methods soon were outdated.

IDS such as Intrusion Detection Systems plus IPS like Intrusion Prevention Systems grew during the 2000s. Malicious activity was found through network traffic analysis. Even despite their advancement, these systems did advance though still reported high false-positive rates beyond failing to detect any previously unseen attacks. Then platforms for Security Information and Event Management (SIEM) surfaced to aggregate and analyze logs across networks. SIEM tools improved upon visibility yet rule-based logic limited those tools also requiring a lot of human work for real perceptions from a ton of data.

The rise of Artificial Intelligence (AI) and machine learning (ML) has marked since a turning point because it shifted the cybersecurity model from reactive defense to predictive, intelligence-driven protection. AI allows continuing education and flexibility. It also has an ability for it to forecast any potential threats via an analysis of behavioral patterns plus contextual data, unlike static, rule-based models.

AI-driven predictive models represent an economic imperative along with a technological necessity. Due to the fact that organizations fail to adopt proactive defense strategies, the global average cost of a data breach in 2023 exceeded $4.45 million, and this highlights their financial burden. Reactive models often drain resources since they overwhelm security teams through false alarms so they contribute toward alert fatigue also delayed responses. High-risk events get priority through predictive analytics using context-aware recommendations lowering inefficiencies. This change streamlines staff abilities and increases company flexibility. Also, this kind of shift ensures compliance with a set of regulatory standards.

Within this transformative landscape, a pivotal role is indeed played by predictive analytics. It enables security systems in order to forecast potential attack vectors plus assess the probability of vulnerabilities being exploited. It also identifies early indicators for emerging threats. Predictive models become adaptive defense systems that decide in real time when analysts couple it with risk intelligence making people aware of context by analyzing environmental factors organizational assets and the broader threat landscape.

Here AI-driven cybersecurity explores more of the convergence of both predictive analytics and risk intelligence. It stresses how hybrid machine learning models detect anomalies within real time and risk-aware intelligence can anticipate and reduce threats. When they do so the discussion passes security's conventional limitations. The discussion then presents toward a vision of intelligence-based cybersecurity ecosystems that proactively defend also anticipate challenges (Sarker et al.,2021).

2. FOUNDATIONS OF PREDICTIVE ANALYTICS IN CYBERSECURITY

Cybersecurity has gone through multiple generations of evolution in response to increasing digital threat sophistication. In the early 2000s, organizations depended on perimeter defenses such as firewalls, antivirus, and signature-based intrusion detection systems. Such tools were effective against known threats but proved helpless when attackers turned to polymorphic malware, living-off-the-land techniques, and zero-day exploits. As enterprise networks expanded through the adoption of cloud environments, mobile integration, and IoT devices, the volume of generated security logs and alerts went well beyond the capacity of manual analysis.

Big-data technologies emerged during 2015-2020 and enabled organizations to collect and process substantial amounts of telemetry data. However, the scarcity of intelligent automation restricted their value until the development and deployment of machine learning and AI-based models could be undertaken for analyzing behaviour patterns, detecting anomalies, and offering adaptive security insights. Starting in 2020, cyberattacks began more and more to rely on automation, AI-generated phishing content, ransomware-as-a-service, and large-scale botnets. These changes spotlight the increasing need for predictive intelligence-identifying threats while they are still in the reconnaissance or early behaviour stage, rather than post-breach (Karpatou et al., 2025).

Recent studies highlight how predictive analytics, enhanced by contextual risk intelligence, becomes a necessity for cyber defence in modern times, providing organizations with the means to shift from reactive incident handling to proactive threat anticipation.

2.1 Understanding Predictive Analytics in Cybersecurity

Predictive analytics can be defined as the forecasting of potential security incidents through the use of machine learning along with big data techniques and statistical modeling. In cybersecurity, it involves the continuous analysis of global threat intelligence feeds, endpoint behavior, system vulnerabilities, and network traffic logs. Advanced algorithms process these datasets so they can identify anomalies as well as assess probabilities of attack along with generating actionable perceptions for security teams (Duary et al., 2024).

Predictive modelling allows for the identification of threats. One such type of threat is phishing campaigns. Historical phishing emails, language patterns, and delivery mechanisms can be parsed and modelled to predict new phishing schemes and to highlight suspicious communications before an end user is compromised. Predictive analytics is also used in malware outbreaks and insider threats. Coordinated distributed denial-of-service attacks are being predicted with increasing frequency. (Chowdhury et al., 2024).

2.2 Key Components of Predictive Analytics

Several interdependent components form cybersecurity's predictive analytics basis:

1. Data collection and Integration - Predictive systems rely upon massive and heterogeneous data sources now. These sources include system logs, authentication records, with firewall data, also external intelligence feeds. Integration of these datasets ensures a view of the threat landscape that is thorough.
2. Feature Engineering and Selection - Predictive models are effective if features with quality are extracted from raw data. Login frequency may act as a predictive feature. Unusual geolocation patterns or file access times can also be predictive features for insider threat detection.
3. **Model Development and Training** – Logistic regression decision trees support vector machines random forests and deep neural networks are algorithms for predictive analytics. To choose a model depends on the uses for which you use it, on the amount of data that you have, and on whether you need interpretability more than you need accuracy.

4. Evaluation and Validation - Detection accuracy, false positives, together with scalability are assessed through continuously testing predictive models with benchmark datasets. Adversarial testing and cross-validation techniques ensure robustness.
5. Feedback and Adaptation - Modern predictive systems integrate with feedback loops. Because new threats emerge, these loops allow models to evolve. This flexibility aids detection of new attack vectors and zero-day vulnerabilities.

In 2024 and 2025, predictive analytics gained greater adoption due to improvements in anomaly-based intrusion detection and adversarial-resilient learning models. Recent work demonstrates how transformer-based architectures and graph neural networks outperform traditional ML approaches for identifying coordinated multi-vector attacks (Habeeb, 2024).

2.3 Machine Learning Techniques for Prediction

The success of predictive analytics in cybersecurity largely depends upon the way that someone applies machine learning. Techniques in supervised learning classify types of known threats like that of the identification of if a file is benign or malicious. On the other hand, unsupervised learning identifies anomalies within network traffic or user behavior when they deviate from established baselines, which enables people to detect unknown threats. Combined methods give still more exactness. These approaches combine supervised with unsupervised learning for resilience. Attackers often move in a lateral way from one compromised system and on to another. This process here, when it is viewed in isolation, may appear normal. However, clustering techniques can reveal unusual correlations between multiple systems, so that provides early warning of an advanced intrusion.

2.4 Role of Big Data and Real-Time Analytics

Before big-data platforms were invented, organizations wrestled with how to process large, dispersed security telemetry. Relational databases and batch jobs of yesteryear weren't designed for the velocity and variety of today's network traffic, login logs, and endpoint events. And as cyberattacks became automated and accelerated, security teams required systems that could analyze fast-moving data streams in real time. This created predictive analytics driven by big data, providing the ability to achieve scalable, continuous threat monitoring.

The explosion of digital data increases the challenge as well as the opportunity for cybersecurity predictive analytics. Enterprises generate terabytes of security-relevant data every second, and this data extends from login attempts and file transfers toward IoT device activity. Usual methods for processing cannot handle this scale in real time. Hadoop and Spark are modern big data frameworks enabling efficient processing of high-volume, high-velocity information streams.

Real-time analytics ensures that threats are detected in a matter of milliseconds. This differs from detections after hours or days. Financial institutions depend greatly on predictive models operating in real-time to spot fraudulent transactions via analysis of strange spending habits. In cybersecurity terms, this means to stop any data exfiltration and ransomware encryption processes just as they happen (Prokopowicz et al., 2023).

2.5 Limitations and Considerations

Despite its potential, predictive analytics has some limitations still. For inaccurate predictions, it can result from biased, incomplete, or from outdated data since the models are only as reliable as the data on which they are trained. Also, adversaries increasingly use machine learning attacks. They craft inputs specifically designed for fooling predictive systems. Lastly, organizations must balance the need for predictive power along with explainability because they must ensure that human analysts are able to understand as well as trust the outputs of predictive models.

In conclusion, By offering early threat detection, reducing noise for analysts, and enabling proactive risk management, predictive analytics empowers organizations to allocate resources effectively and scale protection across dynamic environments.

Predictive analytics founds a broader movement directed proactively toward cybersecurity now. Organizations are able to reduce in a large way their exposure to the evolving threats by a shifting of the focus to "anticipate and prevent" from "detect and respond." This transformation is not merely of a technological nature but is calculated, and it demands that enterprises embrace the security postures that focus on intelligence and on data.

3. RISK INTELLIGENCE AND CONTEXTUAL AWARENESS

While predictive analytics enables organizations to forecast potential threats, it is understanding what matters most to the organization where cybersecurity defense's true value also lies, not only in predicting what could happen. Risk intelligence becomes quite a critical tool. It is helpful here. Risk intelligence makes people aware within contexts so that they can interpret signals that are predictive, and prioritize threats before responding with security that is proportionate. Essentially, it transforms raw predictions so that they align actionably to business objectives, regulatory obligations, also operational resilience.

3.1 Defining Risk Intelligence in Cybersecurity

Risk intelligence may be defined as the process where people systematically collect, analyze, and contextualize threat data to assess cyber incidents' likelihood and potential impact. It goes beyond customary threat intelligence now. Often threat intelligence focuses on external opponent information that is customary, incorporating internal organizational context as well as asset criticality plus business processes (Islam et al., 2024).

That is, until risk intelligence. Detecting that a vulnerability is present on a network helps, but risk intelligence goes one step further. Is this vulnerability found on a mission-critical financial server? Does it involve sensitive personally identifiable data protected by GDPR? Is it currently exploited in the wild? By providing those answers, risk intelligence helps make sure limited security resources are used in spots where there will be maximum risk reduction.

3.2 Sources of Risk Intelligence

Risk intelligence draws on diverse data, internally as well as externally sourcing data as shown in Figure 1.

- **Threat Intelligence Feeds** - Real-time updates that are about opponent tactics, techniques, and procedures (TTPs), indicators of compromise (IOCs), malware signatures, and known vulnerabilities are those that are provided by external feeds.
- **Behavioural Analytics** - Unusual login locations and also abnormal data transfers are deviations that are tracked by user and entity behavior analytics (UEBA) from normal activity; it is possibly signalling compromised accounts and insider threats.
- **Environmental Context** - Through integrated geopolitical factors, industry-specific risks, and regulatory requirements, broader security implications are understood. Because of the overall value of electronic health records (EHRs), healthcare organizations do face some heightened risks.
- **Business Asset Mapping** - Internal reviews assess business resources. This ranking has criticality as its basis. Systems supporting core services, intellectual property, or customer data receive higher risk prioritization. Such a ranking seems standard for these systems.

Figure 1. Predictive Analytics and Risk Intelligence Workflow

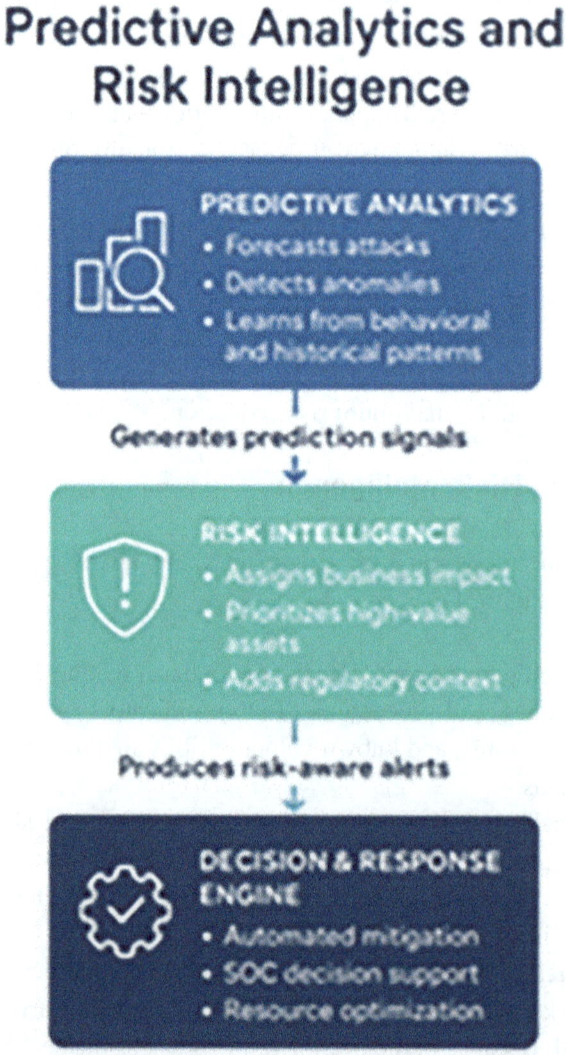
Predictive Analytics and Risk Intelligence
PREDICTIVE ANALYTICS
• Forecasts attacks
• Detects anomalies
• Learns from behavioral and historical patterns
Generates prediction signals
RISK INTELLIGENCE
• Assigns business impact
• Prioritizes high-value assets
• Adds regulatory context
Produces risk-aware alerts
DECISION & RESPONSE ENGINE
• Automated mitigation
• SOC decision support
• Resource optimization

Risk intelligence combines these sources so it goes past detection toward prioritization then decision-making letting organizations center on key threats.

3.3 Contextual Awareness in Action

Contextual awareness refers to the ability of people to have an understanding when interpreting cybersecurity signals in places where these signals occur (Abuabid, 2025).

Picture a situation where predictive analytics spots strange outgoing traffic from a computer. Contextual awareness adds vital layers into cybersecurity. Is this workstation merely a developer's test machine, or does it host customer payment data? Is the anomalous traffic directed toward a trusted third-party partner, or toward a known malicious IP address?

By answering such contextual questions, risk intelligence ensures that analysts focus on high-impact incidents rather than wasting effort on harmless anomalies.

3.4 Case Study: Prioritizing Threats with Risk Intelligence

A lender once possessed intrusion detection systems generating thousands of alerts each day. These detections proved accurate often, though many involved assets of low value or non-critical anomalies. By implementing risk intelligence, the institution began to correlate alerts along with asset criticality, external threat feeds, plus opponent intent. This approach revealed that it was less than 5% of alerts posing genuine risks to high-value systems. Because of all this, analysts could then reallocate resources to the defending of payment gateways and of sensitive data servers. Overall resilience improved, with the institution reducing both response time and operational costs.

3.5 Challenges in Implementing Risk Intelligence

Despite its promise, organizations often face challenges in adopting risk intelligence effectively:

- Data Overload: Because multiple threat feeds with internal logs are integrated, overwhelming data volumes can be created without proper filtering.
- A thorough view of assets' criticality is absent from many organizations plus how businesses depend on them.
- Concerning Skill Shortages: Analysts with the ability to skillfully interpret risk intelligence as well as operationalize it remain actually in short supply.
- It can be detailed to integrate risk intelligence with current SIEM, SOAR, and endpoint solutions regarding alignment.

We must balance automation with advanced analytics plus human expertise. These actions are required in order to address all of these challenges.

3.6 Risk Intelligence as a Strategic Enabler

Ultimately, risk intelligence transforms cybersecurity into resilience with planned enablement of business continuity. With risk intelligence using predictive analytics, organizations can foresee how likely an attack is and its importance. This convergence enables resources to be allocated with more efficiency, executives to receive risk reports with more accuracy, and entities to comply with international regulatory frameworks with more strength (Martiri et al., 2025).

As cyber threats grow more advanced, contextual awareness will be indispensable in ensuring that predictive signals defend actively. As this foundation sets the stage, cybersecurity that is intelligence-driven evolves into an ecosystem that is proactive and adaptive. The sections that are subsequent discuss all of the hybrid models with real-time detection mechanisms evolving from this foundation.

4. HYBRID LEARNING MODELS FOR THREAT PREDICTION

The perpetually dynamic nature of cyber threats requires adaptive models to predict cyber attacks with relative accuracy. Individual machine learning models fail, for many attacks differ in novelty as well as complexity. Hybrid models incorporating the combination of supervised, unsupervised, as well as semi-supervised models, gain the advantages afforded by each type, while compensating for the shortcomings, offering enhanced accurate threat prediction.

Supervised learning trains models with labelled data to discover known threats. This is applied most commonly for the identification of malware, intrusion detection, phishing using decision trees, SVMs, random forests, and deep neural networks. Though accurate for known attacks, it fails to deal with zero-day attacks as it requires large, up-to-date labeled data.

Unsupervised learning analyzes unlabelled data for concealed structure or for identifying anomalies, so it is key to recognizing unidentified or zero-day attacks. Such algorithms as k-means clustering, PCA, or autoencoders identify odd network traffic, behaviour anomalies for the user, or botnet sets. Flexibility is its forte but may give high false positives by the reason for label non-availability. Semi-supervised learning combines small labelled datasets with large unlabeled data, improving detection when labelled data is scarce. Reinforcement learning adapts defense strategies through feedback, dynamically adjusting firewalls or access controls. Together, they enable more flexible and adaptive cybersecurity solutions.

4.1 Hybrid Models: The Best of Both Worlds

Hybrid learning models unite unsupervised with supervised methods toward maximizing adaptability and detection accuracy as shown in Figure 2. For instance:

- Supervised + Unsupervised: For both known threats plus unknown threats, an anomaly detector unsupervised monitors unusual activity, and a classifier supervised detects known malware.
- Semi-Supervised + Reinforcement: Initial detection accuracy with semi-supervised models is improved. The response strategy is adapted through time due to reinforcement learning being used.
- Ensemble Approaches: Multiple models such as neural networks, SVMs, and random forests are combined within Ensemble Approaches for ensuring predictions that are stronger, reducing bias and variance.

APTs are detected particularly effectively by hybrid models. APTs will often combine some known techniques and will also behave in stealth and in unseen ways. These evolving attack chains become visible comprehensively through the leveraging of unlabeled and labelled perceptions by using these models (Al-Taleb et al., 2022).

Figure 2. Hybrid Ensemble Model for Risk Prioritization

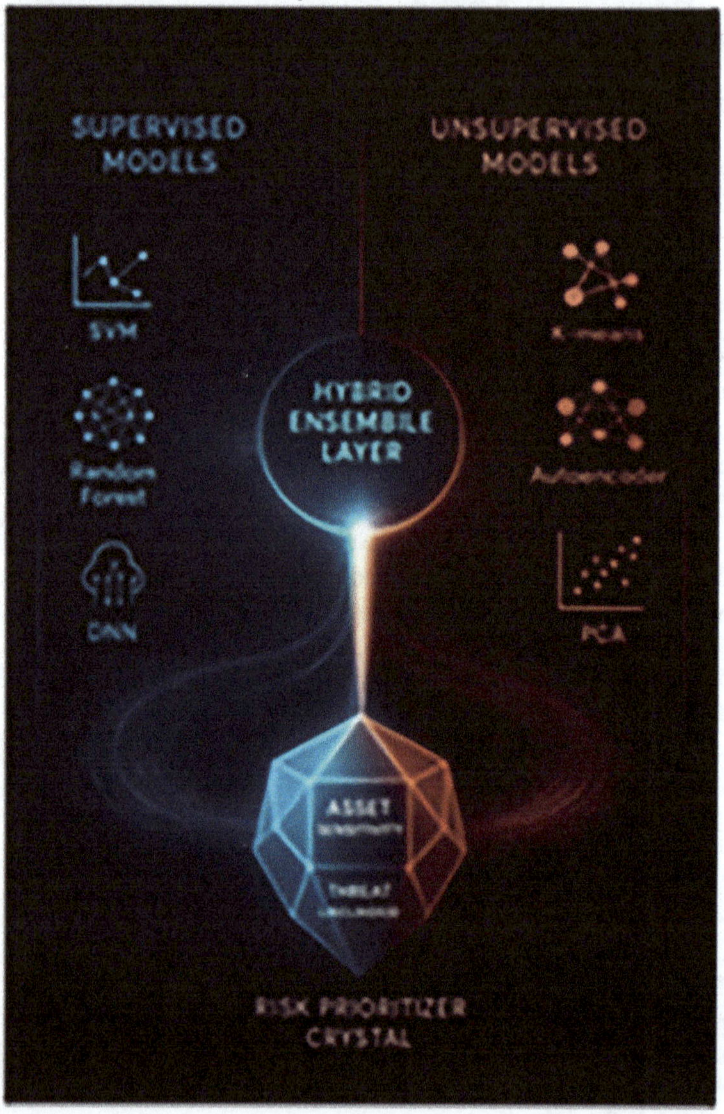

4.2 Real-World Applications of Hybrid Models

The practical value of hybrid models appears in many fields:

- Zero-Day Exploit Detection: Anomaly detection along with supervised learning identifies unusual system calls that deviate from normal patterns, even when labels did not previously exist.
- Insider Threat Detection: In order to flag risky insiders, hybrid approaches analyze known insider attack behaviors in a supervised manner as well as user activity baselines unsupervised.
- Cloud Security: Massive amounts of both structured and also unstructured data are generated within cloud environments. Hybrid models provide a balance between scalability also precision. This equilibrium allows discovery of malicious acts and faulty setups early.

For example, the Microsoft Azure Security Center learns via hybrid methods in order to detect known threats through supervision and to detect suspicious behaviors through anomalies, thereby protecting multi-tenant environments at scale (Al-Taleb et al., 2022).

4.3 Towards Context-Aware Hybrid Prediction

Hybrid models' future depends on contextual risk intelligence integrated into workflows. Risk-aware predictive engines become hybrid models. They align machine learning predictions to asset criticality, to regulatory requirements, together with business priorities. This integration ensures that organizations not only detect anomalies but also understand their importance so they respond proportionately.

Ultimately, hybrid learning models evolve toward AI-driven cybersecurity. This evolution is critical. They provide a thorough toolkit through modern threat prediction by blending semi-supervised efficiency, reinforcement learning adaptability, unsupervised adaptability, and supervised precision. Cybersecurity strategies of resilience and proactivity will rely on hybrid approaches as adversaries innovate.

5. REAL-TIME THREAT ANTICIPATION AND ANOMALY DETECTION

Speed and sophistication of modern cyber attacks demand not just predictive abilities but real-time operation capabilities too. Most accurate of predictions no longer matter once they follow after a breach has already occurred. To meet such a challenge, organizations are just beginning to deploy real-time threat anticipation and adaptive anomaly detection in their cybersecurity practices. By exploiting high-velocity data streams, machine-learned models, and contextual knowledge, such a methodology can identify and respond to threats once they happen in real time.

5.1 The Need for Real-Time Capabilities

Cyberattacks like ransomware, advanced persistent threats (APTs), also distributed denial-of-service (DDoS) attacks may escalate within seconds. Models such as those for customary log analysis or batch processing are simply not sufficient. They may carry perceptions for a matter of days or hours. Real-time analytics addresses this gap because of how it processes continuous data flows from endpoints, from networks, and from cloud environments. Damage is avoided via this processing for early work as shown in Figure 3.

Organizations can notice file encryption rates which are unusual as ransomware attacks do start and do halt the process before data loss becomes common. For login pattern monitoring in real time, you can identify credential-stuffing attempts before account compromise (Khalaf et al., 2025).

Figure 3. Real-Time Security Analytics and SOAR Pipeline

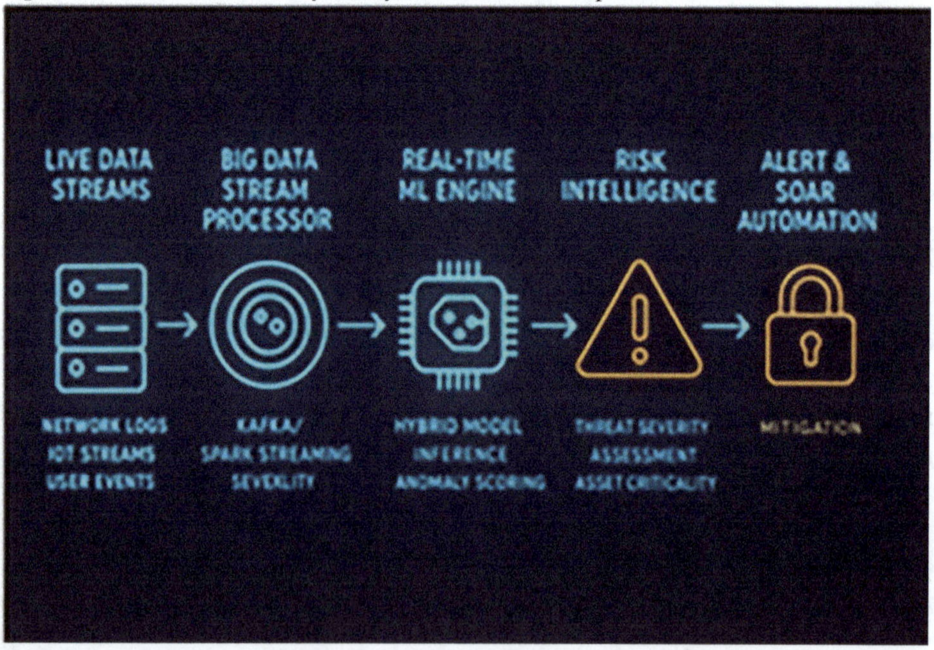

5.2 Key Technologies Enabling Real-Time Analytics

Real-time anticipation relies on a blend of technologies and methodologies:

- Tools such as Apache Kafka, Flink, and Spark Streaming enable the continuous ingestion and also the processing of logs, telemetry, and sensor data.
- CEP engines detect patterns indicating coordinated attacks correlating multiple events across systems.
- Modelled into graphs, network along with user activities reveal anomalies such as privilege escalation or lateral movement as node relationships are analyzed.
- Edge Computing is local processing inside IoT and industrial systems in order to ensure anomalies get flagged instantly, without relying solely upon cloud analysis.

Organizations can with ease transform huge volumes of raw data into actionable threat intelligence. These technologies are enabling results within a real time frame.

5.3 Adaptive Anomaly Detection

Anomaly detection is needed for identifying threats that stray from usual baselines. Anomaly detection does highlight attacks that are previously unseen, so it is of value for zero-day exploits as well as insider threats unlike signature-based methods, which are only able to catch known threats.

Adaptive anomaly detection takes this a step further by continuously updating baselines so they then reflect how user behaviour as well as system dynamics evolve. Adaptive models, for example, adjust expectations if an employee starts work from a new area. As a result of that, false positives are now reduced. Concurrently, they are sensitive enough toward malicious anomaly detection like atypical privilege escalation (Goswami, 2024).

5.4 Application Domains

Real-time anticipation and anomaly detection have broad applications across industries:

- Financial Services: You are able to find fake transactions quickly when you check strange spending habits.
- Healthcare: Access monitoring of electronic health records (EHRs) prevents tampering or forbidden use.
- Cloud Security: Misconfigurations and forbidden access are identified inside multi-tenant cloud environments.

- Critical infrastructure is indeed a vital concern with it involving the protection of industrial control systems and of IoT devices. Unusual action cannot create disturbances for such tools.

In each case, being able to instantly intervene may mean the difference of containing an incident as well as breaching catastrophically.

5.5 Real-Time Threat Detection and Proactive Cybersecurity

The contemporary cyberattacks require not only predictive intelligence but also real-time response. Adaptive anomaly detection with predictive analytics allows businesses to identify attacks in real-time, forecast adversary behaviour, and act before the breach spirals out of control. Top advantages are real-time intervention, identification of zero-day threats, automated priority, and robust operations with minimal down-time.

It challenges high-velocity data processing, false positives due to imperfect models, attackers masquerading normal traffic, and high infrastructure and compute costs. Balancing human oversight, automation, and ongoing refinement of models is needed (Khalaf et al., 2025).

By integrating risk intelligence, alerts are contextualized so analysts can distinguish harmless anomalies from mission-critical threats. Near-real-time detection combined with predictive analytics and contextual awareness establishes a proactive, intelligence-driven cyber defence with timely, effective interventions.

As its operational backbone, AI-driven cybersecurity anticipates real-time threats also detects anomalies. That is the conclusion. They make certain that predictive perceptions can translate into more timely interventions and this also reduces the window of opportunity for most attackers. Digital ecosystems turn more wide-ranging as well as complex. If they can detect and respond instantly, cybersecurity frameworks of the future will be resilient.

6. METRICS, EVALUATION, AND BENCHMARKING

Predictive analytics as well as risk intelligence models in cybersecurity perform with effectiveness only as they do perform within real-world scenarios. Firms need rigid standards to confirm dependability. Evaluation methods and also benchmarking datasets are indeed needed. These mechanisms validate whether models effectively scale across diverse environments, minimize false positives, and can accurately detect threats. Without systematic evaluation, the most advanced algorithms risk becoming misleading or ineffective (Dasso et al, 2016).

6.1 Importance of Evaluation in Cybersecurity Models

Unlike customary software systems, cybersecurity models operate in adversarial environments where attackers adapt their tactics constantly. Therefore, someone should not evaluate something merely as a one-time task. They should handle it continuously instead. Benchmarking can offer value to organizations to:

- Compare in an objective way different machine learning models.
- Assess precision within detection with respect to expense within operations.
- Resilience toward adversarial attacks along with zero-day threats can be measured.
- For analysts and stakeholders, transparent performance reporting builds a sense of trust.

6.2 Common Performance Metrics

Several metrics are widely used to evaluate predictive models in cybersecurity:

- Accuracy: Measures the proportion for correct predictions but might mislead in imbalanced datasets where benign traffic dominates.
- Precision: Detected threats that are truly malicious shown as a percentage. High precision minimizes false positives.
- Sensitivity or Recall is the percentage that tells of actual threats that are successfully identified. Attacks that are missed are reduced by a high recall.
- F1-Score: Precision and recall's harmonic mean. This provides for a balanced measure.
- False Positive Rate (FPR): Quite excessive false positives are vitally important, as indeed they lead to analyst alert fatigue.
- Area Under the ROC Curve AUC-ROC evaluates the trade-off linking true positive with false positive rates. This evaluation is conducted throughout thresholds (Raza et al, 2024).

Intrusion detection systems may still be impractical if irrelevant alerts overwhelm analysts given a 99% accuracy model.

Benchmark datasets have a central role when evaluators evaluate cybersecurity models. Commonly used datasets are NSL-KDD, DARPA, UNSW-NB15, CIC-IDS2017 and CICIDS2018.

These datasets are what enable reproducibility and standard comparisons across all research efforts. However, real-world deployment is often bespoke. This need arises because attackers might use unlisted tactics.

6.3 Real-World Evaluation Challenges

Despite the availability of metrics and datasets, several challenges complicate evaluation:

- Data Imbalance: Cybersecurity data often presents a skew, in which malicious samples are outnumbered to a great extent by benign traffic.
- Since attack strategies change, historical benchmarks represent present-day threats less well.
- Attackers intentionally craft inputs misleading models therefore resilience testing remains a necessity.
- Notably in cloud as well as IoT environments, models must be evaluated within high-throughput conditions.

For instance, an intrusion detection system performs well within a lab setting. The same system may fail with a financial institution's high-velocity data streams (Husak et al, 2021).

6.4 Human-Centric Evaluation

Beyond technical metrics, evaluators should also regard the human element. Analysts often decide according to what models output, so to interpret with trust models matters just as much as accuracy. Security teams may not accept models with high detection rates. The reason for this is on account of these models producing results that are opaque. Explainable AI or XAI techniques such as SHAP and also LIME increasingly integrate into cybersecurity models in order to clarify the reasons why they generated certain alerts.

6.5 Towards Standardized Benchmarks

The cybersecurity community gradually moves in the direction of frameworks for evaluating standards. ATT&CK, frameworks that map opponent tactics, techniques, as well as procedures, were introduced by organizations such as MITRE. Predictive models can be tested against realistic attack scenarios via aligning evaluation with those frameworks. Testing will go further than abstract datasets alone.

Furthermore, hybrid evaluations gain increasing appeal through combining live traffic simulations plus offline dataset testing. Red team, blue team exercises where ethical hackers attempt bypassing AI-driven defences also provide model robustness perceptions. To conclude, metrics, evaluation, as well as benchmarking validates the effectiveness of predictive analytics and risk intelligence in cybersecurity.

Organizations can ensure model accuracy through leveraging diverse performance metrics, realistic datasets, and standardized frameworks. In this way, practicality and scalability and trustworthiness of models are also ensured. Continuous evaluation remains important for it adapts to the ever-changing threat landscape while ensuring predictive models evolve along with opponent tactics.

7. CHALLENGES, RISKS, AND ETHICAL CONCERNS

As predictive analytics and risk intelligence become central within AI-driven cybersecurity, they both offer opportunities and complicate matters. These technologies bring meaningful challenges involving technical limitations, operational risks, together with ethical considerations, despite offering unprecedented accuracy along with adaptability. AI-based defenses have to be both effective and also trustworthy. Resolution of such items is vital to guarantee that aim (Ilieva et al., 2024).

7.1 Technical and Operational Challenges

Adoption of predictive and risk-aware cybersecurity systems has severe technical challenges. Methods require enormous quantities of high-quality data, but cybersecurity data are often noisy, imbalanced, or incomplete, which degrades the quality of outcomes. Threat environments are dynamic with frequent retraining required to deal with concept drift, as attacks by adversaries reveal weaknesses in models. Integration with existing predictive systems and prevailing SIEM, SOAR, and endpoint technologies increases the complexity manyfold, thereby retarding rollout (Kayode et al., 2025).

Operationally, high alert volumes can flood security teams, resulting in missed threats, while real-time and hybrid models for these approaches require high computational power, resulting in expensive deployments for smaller enterprises. Scaling models across wide distributed networks or IoT environments is not easy, and over trust in automation will diminish human supervision, resulting in blindness when models fail or when attackers imitate ordinary behaviour.

7.2 Ethical and Privacy Concerns

Beyond technical and operational issues, AI-driven cybersecurity raises pressing ethical questions:

- Data Privacy: Predictive systems often must monitor user activity in detail, thus concerns arise about surveillance and regulations such as GDPR demand compliance.
- Training data reflecting biases can create bias along with fairness problems. When biases focus heavily on certain geographies or attack types, the model may unfairly underrepresent or overrepresent risks within specific contexts.
- A lot of AI models, most of all the deep learning systems, function just like "black boxes" that are without explainability. Thus, organizations may have to battle to justify them to stakeholders or regulators.
- For defence, predictive models employing Dual Use of Technology could be exploited by attackers in order to design evasive threats (Kaushik et al., 2024).

7.3 Human-Centric Challenges

People remain at the core of cybersecurity, and human factors can either strengthen or weaken AI-driven defenses:

- Skill Shortages: Analysts who can interpret predictive outputs as well as assess contextual risk intelligence are in short supply.
- Security teams must understand conclusions of models: Trust and Interpretability. The valuable tools of ours may be underused by people. This underuse may result because of a lack of trust.
- Resistance to Change: Shifting from reactive models to predictive security ones does require a cultural change within organizations, and stakeholders who are accustomed to customary methods may well resist this.

7.4 Regulatory and Compliance Issues

As AI becomes more embedded in cybersecurity, regulatory scrutiny is increasing.

- Organizations must make certain predictive systems comply with HIPAA as well as NIST guidelines. Compliance Standards include adherence to global regulations such as GDPR.
- In order to validate that organizations actually are making fair and also lawful decisions, regulators increasingly do demand explainable and auditable models.
- Liability: Determining who is accountable when AI systems fail since algorithms are flawed or someone inadequately oversees them remains a legal challenge that someone has not resolved.

In summary, meaningful risks exist in cybersecurity if predictive analytics as well as risk intelligence are adopted. Technical limitations, operational concerns, and ethical issues pose barriers against effective implementation. Data quality, scalability, privacy, adversarial attacks, false positives, and transparency are these limitations. Addressing these challenges requires that we not only innovate technologically but that we also govern with consideration, oversee humans, and adhere to standards that are ethical. These worries must be decreased and recognized for organizations to completely get AI cybersecurity's potential while keeping trust, fairness, and resilience.

8. FUTURE DIRECTIONS AND CONCLUSION

The convergence of predictive analytics as well as risk intelligence already redefines cyber security when defence strategies shift from reactive detection to proactive anticipation. However, AI-driven cybersecurity will become even more advanced from now. The development and the deployment of predictive intelligence will continue to be shaped by the technologies that emerge, by the methodologies that are new, and by the threat landscapes that evolve. This section explores some key future directions that exist. Predictive analytics and risk intelligence transform so in this section reflects on that role then concludes the discussion.

8.1 Integration with Extended Detection and Response (XDR)

Future cybersecurity ecosystems are progressing from customary SIEM as well as SOAR systems to Extended Detection and Response (XDR) platforms. XDR has data integrated within endpoints, networks, cloud services, and applications. The result is as a unified defense system is. End-to-end visibility as well as anticipating multi-vector attacks is now enabled by predictive analytics that is embedded into XDR. Risk intelligence further prioritizes responses since it focuses on the most critical assets, which ensures protection has both breadth and depth.

8.2 Human-AI Collaboration in Cybersecurity Future

Human, AI collaboration remains central to cybersecurity's future. Automation speeds up and increases accuracy, yet human analysts judge context, ethically oversee, and are accountable. Operational and ethical considerations, plus algorithmic predictions, guide decisions that human-in-the-loop security models ensure. Explainable AI (XAI) techniques like SHAP and LIME improve transparency. Analysts can then interpret model outputs also to reduce false positives. This fosters trust within predictive systems as it ensures compliance regarding regulations. Decision-making strengthens too in industries such as medical care, finance, defence, and infrastructure. We must govern in an ethical way, be very transparent, and be fully accountable in order to maintain confidence. This maintenance is needed by cybersecurity solutions using AI (Maennel & Maennel 2024).

Federated learning as well as privacy-preserving AI will increasingly leverage future cybersecurity of strategies. Federated approaches do enable collaboration between organizations while also maintaining privacy as well as compliance regarding regulations like GDPR or HIPAA via the training of models across distributed devices without centralizing sensitive data. Data are further secured by differential privacy and homomorphic encryption (Khan et al,2024). Proactive defence strategies let organizations lure adversaries in addition to these. Cyber deception using honeypots decoy environments together with honeytokens also lets them gather intelligence on tactics and buy time to strengthen defence.

More broadly, predictive analytics along with risk intelligence can help national and global cybersecurity efforts. AI-powered collaborative intelligence-sharing platforms can help governments and operators to counter cyber-espionage reduce risks that arise from cyber warfare, and anticipate future threats. For providing of scalable solutions, these systems resemble early-warning networks such as epidemiology ones, and provide scalable solutions for global threat monitoring (Karunamurthy et al., 2023).

8.3 Challenges Ahead in Future Adoption

Despite such promising directions, challenges still will appear all along the path forward. Smaller organizations still must maintain cost-effectiveness, and ensuring interoperability across diverse platforms requires addressing of adversarial machine learning threats. As predictive systems grow more powerful, ethical as well as legal debates with respect to surveillance, accountability, also cross-border data sharing will strengthen. These challenges require governance frameworks that carefully evolve alongside technology (George, 2024).

Table 1. Consolidated Summary of Findings in Predictive Analytics & Risk Intelligence

Chapter Area	Key Findings	Benefits	Challenges
Evolution of Cybersecurity	Shift from reactive to proactive; AI enables prediction	Reduced breach impact; faster response	Legacy systems, alert overload
Predictive Analytics	ML models forecast threats, detect anomalies, analyze behaviour	Early detection; prevention of attacks	Data imbalance, adversarial ML
Big Data & Real-Time Analytics	High-velocity processing; Hadoop/Spark handle large logs	Millisecond detection; stops ransomware early	High compute cost
Risk Intelligence	Adds context: asset value, compliance, attacker intent	Prioritized alerts; smarter decisions	Requires deep organizational mapping
Hybrid ML Models	Supervised+ unsupervised + semi-supervised + RL	Detects APTs, unknown threats	Model complexity
Real-Time Detection	Enables instant anomaly recognition and response	Prevents rapid-attacks like ransomware	False positives, scaling
Model Evaluation	Metrics like F1, ROC-AUC, precision/recall used	Transparent performance	Dataset limitations
Ethical & Privacy Issues	Bias, surveillance risk, AI explainability	Trusted AI, compliance	Privacy laws, black-box ML
Future Directions	XDR, federated learning, deception tech	More integrated security	Cost & interoperability

9. CONCLUSION

The adventure from reactive cybersecurity models signals a shift in model to proactive, predictive, and intelligence-driven digital defence ecosystems. Predictive analytics sees emerging threats, as risk intelligence provides context to these perceptions, which ensures that organizations focus on what matters most. Together, they can defend with adaptation as well as with tactics in real-time, which can improve resilience since it risks operations even less as shown in Table 1.

Predictive intelligence will be integrated alongside technologies for instance XDR, federated learning, and ethical AI. This integration will strengthen defences against conventional cybercrime along with state-sponsored adversaries. Ethical collaboration, explanation, and governance by humans and AIs will stay critical for ensuring transparent, trusted systems aligned with social values.

Briefly, predictive analytics and risk intelligence improve cybersecurity strategies. They stand as basic foundations of tomorrow's digital defence world. Organizations and also nations alike can build up resilient infrastructures that are capable of withstanding all of tomorrow's evolving cyber threats through embracing each of these approaches in a responsible way.

REFERENCES

Abuabid, A. A. (2025). A data-driven approach to cybersecurity situational awareness: Insights from machine learning. *Journal of Innovative Digital Transformation*, *2*, 131–155. DOI: 10.1108/jidt-03-2025-0013

Al-Taleb, N., & Saqib, N. A. (2022). Towards a hybrid machine learning model for intelligent cyber threat identification in smart city environments. *Applied Sciences (Basel, Switzerland)*, *12*(4), 1863.

Chowdhury, R. H., Prince, N. U., Abdullah, S. M., & Mim, L. A. (2024). The role of predictive analytics in cybersecurity: Detecting and preventing threats. *World Journal of Advanced Research and Reviews*, *23*(2), 1615–1623.

Dasso, A., Funes, A., Montejano, G., Riesco, D., Uzal, R., & Debnath, N. (2016, March). Model-based evaluation of cybersecurity implementations. In *Information Technology: New Generations: 13th International Conference on Information Technology* (pp. 303–313). Springer International Publishing.

Duary, S., Choudhury, P., Mishra, S., Sharma, V., Rao, D. D., & Aderemi, A. P. (2024, February). Cybersecurity threats detection in intelligent networks using predictive analytics approaches. In *2024 4th International Conference on Innovative Practices in Technology and Management (ICIPTM)* (pp. 1–5). IEEE.

George, A. S. (2024). Emerging trends in AI-driven cybersecurity: An in-depth analysis. *Partners Universal Innovative Research Publication*, *2*(4), 15–28.

Goswami, M. (2024). AI-based anomaly detection for real-time cybersecurity. International journal of research and review techniques, 3(1), 45-53.

Habeeb, M. S. (2024). Predictive analytics and cybersecurity. In *Intelligent techniques for predictive data analytics* (pp. 151–169). Wiley., DOI: 10.1002/9781394227990.ch8

Husak, M., Bartoš, V., Sokol, P., & Gajdoš, A. (2021). Predictive methods in cyber defense: Current experience and research challenges. *Future Generation Computer Systems*, *115*, 517–530.

Ilieva, R., & Stoilova, G. (2024, September). Challenges of AI-driven cybersecurity. In *2024 XXXIII International Scientific Conference Electronics (ET)* (pp. 1–4). IEEE.

Islam, S. A. M., Bari, M. S., Sarkar, A., Khan, A. J. M. O. R., & Paul, R. (2024). AI-powered threat intelligence: Revolutionizing cybersecurity with proactive risk management for critical sectors. [JAIGS]. *Journal of Artificial Intelligence General Science*, *7*(1), 1–8. DOI: 10.60087/jaigs.v7i01.291

Karpatou, P. A. (2025). *The evolution of cybersecurity threats & the rise of artificial intelligence* (Bachelor's thesis, University of Piraeus). Dione: Institutional Repository of the University of Piraeus. https://dione.lib.unipi.gr/xmlui/handle/unipi/17786

Karunamurthy, A., Kiruthivasan, R., & Gauthamkrishna, S. (2023). Human-in-the-loop intelligence: Advancing ai-centric cybersecurity for the future. Quing. *International Journal of Multidisciplinary Scientific Research and Development*, *2*(3), 20–43.

Kaushik, K., Khan, A., Kumari, A., Sharma, I., & Dubey, R. (2024). Ethical considerations in AI-based cybersecurity. In *Next-generation cybersecurity: AI, ML, and blockchain* (pp. 437–470). Springer Nature Singapore.

Kayode, B., Adebola, N. T., & Akerele, S. (2025). The state of AI-driven cybersecurity: Trends, challenges, and opportunities. *Journal of Artificial Intelligence. Machine Learning & Data Science*, *3*(2), 2731–2739.

Khalaf, N. Z., Al Barazanchi, I. I., Radhi, A. D., Parihar, S., Shah, P., & Sekhar, R. (2025). Development of real-time threat detection systems with AI-driven cybersecurity in critical infrastructure. *Mesopotamian Journal of CyberSecurity*, *5*(2), 501–513.

Khan, O. U., Abdullah, S. M., Olajide, A. O., Sani, A. I., Faisal, S. M. W., Ogunola, A. A., & Lee, M. D. (2024). The future of cybersecurity: Leveraging artificial intelligence to combat evolving threats and enhance digital defense strategies. *Journal of Computational Analysis and Applications*, *33*(8).

Maennel, K., & Maennel, O. M. (2024, December). Human-AI collaboration and cyber security training: Learning analytics opportunities and challenges. In *2024 17th International Conference on Security of Information and Networks (SIN)* (pp. 1–8). IEEE.

Martiri, E., Vajjhala, N. R., & Dalipi, F. (Eds.). (2025). *AI-enabled threat intelligence and cyber risk assessment* (1st ed.). CRC Press., DOI: 10.1201/9781003504979

Prokopowicz, D., Gołębiowska, A., & Such-Pyrgiel, M. (2023). The role of big data and data science in the context of information security and cybersecurity. *Journal of Modern Science*, *53*(4), 9–42. DOI: 10.13166/jms/177036

Raza, A., Ali, A. K. S., & Hussain, A. A. (2024). AI-driven approaches to cyber and information security: Machine learning algorithms for threat prediction and anomaly detection. *Spectrum of Engineering Sciences*, *2*(4), 565–573.

Sarker, I. H., Furhad, M. H., & Nowrozy, R. (2021). Ai-driven cybersecurity: An overview, security intelligence modeling and research directions. *SN Computer Science*, *2*(3), 173. PMID: 33778771

Chapter 9

Hybrid Systems Combining Neuroscience, AI, and Blockchain for Secure Environments

Anupama Sen
https://orcid.org/0009-0008-4806-0738
Brainware University, India

Saptarshi Kumar Sarkar
https://orcid.org/0009-0004-1786-8284
Brainware University, India

Amitava Podder
https://orcid.org/0009-0004-9268-3781
Brainware University, India

ABSTRACT

Traditional cybersecurity models cannot keep up with current threats and our increasingly complicated digital landscape. This article proposed a potential hybrid architecture that could unify neuroscience technology, artificial intelligence (AI), and blockchain. Neuroscience allows for biometric identification in real-time through brain-computer interfaces (BCIs) or electroencephalography (EEG). AI provides the effective usage of adaptive defense, behaviour profiling, and autonomous detection. Blockchain provides secure transparency, decentralisation, and an immutable ledger. This architecture relationship uses a tri-layer system of sensing (neuro data), intelligence (AI analytics), and ledger (blockchain security). Real-world use cases include BCI-controllable devices, AI-driven energy management systems (smart grids), and

DOI: 10.4018/979-8-3373-5012-7.ch009

federated learning in healthcare. There are still latency, privacy, and scalability hurdles that need to be overcome, but with the advent of quantum computing and advanced neural interfaces, positive opportunities for overcoming challenges exist.

1. INTRODUCTION

There has been a complete change in the way societies use technology, information and infrastructure in the digital age. In the realms of healthcare, defense, finance, education, and urban development, the digital systems have become an inseparable part of the operation of critical services with the increased security guaranteed. The advent of the cloud computing, edge devices, and Internet of Things (IoT), has increased on this transformation rate, generating enormous amounts of data that are processed, transmitted, and stored at rates that have never been experienced before. But it has also drawn us all the more to the advanced cyber threat exposure due to this degree of interconnectedness and reliance on data. The extended attack surface followed by the complexity of the new digital ecosystem is gravely threatening conventional security paradigns (Mohammadi et al., 2021). Legacy security mechanisms (e.g. static firewalls, authentication based on passwords, signature-based IDS) are important, but increasingly inadequate to face dynamic and multi-vector attacks. Because of the rapidly developing technologies, such as artificial intelligence, polymorphic malware, and synchronized cyber-physical actions, adversaries can nowadays make use of the vulnerabilities within the systems to their own advantage (Shekhar et al., 2024). The security infrastructures are slowly becoming obsolete, as they can no longer achieve an appropriate level of protection against threats that have become more intelligent, stealthy and persistent. Besides, most of the traditional systems are reactionary and act only after the danger has been identified, whereas this process, in situations with a high level of speed, may come too late and allow millions of dollars to be lost due to the necessity to respond to emergencies, instead of being saved due to the use of preventative measures (Europol, 2025). As such challenges arise, it has also become increasingly clear that cybersecurity would need to become proactive, intelligent, and decentralized systems. As a result of this, there has been a rising interest in neuroscience, artificial intelligence (AI), and blockchain convergence as the foundation of establishing a new type of hybrid security forms. Neuroscience enhances the understanding of mental procedures and neural actions that can be used to build brain-based user authentication systems guided by user attention, a behavioral intention, and brain activity (Kasralikar et al., 2025). Artificial intelligence provides advanced means of processing complicated information, identifying a pattern, tracking an abnormality, and exercising independent decisions immediately (Shinde et al., 2022). Blockchain enables integrity, auditable, and transparent policy enforcement of data through smart contracts with decentralized security platforms (Adeshina, 2025). The convergence of these areas has the potential of transforming the design of secure systems by establishing systems not just reactionary, but predictive, adaptive as well as tamper resistant.

1.1 Background and Motivation

With increasing levels of digitalization experienced all over the world, a great variety of services and systems have been found to use networked digital environments to provide their operation and manage data. These involve electronic health records, robotic defense systems, decentralized finance systems, and smart city systems. As mass digitization occurs, an enormous amount of personal, biometric, behavioral, and operational data is already being produced, which expands the attack conduit significantly in the hands of bad actors. At the same time, the ways used by cyber criminals have become more advanced, introducing advanced persistent threat (APT) strategies, AI-generated phishing content, social engineering, and zero-day exploit techniques (Shekhar et al., 2024). The conventional security systems tend to be linear and unresponsive. Firewalls run on predetermined rules and antivirus programs use known signatures of threats and broken system passwords by memorizing the credentials which can be stolen easily or cracked. On the contrary, adversarial actions have transformed to be fluid, adaptive and context-sensitive. The only way to address these risks is to ensure that security systems become intelligent agents able not only to detect threats but also foresee them, learn during response interactions, and trigger countermeasures themselves (Li et al., 2023). Combining neuroscience, AI, and blockchain is a special chance to meet these needs. Neuroscience can be used to create next generation biometrics based on the cognitive and neural signal patterns (Kasralikar et al., 2025).

AI makes it possible to interpret and act upon these signals in real time (Shinde et al., 2022). The data and decision steps are secured on blockchain through an un-modifiable decentralized ledger (Adeshina, 2025). Such and such technologies combined can be turned into hybrid systems that can produce secure, intelligent, self-administering environments.

1.2 Limitations of Conventional Security Systems

After decades of optimization, traditional security controls show fatal flaws in how they respond to the current changing threat environment. A key shortcoming of them is the fact that they are based on rules and are therefore, static. Antivirus programs and intrusion detection systems can only detect known threats and as such systems remain very susceptible to new variants (Scarfone & Souppaya, 2007).

Password based (or token based) authentication systems remain highly vulnerable despite their popularity. Passwords (credentials) are phishable, guessable or stealable, and even two-factor authentication is vulnerable to SIM-swapping or social engineering. Besides, many identity and access management systems are based on centralized architecture, which makes them alluring single points of failure and, thus, potential sources of largescale breaches and operational lockdowns in the event of a hack (Shekhar et al., 2024). The other vulnerability is that of the latency of detection followed by response. Old systems tend to rely on human action or programmed responses, creating delays, which may be lethal during a rapid attack. Such industries, as independent land management or high-frequency trading can be affected even by delaying milliseconds due to their disastrous impacts (Europol, 2025). Moreover, the current computing conditions with BYOD policies, remote work, edge computing, and decentralized applications make perimeter-based security models inapplicable virtually in any way. The disjointed security tools in most cases are not integrated to work collaboratively and prompt sophisticated defense and detection. Data privacy and surveillance and other ethical and legal issues with concentrated state power to monitor biometrics adds another dimension of complexity to deployment and makes dynamic and distributed and interdisciplinary approaches to security a necessity.

1.3 Need for a Multidisciplinary Approach

Since the outlined shortcomings exist, the future-proof cybersecurity requires a multidisciplinary approach to ensuring cybersecurity by combining neuroscience, AI, and blockchain. With neuroscience, it is possible to provide secure authentication and behavioral analysis in real-time with the monitoring of brainwaves, monitoring of attention, and assessment of the cognitive state, which are resilient to biometrics and hard to replicate or spoof (Abo Alzahab, 2025). Artificial intelligence will have the computational capabilities to analyze the data streams of the moment, identify abnormalities, educate itself on new or emerging threats, and introduce automated responses (Li et al., 2023). Blockchain makes all data, actions and decisions immutable and decentralized, thus supporting trustless interaction, execution policy enforcement through smart contracts, and clear audit trails (Adeshina, 2025).

1.4 Objectives and Scope of the Paper

The objective of this paper is to explore the hybrid system that incorporates neuroscience, AI, and blockchain in order to improve security in digital settings. It examines the unit contributions in each of the domains and looks into the synergies. This paper lays out a three-layered architecture that consists of a sensing layer (neurodata capture), an intelligence layer (AI-based analysis and management), and a ledger layer (blockchain-based storing and enforcing). Applicable use cases are considered in the fields of healthcare, defense, smart infrastructure and cybersecurity to display flexibility and effectiveness. Technical, ethical, and regulatory concerns are also described in the paper, as well as future improvements that could be made in this multidisciplinary approach, including quantum cryptography and neuromorphic computing as possible avenues of further development.

2. CORE TECHNOLOGY FOUNDATIONS

The architecture of hybrid systems for secure environments relies on a deep understanding of the three foundational pillars: neuroscience, artificial intelligence (AI), and blockchain technology. Each discipline contributes distinct functional and conceptual strengths that, when integrated, provide a comprehensive framework for intelligent, adaptive, and decentralized security. This section provides an in-depth exploration of the fundamental principles, existing technological capabilities, and relevance of each of these domains in the context of cybersecurity and secure system design.

2.1 Overview of Neuroscience in Computing

Neuroscience or the science of nervous system or brain is a traditional part of biomedical area. Nevertheless, recent developments have transferred its influence into the computational field introduces interdisciplinary fields of cognitive neuroscience, neuroinformatics, and brain-computer interfaces (BCIs). These apps will help utilize the neural activation to interact with the computer systems and security purposes. In modern neuroscience, more sophisticated signal acquisition devices, e.g. electroencephalography (EEG), magnetoencephalography (MEG) and functional magnetic resonance imaging (fMRI) are employed to acquire real-time brain activity. These instruments enable investigators to record fine-grade times and spatial operations of psychological behavior, motivation, and emotive conditions (Shinde et al., 2022). Cognitive biometrics is one of the most exciting avenues of neuroscience as applied to the design of secure systems. They are the biometrics based on the unique traits of the brainwave patterns or neural response of the person. Neural patterns are naturally more difficult to fake or replicate as opposed to other common physical methods of biometrics like fingerprints or facial recognition. Consequently, EEG-based authentication systems have become an emerging front in the realm of identity verification security. In addition, neuroscience can also be applied to create adaptive interfaces that react according to the cognition of the user. Where the consequences of failure are high, as in a military situation or when making clinical decisions, systems able to detect stress, fatigue or attention states in real time allow safer and more reliable results. These understandings make neuroscience an important part of the layer of the hybrid architecture sensing and personalization.

2.2 Artificial Intelligence and Its Role in Security

The cognitive processing core of the hybrid security system is through Artificial Intelligence and more specifically machine learning and deep learning. AI replicates human thinking where machines can learn through experience, adjust to new stimuli and perform complex activities of decision making. Introducing AI into cybersecurity systems helps resolve one of the most acute flaws of the traditional systems when it comes to adapting to unexpected threats on the fly. The set of available AI technologies in the market is rich and comprising of supervised learning, unsupervised learning, reinforcement learning, and deep neural networks. Such models can consume large sets of unstructured data, e.g. network logs, behavioural telemetry, and even biometric data, and identify patterns supportive of normal or abnormal behaviour. As an example, an approach based on training AI on patterns of EEG can isolate the difference between the behavior of an authentic user and coercion, impersonation, or cognitive duress. The applications of AI in security settings are anomaly detection, user behaviour analytics (UBA), and threat intelligence aggregation. AI-powered real-time inference engines have the capacity to process thousands of events every second, recognize when conditions have departed set baselines, and take action on their own to contain the problem. Such real-time capability of operations is essential in areas such as financial transactions, critical infrastructure and healthcare delivery systems (Gwala, 2025). In addition, AI facilitates simulation and predictive modelling. Valuable training can be performed by simulating an attack scenario or threat vectors using AI to evaluate a systems vulnerabilities and advise on proactive counter actions. This is why AI is not only a defence mechanism but a system analysis engine that increases system resilience. Even in hybrid architecture, AI connects raw neural signals (neuroscience) and secure decision execution (blockchain). The intelligence layer of the system depends on its capability to interpret dynamic, multi-modal inputs and produce actions that can be interpreted.

2.3 Blockchain Technology for Secure Systems

Intended as the foundation of cryptocurrencies, blockchain is undergoing a very fast transition to become a fundamental technology of tamper-proof decentralized data. A blockchain is more or less like a distributed ledger that has a chain of cryptographically secured records, or block, that are kept on a network of nodes. Such decentralized mechanism does not involve central authorities, has transparency, immutability, and consensus. Blockchain resolves some of the fundamental challenges in secure systems. First, it guarantees the integrity of data with its cryptographic mechanisms. When information is on the blockchain, it becomes close to impossible to change with approval of most nodes. This particular property finds application mostly in places where authenticity and traceability of records are paramount, examples being in healthcare audits, military logs, or in forensics.

Second, blockchain will allow identity and access management using decentralized identifiers (DIDs), public-key infrastructure (PKI), and smart contracts. These systems enable characteristics to validate identities, control authorizations as well as implement policies without having to depend on central servers subject to compromises. Third, security response can be automated using smart contracts included into the blockchain. These are contracts that are codes that are self-executing and thus cause actions when there are certain conditions. As an example, in the event that an AI system signals something out of the ordinary in brainwave activity that indicates that the user is being impersonated, a smart contract would respond by removing the ability to access the system and contact authorities in real time. Second, blockchain has an important application in terms of data sharing and model approval in the AI processes. In federated learning a system using which the machine learning models are trained on multiple devices that are not centralized can use blockchain to track and verify contributions, secure intellectual property and make sure that the updates to the model are genuine and transparent. The use of blockchain in the hybrid approach is not limited only to the security of data, but its related features to ensure distributed trust, transparency of processes, and automatic enforcement of AI-based decisions.

2.4 Comparative Strengths and Integration Rationale

All three technologies under discussion have unique advantages to table. Neuroscience provides detail in cognitive signal harvest and real-time biometric detection. AI brings the computational backbone to the ability to derive insights out of the large and complex data, create actionable intelligence and have predictive power. Blockchain on the other hand provides the foundation of safe, unchangeable and non-centralized transaction record and policy execution. A combination of these technologies has synergistic effects. When BCI data and/or EEG data are analyzed using AI, they can be translated into some sort of identity verification, cognitive load, or anomaly identification. When these insights are hidden and preserved on the blockchain, they provide an impregnable audit path to improve the level of transparency and compliance in the system. AI analysis can be used to automate response through the Smart contracts, providing response in time and reliable way (Abo Alzahab, 2025).

In addition, some of the most serious drawbacks of traditional systems are resolved through the integration. It does not focus on password and static credentials security but shifts to cognitive biometrics. It transforms a reactive rule-based policies to smart intelligent response. And it does away with points of attrition by making use of decentralized blockchain protocols which results in the increased resiliency on the system. So the reasons to combine neuroscience, AI, and blockchain are not only additive but multiplicative: the combination yields more than the individual elements. It enables designing secure environments that are both physically fortified and environmentally conscious, ethically in line, and flexible to the fast changing digital frontier.

3. CONVERGENCE OF NEUROSCIENCE AND ARTIFICIAL INTELLIGENCE

The pairing of neuroscience and artificial intelligence is another revolutionary step toward creating intelligent security systems. The field of neuroscience can give information on the cognitive processes of the human brain, how it responds to situations behaviorally, including its neural traces, whereas the field of artificial intelligence can offer a tool of computation which includes pattern recognition, learning, and decision-making without the influence of worldly command. The combination of these two fields together allows the development of systems that will be able to decipher complicated brain activity in real-time, allowing new forms of user authentication, response to threats in real-time, and getting behavioral profiles. Such convergence will present a change in traditional predominantly machine centered security solutions to a bio-cognitive framework focusing on exploiting human brains natural uniqueness and complexity.

3.1 Cognitive Neuroscience and Computational Modelling

Cognitive neuroscience is an effort to comprehend the structural representation of mental processes in the brain including perception, memory, decision-making and emotion. With the availability of technological advancements such as neuroimaging tools through methods such as electroencephalography (EEG), functional magnetic resonance imaging (fMRI) and magnetoencephalography (MEG) researchers are able to monitor and measure neural activity whilst engaged in definite states of mind. The data, formerly restricted to clinical or experimental contexts, are being more frequently utilized as the input to machine learning models in order to build computational models of human cognition. Neural networks and the use of deep learning algorithms have performed extremely well, especially in modelling complex and nonlinear patterns (Li et al., 2023). Applying them to the data of cognitive neuroscience, AI can create predictive models that train to differentiate between various mental states, levels of attention or emotional reactions by patterns of neural signals. Its integration enables intelligent systems to be designed which can understand the thought and actions of users at a cognition level than on mere mechanical or written inputs. Within the security framework, this is the ability to perform real-time monitoring of cognitive anomalies that could suggest stress, coercion, distraction, and malice.

As an example, AI networks trained on neural activity data would be able to know when the user is being coerced into a task or other scenarios where the user has found themselves with less than desirable levels of cognitive involvement and trigger adaptive security measures. Combining cognitive neuroscience and AI is establishing new frontiers in security systems and intelligence that perceive and reason similarly to human beings as a result of translating raw neural data into computational models of thought and behaviour.

3.2 Brainwave-Based Biometrics and Behavioral Authentication

The conventional biometrics systems use the physical characteristics like fingerprints, facial aspects, or the Iris patterns to authenticate users. Although these techniques have become better with advancements, they lack resilience to spoofing, cloning and privacy issues. A far safer and uncalendarable choice is brainwave-based biometrics premised on personal activity patterns of the brain. Electroencephalography (EEG) is one of the most readily available techniques of recording real-time electrical activity recorded on the scalp, and representing the processes occurring in the brain. Every person has individual signs of the brain (neural) when it comes to the reaction on different frequency bands (alpha, beta, gamma, and so on) on particular stimulus or action. These signatures are capable of functioning as biometrics identifiers, similar to a cognitive fingerprint. Together with AI algorithms that are able to classify EEG patterns, this method makes secure authentication, which is hard to forge or imitate (Scarfone & Souppaya, 2007). Behavioral authentication also broadens this concept by taking into consideration the dynamics of user-system interaction. The changes in neural patterns belonging to the behavioral changes (e.g. level of attention, mental load, or emotion) can be analyzed by AI to perform the task of verifying the user identity and attempting to detect the anomalies continuously. As another example, the sudden shift in neural activity when opening a sensitive file can result in a multi-factor verification procedure or access disabilities of certain privileges. In contrast to the static nature of biometrics, ways based on brainwaves are dynamic and context-aware, i.e., they do not simply identify users, but also offer information about how they currently are interacting with a system in hand. This forms a continuous and adaptive authentication model where an impersonation, the stolen credentials, or unauthorized access are minimized, especially on high-security facilities like a defence facility, a critical infrastructure, or a digital forensic platform.

3.3 Enhancing Brain-Computer Interfaces through AI

Brain-computer interfaces (BCIs) represent an apparatus/system which allows a direct communication between the human brain and an external device, and circumventing the canonical neuromuscular pathways. First built around the needs of helping people with motor disabilities, BCIs are increasingly used in the field of games, cognitive training, prosthetics manipulation, and human augmentation. The combination of BCIs and AI highly boost their intelligence, reliability, and response. AI is essential in interpreting non-stationary, complex signals recorded by BCIs. Raw neural data is also naturally high-dimensional, time-dependent, and noisy, and it is difficult to interpret sensibly without complex processing. Markov model, especially based on recurrent neural networks (RNNs), long short-term memory (LSTM) and convolutional neural networks (CNNs) can perform well in identifying spatiotemporal patterns of a neural signal (Mohammadi et al., 2021). The models are capable of classifying mental commands, forecasting intent, and live-time adaptation of control systems. As BCIs get more specific and popular, their application to security-sensitive tasks gets ever more viable. BCIs can be used in the military by enabling soldiers to remotely operate drone, vehicles, or communication systems by solely using their minds, reducing the use of manual labor and enhancing a high degree of situation awareness. BCIs with AI may help to have secure interaction with the system by determining the user intent through real-time brain activity and providing a secure interaction by removing the opportunity or chance of unauthorized/coercive interaction.

3.4 Real-Time Neural Monitoring and Adaptive Security

Due to the changing nature of security risks in the digital world, there is also the need to have a system that is able to observe how a given user behaves online and can adjust itself to counter these threats. Wearable EEG technology and AI-mediated cognitive analytics allow real-time neural monitoring, which could become an effective way of determining whether a person is tired, under stress, lying, or has other any intentions. The feature is crucial when objects that have to be carefully monitored are in conditions that demand continuous observation, i.e. air traffic control, military command centre or critical infrastructure control. This process of streaming analysis to identify neural aberrations that characterize a users normal line will allow the AI to infer conditions that range between compromised attention, emotional imbalance and consent violation (by knowing that unauthorized behaviour has been identified). As an example, a system that identifies diminished cognitive engagement when running important machinery may raise warnings, trigger emergency procedures or even shut the program down in, hopefully, temporarily until an understanding and awake user takes control. Contextual neural inputs can also provide inputs to adaptive security protocols. Adaptive systems are real-time dynamic systems that instead of using fixed thresholds or making binary decisions about the access to a system, they use real-time neural cues. As an illustration, privileges to sensitive information could automatically change depending on the level of stress, location, or attention span of the user. Such adaptive responses not only achieve better security but also augment usability through fewer not needed distractions or fake alarms (Adeshina, 2025). Implementation of such systems with ethics is important. Informed consent, availability of boundaries, and data privacy are critical aspects that have to be adhered to when performing real-time neural monitoring. However, ethically sound development and deployment of such technology would provide a user-conscious, proactive frontier of security which is in concordance with the dynamic and complex nature of human behaviour.

4. SYNERGY BETWEEN AI AND BLOCKCHAIN

The intersection of artificial intelligence (AI) and blockchain is an attractive synergy with the capacity to take advantage of the learning and adaptiveness of AI with the trust, transparency and decentralization of blockchain. Although the technologies have varying value to digital systems on their own, their combination addresses some of the fundamental weaknesses associated with each of the technologies working individually. AI will frequently be faced with explainability, data integrity, and centralized training paradigm that is prone to bias or compromise, and blockchain may be restricted in terms of processing capacity and scalability to execute complicated calculations. In a well thought-out combination, however, AI and blockchain create an intelligent and trustworthy foundation of secure, autonomous, and decentralized systems. The main areas of synergies between these technologies, such as data integrity in the use of machine learning, the deployment of decentralized AI models, federated learning on blockchain, and automated AI-based responses using smart contracts will be discussed in this section.

4.1 Data Integrity for Machine Learning

Machine learning (ML) systems are dependent on data. The performance of AI models depends directly on the quality, consistency, and provenance of the training data as does accuracy and fairness. Unfortunately, in practice, in most cases, datasets employed during training or during inference are susceptible to corruption, manipulation or other forms of tampering, either out of ignorance or with malicious intent. These trades can greatly affect the accuracy of the AI predictions or create potentially hazardous judgments, especially in the important fields of healthcare, finance, and defence. Blockchain solutions to this issue can be described as providing a manner of recording all data transactions in a way that is immutable and verifiable. When information is entered into a blockchain ledger, it can hardly be changed without the agreement of the whole network. This enables traceability of all the data consumed in an AI pipeline to its original source taking into account the integrity of any received data as well as audited compliance standards. Hash value or metadata of these datasets on the blockchain can make it feasible to scout unauthorized modifications, authenticate input and trace through the lineage of the ML cycle transparently. An example could include applying blockchain as a means to validate data in fields that have a compliance or accounting responsibility, e.g., pharmaceutical research, or autonomous systems in the transportation industry: in order to retain a sense of data integrity or the provenance of the data, by utilizing blockchain to establish the validation of a dataset, the entities responsible may ensure that the appropriate stakeholders, such as file authors, may know that the AI model was trained on untouched and ethically sourced data. It would also assist in establishing a trustful relationship with its users, researchers, as well as regulatory bodies as it facilitates complete audit trails of the data-to-decision process.

4.2 Decentralized AI Models and Edge Deployment

The traditional, legacy models of AI are traditionally created and rolled out in centralised settings, where the data of various sources is collated on a central server or cloud system. Although this architecture is computationally cost-effective and simple, it poses a lot of risks, such as single points of failures, vulnerable to cyberattacks, high latency, and privacy issues. One of the main issues of centralized systems is that in privacy-respecting or in vital-valued applications e.g. a control center in the military, smart city, or personal health tracking. Highly distributed AI models are coming into more use to address these anxieties. Such models are then trained and used on remotely located edge devices like IoT sensors, cell phones, or wearable medical devices. Blockchain is critical in this design because it allows secure peer-to-peer, it ensures model update verification, and that it coordinates the activities of distributed agents without using a central authority. At the edge, AI in conjunction with blockchain has a number of advantages. They enable less latency in real-time application, supporting a faster response to data processing. They increase privacy because there is no need in transferring personal information through the internet, which is prone to security threats that are involved in transmission of data in the internet. Besides, orchestrating AI activities using blockchain ensures that all the involved parties act according to some agreed protocols, and any variations or anomalies will be documented irrevocably.

Figure 1. Decentralized AI and Edge Deployment Framework

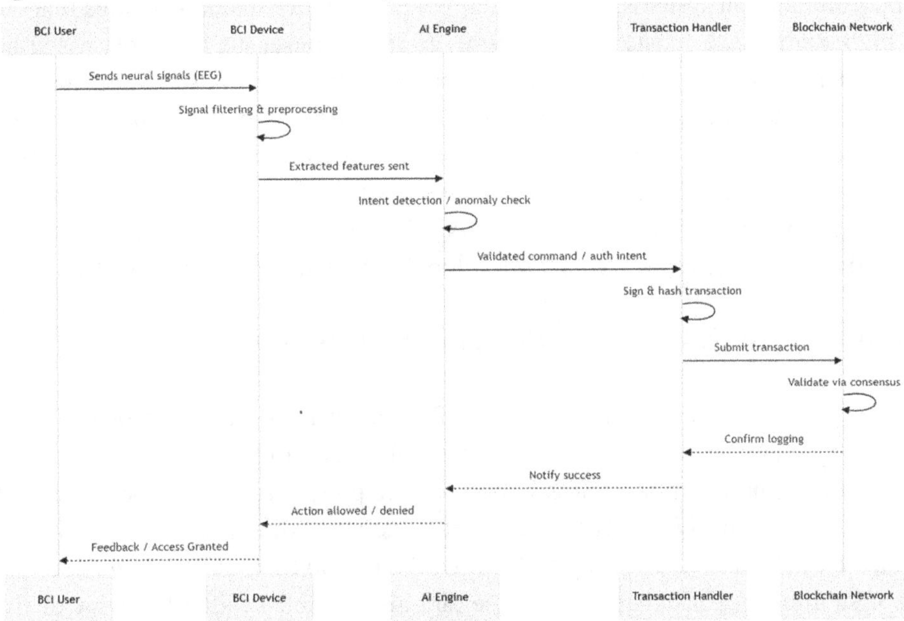

Different sensors, AI, and blockchain-based governance can work together to manage environments and address deviations and compose any actions required, as seen in smart infrastructure, where such a model is especially helpful.

4.3 Federated Learning and Blockchain-Based Aggregation

A new paradigm of machine learning known as federated learning applies to among many devices or organisations so that the trained models can be learned without accessing the underlying data centrally. Participants instead of submitting the data to a central server are allowed to train a local model on locally held data and only the parameters of the model learned are shared. These parameters are summed up to generate an international model. Although federated learning alleviates the issue of privacy, it also brings a coordination problem, trust issue and validation of contributions. Players might make fake updates or distort the models or even be trying to deduce on the data of other participants on the basis of updating models. In this case, block chain will offer a system to facilitate transparency, accountability and trust (Scarfone & Souppaya, 2007). Every part of the federated learning process can be written to a blockchain, because every part of the process can be recorded (model updates, timestamps, device identities and version histories etc.). This unmodifiable record enables validators to audit contributions, ensure that they are genuine and evaluate their effect into the world model. Blockchain is also able to support reputation systems. This can help give preference to contributions that are of high quality and consistency overtime. Further, consensus protocols based on blockchain technology guarantee validation and verification of the updates that can be incorporated into a global model. This aggregation process can be automated using smart contracts that check predetermined conditions, run secure updating logic, and pay rewards or incentives in tokenized form to take part honestly. The combination of federated learning and blockchain therefore provides a very secure and privacy-protective setting to co-develop AI (Mohammadi et al., 2021).

4.4 Smart Contracts for Autonomous AI Responses

The potential application of AI and blockchain is perhaps one of the most promising one, which is the automatization of reaction to the insights produced by AI using smart contracts. Smart contracts are programs on the blockchain that operate autonomously and carry out a set of actions when preset conditions are attained. Such contracts help in the fact that there is no need of human interaction, the system creates faster response time and also establishes the behavior of the system with great reliability. Being combined with AI, smart contracts will make systems switch in reactive to proactive and autonomous ones. An example is when an AI model identifies a network anomaly that an attack is underway, in which case a smart contract is the means to automatically isolate the affected node, send out notifications to administrators, and commence forensic data capture. In another scenario, when an AI model that tracks the health of the patient detects risk levels, a smart contract may issue a signal to the medical team, record events to be reviewed in an audit, and give access to unencrypted patient data as a commentary situation (Kasralikar et al., 2025). Such a combination results in a security domain that uses AI as the sense and processing engine and blockchain with smart contracts as its action and enforcement layer. These systems will not only be faster and reliable, but also transparent and impossible to tamper with since all the decisions and the reasons behind them are still recorded on-chain.

5. INTEGRATION OF NEUROSCIENCE AND BLOCKCHAIN

Neuroscience and blockchain technology are an emergent and largely unstudied area of cybersecurity and digital trust. The understanding of the cognitive process and neural biometrics as provided by neuroscience is unique and helpful but blockchain offers the infrastructure of transparent, secure, and decentralized operations of data management. The integration becomes particularly important in situations where the features of neural data, cognitive authentication, and tamper-evident logging receive top priority. There is an imperative in emerging forms of brain-computer interfaces (BCIs), neuro prosthetics and cognitive monitoring systems that the brain-related information must be handled in an unchangeable, secure and privacy-preserving manner. The subsections below discuss technical, ethical, and architecture implementation issues of neuroscience and blockchain.

5.1 Secure Identity Management Using Cognitive Biometrics

Among the most promising applications of where neuroscience and blockchain can be seen to meet is development of safe and secure system of identity management using cognitive biometrics. In comparison with the classical application of biometrics, like fingerprinting, facial recognition or iris scan, cognitive biometrics applies unique neural signatures (EEG (electroencephalogram) waveforms or attention-related brain responses) to an authentication process. These neural signatures are complicated, each unique to an individual, and nearly impossible to dereplicate/spoof, which makes them perfectly suited to high-security implementation (as fit for crypto algorithms). Incorporating such cognitive biomarkers into blockchain will allow creating a decentralized and tamper-resistant identity management system. When a single user interacts with a system that has BCI configured in it, the data on the EEG or other brain wave reads is obtained and matched with already saved biometrics data records. As opposed to retaining these signatures in a dedicated server, these signatures or hash or encrypted versions of these neural data are deposited in a blockchain ledger (Shekhar et al., 2024). This arrangement has two significant advantages. First, it can guarantee that the process of identity verification would be immutable and traceable, which would make it almost impossible to forge or gain unauthorized access to it. Second, decentralizes the management of biometrics reducing the risk of centralized databases that deal with single-point failures, internal attacks or data breaches in mass. The notion of self-sovereign identity can be applied since each person can be provided with the ability to manage their exclusive cognitive identity through personal keys or crypto tokens. Practically, this method of high-stakes-protecting, blockchain-based, cognitive authentication may be implemented in a high-security setting where a standard password or token would be insufficient (military access, although possibly a miniature labs or digital health platforms).

5.2 Blockchain-Based Logging for BCI Transactions

The brain-computer interface (BCI) technologies are getting more advanced in nature with their usage reported in cerebral prosthetics, long-distance control over devices, and cognitive training tools. Both of these applications are composed of a chain of event connections between inputs in the neural system, and outputs of the system, comprising a trail of raw transactional data of a sensitive and high-stakes kind. In order to make these systems trusted and accountable, one needs to use reliable and unchangeable logging facilities. Blockchain can also fulfill this role well since it is a distributed ledger recording and tracking all BCI transactions, including a brain command to operate a robotic arm or a cognitive input that is used to authenticate the system (Abo Alzahab, 2025). On the other hand, every transaction may be timestamped, encrypted, and written on-chain, which gives a trackable history of user interactions and responses to those interactions. This is particularly useful when there is a need to audit logs in the case of medical applications or defense systems, in order to prove compliance, or to diagnose malfunctions or repel liability suits. As an example, should the neuro prosthetic limb belonging to a patient malfunction or end up taking inaccurate representations, the blockchain log can be used to recreate the decision pathway and discover whether such a problem was caused by the neural action, the AI interpretation layer, or rather the actuator mechanism.

Figure 2. BCI-to-Blockchain Authentication Sequence

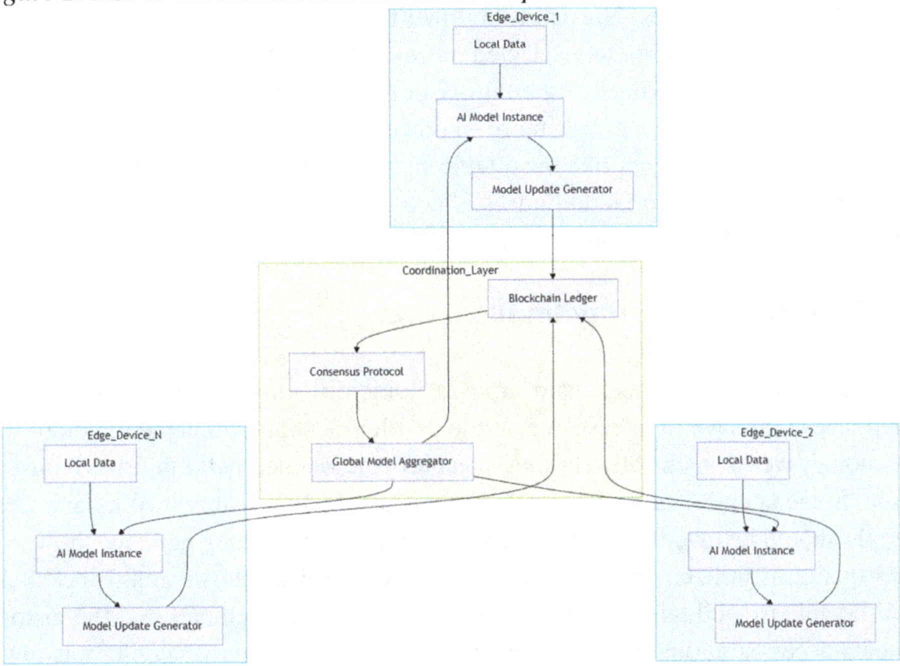

Blockchain is the capability to have multi-stakeholder transparency without jeopardizing ownership of data. The relevant logs are available to the healthcare provider, the regulatory bodies, the patients, and the researchers, where appropriate; they do not change the underlying records. This builds confidence on BCI systems and helps in the regulation of sensitive industries.

5.3 Decentralized Storage and Privacy of Neural Data

Privacy of the neural data is an emerging issue especially as the BCI devices start recording the minute details about what a person is thinking, intending, their emotional disposition and their cognitive performance. Such information is perhaps more sensitive than the conventional biometrics since it spills unconscious activities, mental disorders, or even political affiliations. Keeping data of this kind in centralized capacities makes these data prone to various exploits, such as hacking, electronic surveillance, and commercialization. When used together with decentralized storage systems like IPFS (Inter Planetary File System) or Swarm, blockchain presents still another way of neural data being encrypted, fragmented and distributed. The real neural data is off-chain stored on distributed storage networks, and on-chain only the hash, or pointer to the data, and related access rights are stored. The information is accessed by cryptographic keys and by smart contracts which implement fine-grained privacy policies. Normal users own the data of their neural information and have the option of sending selected pieces to researchers, physicians or secure applications without giving up the controls, or threat of exposure. The decentralized data structure can make a person more empowered and still allow them to adhere to data laws in various places like the GDPR and HIPAA. Also, it enables the ethical development of neurotechnology; this is because clear limits on data ownership, accessibility, and accountability are set.

5.4 Ethical and Security Implications

Neuroscience plus blockchain arouses numerous ethical, legal, and security challenges that have to be resolved so the development and implementation of the technology were responsible. The most notable of these concerns the informed consent issue. Since neural data may reveal highly personal and possibly involuntary data, people should be made very aware of what information is being gathered, how this information is utilized, and who they give access to that information. Blockchain will be able to facilitate this process because consent agreements and the history of data access granting can be entrenched immutably, yet the technology is not a substitute to human-centric ethical governance. The other important issue is the threat of misuse of neural information. The theft or misuse of brain based information may cause privacy infringements never seen before, even using encryption and decentralized storage. Consider, when a cognitive profile is compromised, an opponent may undeveloped drawn backs in behaviour or emotional manipulation. As such, any neuro data systems created on the basis of blockchain should incorporate a military-standard encryption, multi-signature authorization and ongoing security auditing (Gwala, 2025). Also, the permanency of blockchain records begs the question of rectification of data. The irreversibility of blockchain can turn out to be a drawback, in case a user requires to deauthorize access to his or her neural information or amend already registered cognitive prints. Zero-knowledge proofs or other sophisticated cryptographic tools, or privacy-oriented blockchains like Zcash might allow alleviating this tension, but the solutions are at an early stage of development, and careful vetting is necessary. On a societal level, the development of large scale use of brain-data-linked identity systems may result in just new forms of discrimination, surveillance or social stratification. The ethical systems that regulate these integrations require centralizing, open, and culturally aware ethics and require the work of various interdisciplinary groups in the field of technologists, ethicists, legal professors, and those who would be affected.

6. HYBRID ARCHITECTURE FOR SECURE ENVIRONMENTS

The effective and secure combination of such technologies as neuroscience, artificial intelligence (AI), and blockchain demands a thoroughly organized flexible architecture in which all the elements could interact easily. This part includes a proposed cross-functional design that would solve the challenges of addressing the intricacies of the contemporary security and cybersecurity requirements by integrating the strengths of cognitive sensing, intelligent processing, and immutable logging in a synergistic manner. Its architecture consists of three main layers which are sensing layer, intelligence layer, and ledger layer with each of them playing a unique but independent role. Alongside these layers, secure communication protocols and effective access controls allow the system to remain reliable and afford protection to privacy in various spheres of applications.

6.1 Architectural Layers Overview

In the architecture, the modularity and layering is done in such a way as to support the heterogeneity and rapid change of emerging technologies. All layers are working separately, although they can interact with each other at the specific interfaces and via secure protocols. The sensing layer will collect the neuro real-time data on users using devices e.g. EEG sensors or brain-computer interfaces (BCIs). The devices record an electrical or hemodynamic brain activity, which reflects cognitive states, attention levels, emotional responses or intentions of a user. The computational core involves the use of the intelligence layer in which the AI models study the neuro data in real time to determine patterns, anomalies, authenticate a user or activate adaptive responses. This layer should deal with high frequency input data, implement machine learning algorithms and transform complex neural signals into actionable measures. Blockchain layer as a ledger can ensure that all decisions, events, and actions by the system are posted and their history is recorded immutably and transparently. It offends a notion of decentralizing trust, which assists in securing sensitive information, executing smart contracts and enables auditability.

Table 1. Hybrid System Architectural Layers Overview

Layer	Function	Technologies Involved	Privacy & Reliability Role
Sensing Layer	Captures real-time neurodata (EEG, BCI)	EEG sensors, BCIs, neuroimaging devices	Provides unique cognitive identifiers and context-sensitive data
Preprocessing Layer	Filters, normalizes, and encodes neurodata into usable formats	Signal processors, edge filters	Protects raw data and reduces transmission load
Intelligence Layer	Analyzes data for intent detection, anomaly recognition, decision-making	AI/ML models, neural networks	Enables real-time adaptive security responses
Ledger Layer	Logs data transactions immutably and enforces access policies	Blockchain, smart contracts	Ensures auditability, integrity, and decentralized trust
Application Layer	Interfaces with user systems and enforces output actions	APIs, BCI interfaces, system controls	Bridges intelligent responses to real-world applications

Together, these layers form an adaptive security framework capable of responding to real-time threats, enforcing decentralized control, and ensuring data integrity across environments such as smart healthcare systems, military operations, and intelligent infrastructure.

6.2 The Sensing Layer: Neurodata Acquisition

The basis of the hybrid architecture is the sensing layer that is in continuous acquisition of brain activity through non-invasive or minimum invasive implementation of the neurotechnology. Interfaces like electroencephalography (EEG), magnetoencephalography (MEG), and functional near-infrared spectroscopy (fNIRS) are placed to detect cognitive signal of an attention signal, a memory signal, a motor intent signal, or stress signal. They are usually used on the head or as part of an assembled clothing system and convey information to the other architecture through secure information flows. Raw data gathered consists of high-dimensional and frequently noisy neurodata that must be processed by technologies like artifact-removal, normalization, and segmentation of signals in time. The main neural patterns these algorithms extract are then isolated and are available to later analysis, e.g., frequency bands (alpha, beta, theta), signal entropy or event-related potentials (ERPs). This layer can additionally integrate behavioral and environmental sensors, e.g., eye trackers, motion sensors, and voice technology, to supplement neurodata with contextual inputs. As an example, eye trajectory tracking in combination with EEG may be used to improve the guess of user intention or authorship attempts. Notably, the sensing layer should guarantee data fidelity, low latency, and privacy of the user at inception. Lightweight cryptographic protocols are used to encrypt transmission of preprocessed data to the intelligence level to ensure that neither is intercepted nor manipulated.

6.3 The Intelligence Layer: AI-Driven Decision Making

When a neuro data gets processed to a level where intelligence can be interpreted, the intelligence layer uses machine learning and deep learning processes on-demand. This tier becomes the system hub of decision making, transforming raw cognitive signals or feature extracted signals into trusted system actions, user identifications, behavioral evaluations, or alert of the presence of a threat.

Figure 3. Layered Hybrid Architecture for Reliable and Private Neurodata-Driven Systems

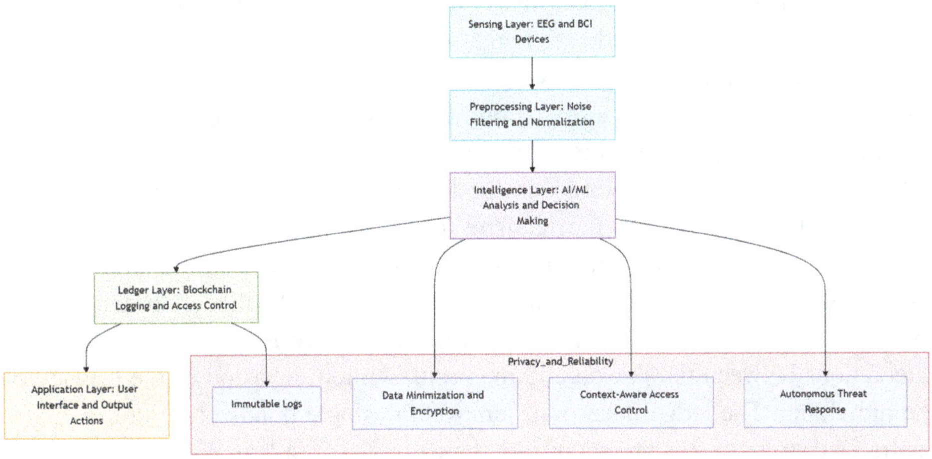

The typical models are CNN, which would help learn spatial features, RNN or LSTM network to model temporal sequences, and SVM to classify the user state. They develop very robust pattern recognition through being trained on labeled neurodata (of different users and tasks). To illustrate the point, take the case where a machine is provided with the brainwave information when logging in and the appropriate, intelligent layer, defines whether the brainwave profile fits the neural biometric specifications of the authorized individual. In a different situation, the system may scan neurodata to detect stress, distraction, or coercion and mark deviations that could imply the possibility of 3.1 an internal threat or the insurgency of the functioning. AI in this layer does not remain the same; it can learn either by reinforcement learning or through federated learning methods, remaining flexible to raw data changes but maintaining data privacy. The results of the decision-making are then recorded to structured events to be transferred further to the ledger layer to have it securely recorded.

6.4 The Ledger Layer: Blockchain for Security and Auditing

The last and most important part of the architecture is the ledger layer, which is based on the blockchain technology. This is because this layer captures all the major events, decisions, transactions and changes in a decentralized not-able-to-modify format that guarantees transparency, trust and tamper resistance. The transfer of every single story (an authorisation of a cognitive identification, a user purpose command, or an AI-initiated abuse notification) is transformed into a block signed cryptographically. The blocks are contributing to a decentralized ledger that is distributed around a network of nodes, it is thus unlikely that the history can be altered or erased without the consensus. Smart contracts are also supported in the ledger layer, and they are automated scripts that carry out security policies on the basis of pre-clayed conditions. As one example, in the event that unauthorized cognitive activity is detected by the AI, a smart contract could be used to instantiate automatic deauthorization of access and inform other applicable admins and create a log record with a digital time-stamp. Moreover, the ledger layer may apply zero-knowledge proofs or differential privacy mechanisms to make sure that the integrity of neural data should be confirmed without disclosing confidential information. In cases where this may be applicable like in the medical field, in healthcare or under legal forensics, it can enable stakeholders and regulators to verify the legitimacy of the interactions between the person and the brain, without invasion of the privacy of the individual. The ledger layer will remove any single points of failure in its decentralized structure, counteract insider threat, and make all decisions of the system verifiable, and compliant with audit and regulatory demands.

6.5 Secure Communication and Access Control

All the layers should have strong and encrypted protocols to facilitate assured operation of the entire architecture. Transport layer security (TLS), secure multi-party computation (SMPC), and blockchain consensus protocols are implemented simultaneously to help detect any potential interception or modification of sensitive data streams, as well as withhold them from the unauthorized interactor. Decentralized access control systems regulate access to system components: be that neurodata, AI decisions, or blockchain records. These are implemented by intelligent contracts and identity verification procedures that are applied under cognitive biometrics, two-column expert, copyright certificates, or digital certificates.

All users or devices within the ecosystem will have their own identity which is registered to the blockchain and they will be given specific context security privileges. To take an example, healthcare provider might be permitted to see the anonymized cognitive data that a patient has, but not to download or export it. The access controls are visible, accountable and manageable with no manual intervention. In addition, the architecture facilitates secure onboarding and revocation, dynamic, user-, device-, and application-level management based on real-time evaluation and measures reflecting changing levels of trust.

7. APPLICATIONS AND USE CASES

The intersection of the neuroscience, artificial intelligence (AI), and blockchain technologies provides a potent model that drives the creation of secure, responsive, and reliant digital systems. Such mixed architectures are particularly useful in fields where people work with sensitive information and critical businesses. In this section, real-life solutions that target a number of sectors with high impact are discussed, including healthcare, defence, smart infrastructure and cybersecurity sectors, and the comparative analysis performed reveals the versatility and benefit of the proposed model.

7.1 Healthcare Systems and Neuro prosthetics

The application of hybrid security systems in the healthcare sphere is one of the most promising ones. The information that is the most sensitive and has a meticulous privacy policy like HIPAA and GDPR is patient data. Neuroscience can also be used to monitor the patient in real time with respect to thought, feeling and neural patterns, especially on more advanced treatment programs such as neuro prostheses or mind computing (BCIs). They may be applied as motor implants in paralyzed people or as brain-controlled prosthetic arms and legs.

The AI algorithms decode neural signals in real-time and can make decisions that change therapy parameters or trigger emergency alerts, whereas blockchain guarantees that those alignments or adjustments in therapy, patient reactions and medical decision making are permanently recorded and thus audit-able. Blockchain also enables safe exchange of data across hospitals, researchers and insurance providers without loss of control over the data and privacy. As an example, smart contracts are able to implement the rule to make data accessible only in case the patient consent has been confirmed on-chain, leaving less opportunity to have data compromised.

The unified model increases the credibility, transparency, and customization of online care systems and makes sure that patients are always in charge of their data, whereas providers enjoy intelligent and adaptive monitoring.

7.2 Defense Systems and Secure Military Interfaces

The defense environment requires quick decision making processes, real-time situational understanding and perfect security of the system. Mixed strategies of defense open up new possibilities since they combine cognitive authentication, threat detection using AI, and logging based on blockchain. Neurotechnology allows direct interaction between soldiers and autonomous functionality that can be drones, autonomous cars or even cyber defence measures. By using BCIs, an individual can command through thought patterns, thus shortening their reaction time and doing more work. These signals constantly run through the process of being interpreted, filtered of noise and mistakes in recognition made by stress or fatigue do not occur with AI. At the same time, blockchain tracks all activity and sensor sensors and decisions in an irreversible ledger, enabling post-factum reviews, responsibility, and strategic auditing. Smart contracts may also be used to provide access to the battle field conditions- re negation of access to classified systems due to current state of mind or correct command authority in real time. Such a combination will not only guarantee secure communication and control, but also robustness against insider attacks or breakage of the system by the adversaries.

7.3 Smart Cities and Urban Infrastructure Management

Smart cities have connected technology to urban planning, transportation, energy, and waste management/emergency services. The additions of the hybrid systems make them facilitate identity authentication, behavior prediction, and infrastructure security by virtue of non-invasive neural sensing and AI analytics. Brainwave authentication enables citizens to communicate with the intelligent systems, including public transport terminals, secure buildings, or voting stations. This removes the option of using physical documents or the mobile device, making systems more all-embracing and safe. The AI can organize the data input across the city in order to organize the traffic flow in the most efficient way possible, minimize energy consumption, and identify abnormalities like a failure of the infrastructure or an emergency event. Blockchain helps to ensure the transparency that essentially means better coordination among agencies with a decentralized and tamper-proof record of decisions, sensor data, and control system adjustments. Including the element of neurocognitive awareness in the work of the governments improves their ability to react quickly to the needs of the people who use them, to allocate resources in the most efficient manner and provide a higher level of safety in the urban environments.

7.4 Cybersecurity and Continuous Authentication

Static credentials and preset rules that are subject to thefts, spoofing, and evasion are used by traditional cybersecurity systems. Hybrid systems present a shift in paradigm by performing behavior-based authentication on a continuous, endless basis and proactive anomaly response. Neuroscience presents more personal cognitive signals like those from EEG-based attention and emotional status monitoring as a source of real-time user verification. They cannot be copied or stolen as in the case of passwords or biometrics. With time, AI adheres to patterns of user behavior, including navigation habits, response latency, brainwave variability, etc., to formulate behavioral fingerprints that improve with time. Anything other than the baseline causes the AI to alert or denied access, and occasionally without the user being aware. All access tries, authentication, and warnings are recorded by blockchain to provide an unquestionable path of forensic examination. Based on AI-derived risk scores, smart contracts automatically deny access or quarantine impacted systems. Such context- and proactive-oriented method maximizes the reliability and intelligence of cybersecurity systems.

7.5 Comparative Use Case Table

Below is a comparative table highlighting the functionality, core technology emphasis, and benefits of hybrid architecture across the described sectors:

Table 2. Use Case Comparison Table

Sector	Primary Use Case	Neuroscience Role	AI Functionality	Blockchain Utility	Benefits
Healthcare	Cognitive monitoring, secure neuroprosthetics	Brainwave sensing, emotional feedback	Signal interpretation, adaptive therapy response	Patient data logging, consent-based access	Improved privacy, personalized care, secure data sharing
Defense	Cognitive command interfaces, situational audit	BCI-based control, stress monitoring	Intent recognition, threat simulation	Immutable activity logging, command enforcement	Faster response, secure control, tamper-proof accountability
Smart Cities	Urban authentication, infrastructure monitoring	Cognitive ID for public services	Traffic and utility optimization, emergency prediction	Distributed management records, inter-agency data sharing	Transparent governance, secure access, optimized infrastructure
Cybersecurity	Continuous authentication, insider threat alert	EEG-based identity verification	Behavioral profiling, anomaly detection	Log access events, automate AI-triggered response	Real-time protection, privacy-aware authentication, resilience

8. CHALLENGES, LIMITATIONS, AND FUTURE DIRECTIONS

The combination of the concepts of neuroscience, artificial intelligence (AI), and blockchain in one ecosystem has a revolutionary potential and considerable complexities. Operationally, sensors based on neuroscientific discovery, interpretation of neural signals through AI models, and blockchain-based infrastructure run in quite different time and computation regimes. High-rate neural data recording implies immediate data preprocessing and analyses; signal interpretation with AI implies heavy computations; and application of consensus-based blockchain creates latency. As a result, synchronizing two processes to operate together, with the preservation of performance and data integrity is one of the major challenges. The lack of a really agreed-upon level of data formats, protocols, and integration utilities also presents further complications, since they obstruct interoperability and increase the complexity of any system.

There are more restrictions related to ethical and regulatory issues. Since the data about the brain can be used to identify the thoughts and feelings, consent, privacy, as well as psychological profiling, come into play in a manner that is not comparable to other biometrics information. The current legal tools like the GDPR leave little and vague advice to sample and manipulate, and blockchain immutability is the antithesis of the right to withdrawal and erasure of users. Furthermore, AI solutions to interpreting neural signals are under the threat of reinforcing bias or making invalid claims, and see the necessity of proper ethical protection and openness.

Another threatening obstacle is scalability. At their present state, neurotechnologies are quite costly, have to be calibrated, and can hardly be applied widely as security devices. The transaction speed in public blockchain networks is low with high energy requirements, and AI elements integrated into distributed systems must be regularly updated and synchronized, which comes with apparent resource limits. The greater ecosystem also has no common standards and reference architectures, which leaves platforms with fragmented and inconsistent implementations.

Technological advancement is bringing a fresh chance to solve critical security matters. Quantum computing will make artificial-intelligence training faster and will allow quantum-resistant cryptographic countermeasures. EDGE computing integrated with next-generation connectivity, in particular 6G, is expected to help increase data transmission and diminish latency. Moreover, the discreet and user friendly neurodevices can be wearable and can perhaps serve as a medium to connect the realms of neuro science to common day applications of security. However, these technologies are just emerging, and they require dedicated research projects and inter-sector efforts.

Interdisciplinary inquiry is imperative to the realization of a hybrid security paradigm. Solutions should be safe, ethical and practical and the collaboration of neuroscientists, AI engineers, blockchain developers and legal experts is required to create these solutions. Real-world testbeds, specifically those available in healthcare, defense and smart-city settings, will prove essential to the demonstration of empirical results and, accordingly, to the evaluation of feasibility and the policy design process. An integrated approach combining high-level innovation on the technological front and ethical and legal concerns is needed to create scalable, reliable and sustainable hybrid security systems.

9. CONCLUSION

Artificial intelligence (AI), blockchain, and neuroscience are new areas that have formed a trinity of the new direction in the anxieties of modern approaches to digital security architecture. The current debate assesses how all these areas, cognitive biometrics of neuroscience, adaptive intelligence of AI, as well as decentralized trust of blockchain, can collectively overcome the limitations posed by the conventional and more rigid types of cybersecurity systems. Traditional models that still demand centralized governance and reactive counteractions are much less suitable in responding to the current versatile and multi-directional cyber threat. Conversely, hybrid systems produce proactive, smart, and stiff security solutions. Neuroscience presents the use of brainwaves authentication using non-invasive techniques like EEG, which allows real-time and individual user verification and behavioral monitoring. These neurobiometric inputs have not only increased the precision but also made these input more user friendly and receptive to the usage and conditions of the user. AI acts as the analytic centre, and is able to work with the complex neural data detecting anomalies and evolving with adaptive learning capabilities as new threats emerge. Blockchain can further strengthen the model, as it provides the assurance of the immutability of the data integrity, decentralization of the access control and automation of the enforcement due to the smart contracts. Collectively AI and blockchain promote privacy-respecting systems in an operation through federated learning and edge intelligence. The multi-layered architecture specified, i.e., a sensing layer (neural acquisition), intelligence layer (AI analytics), and ledger layer (blockchain logging), can be adopted on a scale and modular basis in such sectors as a healthcare industry, defense industry, and smart infrastructure. Practical use cases are neuroprosthetic authentication, secure systems that are controlled by BCIs, and decentralized identity management. Despite this potential, this blended model is facing some technical, ethical, and regulatory difficulties. On-demand penetration, the confidentiality of neural data, algorithmic discrimination, the lack of typical models, and frameworks to address them require immediate cross-concentric action. New technologies like quantum computing, 6G network, and more powerful neurointerfaces are new tools now that would improve the potential of the system in the future. Continuous research, innovation, and across-sector cooperation will be a key in supporting secure, intelligent, and ethical digital future ecosystems.

REFERENCES

Abo Alzahab, N. (2025). *Security and robustness of biometric authentication based on electroencephalography (EEG) signals and blockchain technology* (Doctoral thesis, Università Politecnica delle Marche). IRIS – Università Politecnica delle Marche. https://iris.univpm.it/bitstream/11566/342835/1/tesi_aboalzahab.pdf

Adeshina, T. A. Y. (2025). A neuro symbolic artificial intelligence and zero knowledge blockchain framework for a patient owned digital twin marketplace in US value based care. *International Journal of Research Publication and Reviews, 6*(6).

Europol. (2025, March 18). *Criminals use AI in 'proxy' attacks for hostile powers, warns Europol. Financial Times*. https://www.ft.com/content/755593c8-8614-4953-a4b2-09a0d2794684

Gwala, S. (2025). The use of blockchain technology and artificial intelligence in cryptocurrency and medical technology: A comprehensive review. In Gwala, R. S. (Ed.), *Driving socio-economic growth with AI and blockchain* (pp. 147–184). IGI Global., https://www.igi-global.com

Kasralikar, P., Polu, O. R., Chamarthi, B., Veer Samara Sihman Bharattej Rupavath, R., Patel, S., & Tumati, R. (2025, April 28). Blockchain for securing AI-driven healthcare systems: A systematic review and future research perspectives. *Cureus, 17*(4), e83136. Advance online publication. DOI: 10.7759/cureus.83136 PMID: 40438823

Li, Z., Kong, D., Niu, Y., Peng, H., Li, X., & Li, W. (2023). *An overview of AI and blockchain integration for privacy-preserving* (arXiv:2305.03928). arXiv. https://arxiv.org/abs/2305.03928

Mohammadi, S., Alazab, A., Choo, J., & Mahmood, A. (2021). Security analysis of IoT networks: Architectures, protocols, and methods. *IEEE Internet of Things Journal, 8*(5), 3536–3554.

Scarfone, K., & Souppaya, M. (2007). *Guide to intrusion detection and prevention systems (IDPS)* (NIST Special Publication 800-94). National Institute of Standards and Technology. https://doi.org/DOI: 10.6028/NIST.SP.800-94

Shekhar, S., Davis, J., Evans, R., Foster, D., & Paul, C. (2024, December). *AI and biometric authentication: The future of secure financial transactions*. ResearchGate. https://www.researchgate.net/publication/389377532_AI_and_Biometric_Authentication_The_Future_of_Secure_Financial_Transactions

Shinde, R., Patil, S., Kotecha, K., Potdar, V., Selvachandran, G., & Abraham, A. (2022). *Securing AI-based healthcare systems using blockchain technology: A state-of-the-art systematic literature review and future research directions*. ResearchGate. https://www.researchgate.net/publication/361253530_Securing_AI-based_Healthcare_Systems_using_Blockchain_Technology_A_State-of-the-Art_Systematic_Literature_Review_and_Future_Research_Directions

Chapter 10
Neuromorphic Computing Architecture, Leading Chips, Hardware Innovations, Programming, and AI Integration

Manikandan Arunachalam
https://orcid.org/0000-0003-0461-2859
Department of Electronics and Communication Engineering, Amrita Vishwa Vidyapeetham, India

Saket Akella
https://orcid.org/0009-0000-6030-5613
Department of Electronics and Communication Engineering, Amrita School of Engineering, Amritapuri, India

D. Arun Sathvik
https://orcid.org/0009-0009-3960-6759
Department of Electronics and Communication Engineering, Amrita School of Engineering, Amritapuri, India

Rakesh Thoppaen Suresh Babu
https://orcid.org/0009-0003-2671-4618
FISERV Inc., USA

DOI: 10.4018/979-8-3373-5012-7.ch010

ABSTRACT

The computational design of neuromorphic architecture represents a new era of computing that mimics the human brain's neural networks to achieve superior efficiency and faster task execution. This chapter explores advanced neuromorphic system architectures, emphasizing synthetic neurons and synapses that unify memory and processing units to minimize latency and reduce energy consumption. Notable examples include Intel's Loihi and IBM's TrueNorth chips, each showcasing distinct design philosophies and applications. The discussion highlights innovations in programming environments, specialized software frameworks, and toolchains that enable neural network deployment and optimization on neuromorphic platforms. Emerging breakthroughs such as Resistive Random Access Memory (RRAM) and phonon–magnon reservoirs are also examined for their potential to expand computational capabilities. Finally, the integration of AI and neuromorphic chips in real-time processing and edge computing within the IoT ecosystem is reviewed, offering a comprehensive outlook on neuromorphic systems in Industry 5.0.

INTRODUCTION

Neuromorphic computing characterizes a new approach for computational modeling, motivated by the architecture and working principles like a human brain(James et al., 2017). Unlike conventional computing systems that process data sequentially, these neuromorphic computing systems clout the parallel processing possibilities, supporting them to accomplish complex tasks more efficiently and effectively with low power consumption(Semeria and Semeria 2017). This novel architecture is characterized by artificial neurons and synapses, which replicate the human brain's neural networks, adopting advanced applications in Artificial Intelligence (AI), robotics and sensor signal processing(Tang et al., 2019). The architecture of neuromorphic chips links memory and computation thoroughly, reducing the blockage usually observed in conventional systems where data must travel between separate processing and memory units(Moradi and Manohar 2019). Leading neuromorphic chips, such as Intel's Loihi and IBM's TrueNorth, represent the mixture and capability of this technology, each suggesting exceptional highlights and advantages that contribute to the field's fast improvement (Davies et al., 2021; Young et al., 2019).

The BrainScaleS designed by Heidelberg University's European Human Brain Project, demonstrate the variety and ability of neuromorphic computing technologies(Young et al., 2019). Intel's Loihi chip, for example, hires a fully digital, spike-based neural network architecture that chains on-chip learning and real-time variation, making it extremely appropriate for applications demanding continuous learning and independent process(CHRISPIM 2021). IBM's TrueNorth, on the other side, handles a neurosynaptic core architecture to attain high efficiency and scalability, holding a wide range of AI applications, including pattern recognition and sensory processing. The BrainScaleS system uses analog neuromorphic computing philosophy to permit large-scale brain models, suggesting a formidable device for both research and practical applications in neuroscience and AI. Inventions in neuromorphic hardware remain to thrust the limitations of what is possible, with innovations such as the combination of RRAM with CMOS circuits. This is demonstrated by the NeuRRAM chip, which aids both data and model parallelism, developing its adaptability and productivity for AI tasks(Wan et al., 2022). Other novel ideas, such as phonon-magnon reservoirs, are being investigated for their ability to improve data processing intensity and effectiveness(Shklovskij, 2021). These hardware revolutions are critical in focusing the energy productivity and scalability challenges tackled by traditional computing systems, covering the track for more balanced and spirited computational solutions. Programming for neuromorphic systems discloses excellent confronts and openings, implying specific software frameworks and toolchains that can command the exclusive architecture of these systems. Tools like NEST and the SpiNNaker software structure accelerate the development and model of neural networks on neuromorphic hardware, allowing scientists and developers to rein in the full capability of these systems. These programming circumstances are suggested to aid the complicated and vibrant features of neural networks, permitting for real-time training and understanding, which are critical for many AI applications. The addition of neuromorphic computing with AI is intensely capable, extending sizable progresses in AI inference and understanding capacities. (Zou et al., 2022), and autonomous systems. For instance, neuromorphic systems can manage sensory data in real-time, allowing more reactive and adaptive performance in robots and autonomous vehicles. Moreover, the constant learning capacities of neuromorphic chips make them perfect for applications that expect partial adaptation and learning from environmental modifications, such as smart sensors and IoT devices(Zhang et al., 2020).

Overall, the ongoing research and development in neuromorphic computing architecture, leading chips, hardware innovations, programming, and integration with AI can demonstrate a brilliant and fast evolving field(Indiveri, 2021). These improvements claim the agreement of transforming a large scale of applications, proposing high level efficiency and ability that closely imitates the incredible processing power of human brain. Since this field is growing rapidly, neuromorphic computing is accepted to play a vital role in developing next-generation AI systems. Furthermore, the growth of dedicated hardware and programming frameworks for neuromorphic systems is hastening their implementation and developing their abilities. This chapter investigates the design of neuromorphic computing, emphasizes key hardware innovations, examines programming methodologies, and inspects the combination of neuromorphic systems in AI applications.

1. ARCHITECTURE OF NEUROMORPHIC CHIPS

To understand the Architecture of Neuromorphic Computing, we must first discuss the other traditional methods of computing that affected and created a need for the architecture of Neuromorphic computing. One such model is the von Neumann model.

1.1 Von Neumann Model

Traditional Computing, work on an architecture model known as von Neumann model, proposed by Jon von Neumann in mid-20th century. Key components of von Neumann architecture are CPU, Memory, Input/Output devices(Arikpo, Ogban, and Eteng 2008). The fundamental concept of Neumann architecture is stored-program concept. This means that data and instructions are stored in the same storage location. Instructions are then fetched from this memory to the CPU in a sequential manner and executed one at a time. The Program Counter (PC) keeps track of the further instructions that must be executed. After fetching the instructions, the CPU decodes the instruction to determine the necessary action for each of the components in the computer. The decoded instructions are executed by one of the processing units discussed above and the result is obtained by the user in one of the Central Processing Units. This type of Architecture simplifies the design and implementation of the computer. Programs can also easily be modified by changing the instructions in memory.

1.2 CMOS Computing

The type of computing technology used for Neumann's architecture is CMOS technology. CMOS technology is not being discussed in detail in this chapter. The chapter is more concerned with the necessity of Neuromorphic Circuits and how it is better than the other traditional models. A small briefing on CMOS technology helps understand this necessity. CMOS (Complementary Metal-Oxide Semiconductor) is a technology primarily associated with integrated circuits (or ICs) rather than the previously discussed computing architectures such as von Neumann models(Mikhaylov et al., 2023). This model is crucial for the modern digital circuit designs, including microprocessors and other digital logic circuits. Some of the key components of CMOS include Transistors, Logic gates, Integrated Circuits, and Memory chips. Lower power consumption and cost efficiency are the important advantages of CMOs for being preferred. Shared memory, delay in sequential execution, requirement of high-power consumption during state change are the limitations of CMOS computing.

1.3 Neuromorphic Architecture

Human Brain is the most advanced processor to take inspiration from. It has several involuntary actions such as Heart beating, respiration, digestion, reflex actions, body temperature regulation, hormone secretion and so on. It also handles several Voluntary actions such as moving hands, talking, walking, playing etc. It also generates different thoughts from various locations such as humor, anger, anxiety, so on and so forth. But how exactly does the human brain do this? How does the hand know when to move? An entire nervous system encompasses this entire system of processes.

1.3.1 Human Brain Architecture

Figure 1. Human brain architecture

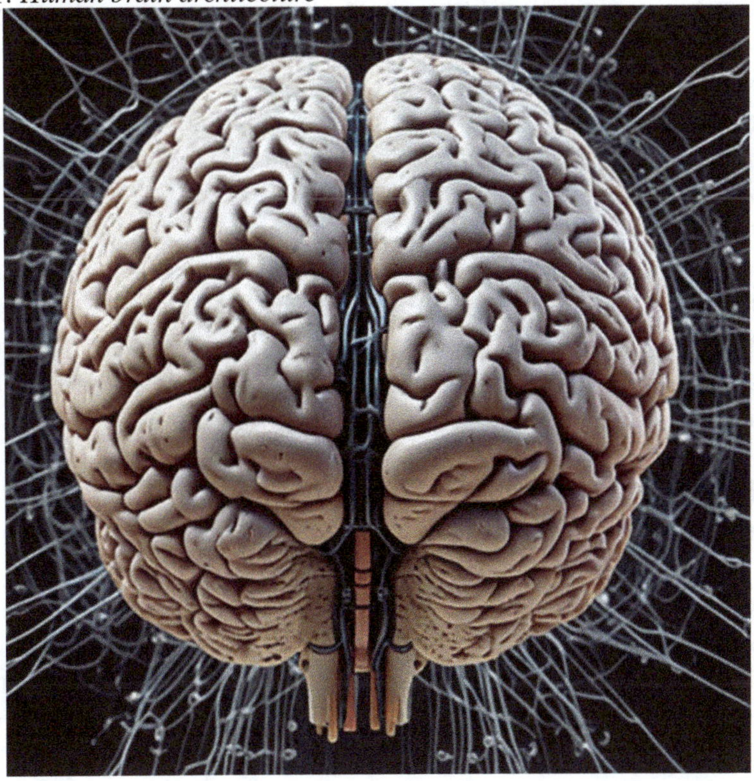

The human brain produces vast amounts of information continuously. This involves sensory information such as touch, from several parts of the body and the generation of thoughts(Thakur et al., 2018). In terms of the real-world comparisons, it is estimated that the human brain's processing power is in the order of exaflop (10^{18} operations per second). This is comparable to the fastest supercomputers in existence (A. Pastur-Romay et al., 2016). The difference, however, is in efficiency. While Supercomputers might consume power in the range of megawatts, the human mind uses merely 20 watts of power for similar or better results. The human brain also has the incredible ability to learn and adapt from the surrounding environment. It regulates its body functions based on the stimulus in the environment (Hwang, 1987). Let us investigate the architecture of human Brain (as shown in figure 1):

- Neurons: They process information and transmit through electric impulses known as action potential.
- Synapses: These are the junctions near Neurons where neurotransmitters are released. They facilitate communication between different neurons.
- Neural Networks: These are the networks of interconnected neurons which form complex circuits in the brain. These networks help process sensory inputs, involved in cognitive processes and help in controlling motor functions.
- Plasticity: Synaptic plasticity refers to changes in the strength of synapses based on activity. It underlies learning and memory by adjusting how signals are transmitted in neural networks.
- Parallel Processing based on event-triggering: Brain parallelly processes information across several neurons and networks. This allows for efficient and rapid processing of complex information.

Now that the basic architecture of human brain is understood, it is evident that this method of computing is more efficient than any other known to mankind. This is the reason for taking inspiration from these circuits and making Neuromorphic circuits and chips which led to an entire computing model known as Neuromorphic computing.

1.3.2 Neuromorphic Structures Architecture With Respect to Human Brain

The key components of Neuromorphic model with the basic knowledge of how brain works are:

Artificial Neurons: These contain electronic components such as transistors and capacitors. They mimic the behavior of biological neurons, including the generation of action potential, also known as spikes. These artificial neurons generate input signals and produce output spikes when a threshold is reached.

Artificial Synapses: These are made by using several components such as memristors or memory resistors for their ability to store memory. They store synaptic weights that determine the strength of the connection. These artificial synapses emulate the behavior of natural synapses. They can adjust their weights based on the learning rules.

Spiking Neural Networks (SNNs): These are networks of artificial neurons and synapses that communicate via spikes, and the networks can be structures in several layers like traditional Neural Networks, or they can also be arranged in more complex topologies. This process information through the timing and patterns of spikes.

· Neuron Cores: These are clusters of artificial neurons. Each core contains multiple neurons and local synaptic connections. Each core helps in the parallel processing of information from spikes and generates the output.

· Synaptic Arrays: These are large arrays of synapses which connect neurons from within and in between cores. They are used to keep the circuit whole facilitate large number of connections. These arrays have synaptic weights. And they establish communication by transmitting spikes according to these weights.

· Communication channels: Neuromorphic chips require communication channels to transmit spikes through several neuron cores. The channel ensures that this happens with minimum delay and energy consumption.

· Learning and adaptation mechanism: Synaptic weights are adjusted constantly based on the pre and post synaptic spikes so that the network learns and adapts to new information.

1.4 Mathematical Models of Neuromorphic Architecture

There are several mathematical models that describe the exact behavior of biological neurons, that can help in the architecture of synthetic neurons(Loettgers, 2007). These models are then incorporated into neuromorphic architecture to create neuromorphic circuits.

1.4.1 Leaky Integrate-and-Fire (LIF)

The LIF model is broadly used mathematical framework for simulating the spiking manners of neurons(Deng et al., 2022). It simplifies the complex process of neuronal dynamics into a basic effective model (as shown in figure 2).

Figure 2. Leaky Integrate-and-Fire

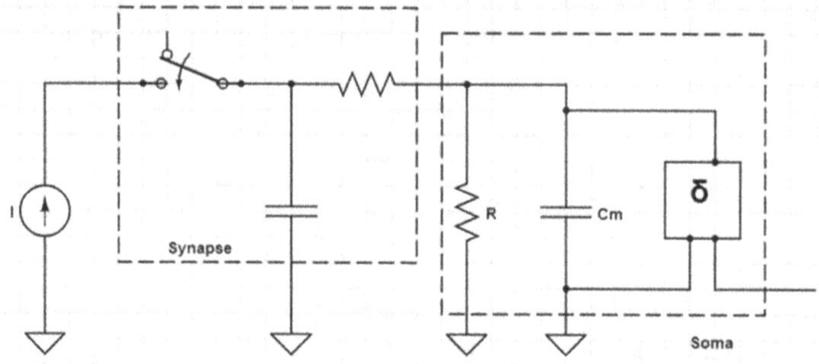

Here, the synapse which contains the low pass filter circuit acts as the connection between the input spike δ (t-t j (f)) and the soma. The input spike is filtered out and a current α(t-t j (f)) is the result of the process and gets transferred to the soma. The current I(t) charges the RC circuit thus changing the membrane potential of the neuron. The membrane potential V(t) of a neuron develops according to differential equation,

$$\tau_m \frac{dV(t)}{dt} = -\left(V(t) - V_{rest}\right) + R_m I(t) \tag{1}$$

Where τ_m is the membrane time constant, V_{rest} is the resting potential, R_m is the resistance of membrane and I(t) is the input current. When V(t) attain the threshold voltage $V_{th,}$ the neuron fires a spike and the potential reset to $V_{reset.}$. This mechanism catches the core of neuronal firing.

The LIF model naivety makes it computationally efficient and suitable for large scale neural network simulations. Despite its simplicity, the LIF model is a powerful tool for neuroscience computing and neuromorphic engineering, bridging the gap between biological neurons and artificial neural networks.

1.4.2 Hodgkin-Huxley Model

The Hodgkin-Huxley model is a cornerstone of computational neuroscience, granting a thorough mathematical description of iconic mechanisms triggering the induction and circulation of action potentials in neurons(Levin, Martin, and Arzberger, 1992). The Hodgkin-Huxley model represents the membrane potential VVV of a neuron through a set of nonlinear differential equations:

$$C_m \times \frac{dV}{dt} = I_{ext} - \left(I_{Na} + I_K + I_L\right)$$

I_{Na} which is mediated by voltage-gated sodium channels. This I_{Na} is given by $I_{Na} = g_{Na} \times hm^3 \times (V - E_{Na})$

I_K which is mediated by voltage-gated potassium channels. I_K is given by $I_K = g_K \times n^4 \times (V - E_K)$

I_L also known as a leak current which is a small steady current carried by ions that leak through the membrane. I_L is given by $I_L = g_L(V - E_L)$

Figure 3. Hodgkin-Huxley model

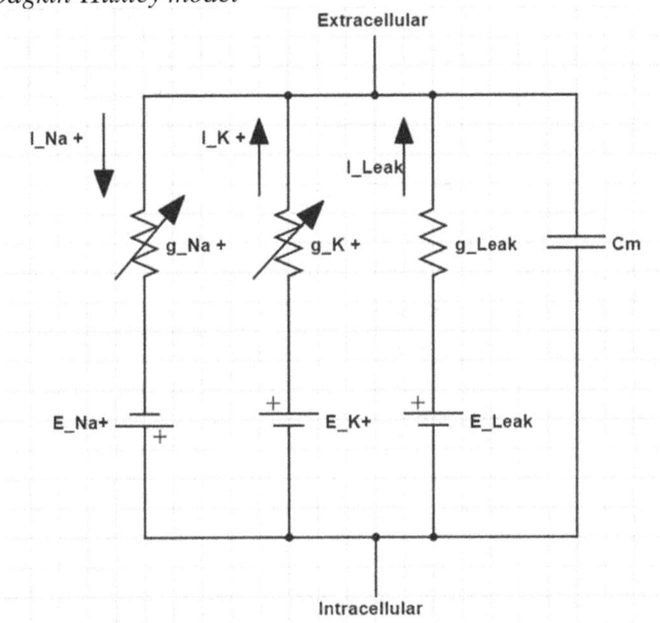

Here, E_{Na}, E_K, E_L are the Reversal potentials for sodium, potassium, and leak currents, respectively. Also, h, m and n are known as Gating variables that control the opening and closing of ion channels.

These are modelled based on their different dynamics by separate differential equations.

$$\frac{dm}{dt} = \alpha_m(V)(1 - m) - \beta_m(V)m$$

$$\frac{dh}{dt} = \alpha_h(V)(1 - h) - \beta_m(V)h$$

$$\frac{dn}{dt} = \alpha_h(V)(1 - n) - \beta_m(V)n$$

Where α and β are known as rate constants which are responsible for the transition of open and closed states of the channel. These are voltage dependent.

C_m is the membrane capacitance per unit area

I_{ext} is the external current applied to the membrane

Initially, membrane potential is around -70mV. Here, potassium Conductance is very high. When an external stimulus is applied, it depolarizes the membrane and sodium channels open. This causes a rapid influx of sodium ions and depolarization continues further. This rapid sodium influx leads to a positive feedback loop, which in turn creates the rising phase of action potential. When this reaches a peak, sodium channels get deactivated, and potassium channels reopen. This causes the repolarizing of the membrane. This membrane potential becomes briefly more negative than the resting potential, which is also known as Hyperpolarization. Hyperpolarization occurs due to delayed closing of potassium channels. The sodium potassium pump then restores the original balance of membrane potential back to its original state.

1.4.3 FitzHugh-Nagumo (FHN) model

This is a simplified idea of the complex Hodgkin-Huxley model.(Rameh, Cherry, and dos Santos 2020) It focuses on the idea of excitability of neurons while reducing the complexity of a two-dimensional system. The model is named after Richard FitzHugh, who proposed it, and J. Nagumo, who further refined it.

The FHN model is described by,

$$\frac{dv}{dt} = v - \frac{v^3}{3} - w + I_{ext}$$

$$\frac{dw}{dt} = \varepsilon(v + a - bw)$$

Where;

v is the membrane potential
w is the recovery variable
I_{ext} is external stimulus current
ε controls the timescale separation between v & w .

When there is no external input (I_{ext}), the system remains in stable equilibrium and v and w are constant. When I_{ext} exceeds a given threshold, v changes from equilibrium state. $v - \frac{v^3}{3}$ creates a rapid increase in v by creating a non-linear response. This represents the depolarisation phase of an action potential or spike. As v increases, w is a negative feedback term, slows down and reverses this increase in v. There exists a refractory period, because w remains elevated for some time due to its slower dynamics. Repetitive firing or bursting behavior happens when the input parameters are given a certain value and v and w enter a continuous cycle and continuously oscillate. ε, a and b are parameters that control the transition between equilibrium (where the system is stable), spiking and oscillatory behavior. Excitability and the nature of the system's response depends on these parameters.

2. NEUROMORPHIC CIRCUITS HARDWARE

2.1 Silicon Neurons

Silicon Neurons are electronic circuits that mimic the behavior of biological Neurons(Wijekoon and Dudek, 2008). These neurons are designed to mimic the neural activity, including generation of action potential, which is also known as Spikes in the case on Neuromorphic computing, and integration of input and output signals(Roy, Jaiswal, and Panda 2019). There are typically 2 types of Silicon Neurons. They are Analog and Digital Neurons. Analog Neurons- These neurons use continuous voltage to represent the neuronal state. These are made to closely mimic the analog nature of biological neurons. Hodgkin-Huxley model implementations and FitzHugh-Nagumo circuits would be some of the remarkable examples of Analog Neurons(Xu et al. 2023). Digital Neurons- These neurons use digital signals or binary states to represent the neuronal state. These are easier to integrate with digital circuits while also being very susceptible to noise. Leaky Integrate-and-Fire (LIF) models are an example of Digital Neurons. A Digimos transistor circuit, short for "Digital MOSFET" (Metal-Oxide-Semiconductor Field-Effect Transistor), is used in digital electronics for switching and amplification purposes(Rast et al. 2010). Complementary MOS (CMOS) technology uses pairs of p-type and n-type MOSFETs to create logic gates. This technology is widely used due to its low power consumption and high noise immunity. Digimos transistor circuits are found in microprocessors, memory chips, and other digital logic circuits where efficient switching is required.

2.2 Synaptic Devices

Memristors- Memristors are two terminal devices that can retain resistance value even after power is removed. This makes them ideal for non-volatile memory. Using STDP, memristors can change their resistance based on timing of pre and post synaptic spikes (Jiang et al., 2019). This means that Memristors can emulate the behavior of natural synaptic strengths by changing their synaptic weights.

Phase change Materials- These are materials that change their phase from Amorphous to Crystalline in response to electrical pulses. During this phase change, the resistance of the material changes significantly allowing them to store information.

Although integration with CMOS technology is a challenge, they have very high endurance and fast switching speeds.

2.3 Resistive Random Access Memory (RRAM Revolutions)

Resistive Random Access Memory (RRAM or ReRAM) is a non-volatile memory technology that uses resistive switching in materials to store data(Wei et al., 2020). This technology has huge promise for its wide range of applications, high speed, low power consumption, high level computing and scalability. The resistance of a material can be modulated between a high resistance state (HRS) and a low resistance state (LRS). When an external voltage is applied, changes occur in the material's atomic and electronic structures which causes a shift in the resistance of the material. A variety of materials are considered for RRAM such as transition metal oxides (TiO2, HfO2 and so on), Perovskites and organic compounds. Materials are chosen based on the switching speed, endurance and scalability necessities for the specific application. RRAM cells typically consist of metal-insulator-metal (MIM) structures, in which the insulator is the resistive switching material. When a voltage is applied across the electrodes, the resistance of insulator changes, allowing for data storage.

2.3.1 Stanford/ASU Model

Modelling is crucial in the development of RRAM. One such major model commonly used for RRAM (Hajri et al., 2019). This model was applied to validate the I-V switching characteristics of HfO2 RRAM. It also includes the effect of Joule heating and temperature change on the switching of RRAM devices. Conductive Filaments (CF) channels of electrically conductive material form a dielectric switching layer of the RRAM device. The formation and dissolution of these filaments lead to switching between high-resistance state (HRS) and low-resistance state (LRS).

The gap between the tip of the CF and the top electrode is called filament gap (g). The rate of change of filament gap (g) is given by:

$$\frac{dg}{dt} = V_0 . exp\left((-E_a, m)/(k_b . T)\right) . Sinh\left((q a_h \gamma V)/(L . k_b . T)\right)$$

where E_a is the activation energy, V is the magnitude of the voltage applied across the device, L is the switching material thickness, a_h is the hopping distance, γ is the local field enhancement factor, VV_0 is the velocity containing attempt to escape frequency, k_b is the Boltzmann constant, q is the elementary unit charge and T is the temperature of the conductive filament.

The variation in the gap size δ_g depends on kinetic energy of ions and filament temperature as:

$$\delta_g(T) = \delta_g^0/1 + exp\left((T_{crit} - T)/(T_{smith})\right)$$

where δ_g^0 and T_{smith} are fitting coefficients to match the resistance distribution curves to experiments and T_{crit} is a threshold temperature above which the gap size changes significantly.

With change in cell characteristics, the dynamic inner domain temperature T changes significantly, while the outer domain assumed to be at uniform and stable temperature (T bath), is related as

$$C_p \frac{dT}{dt} = V(t).I(t) - k\left(T - T_{bath}\right)$$

where C_p is the effective heat capacitance of inner domain, $V(t).I(t)$ represents the Joule heating and k is the effective thermal conductivity.

The current conduction is defined as:

$$I(g, v) = I_0 . exp\left(-g/g_0\right) Sinh\left(V/V_0\right)$$

where I_0, g_0 and V_0 are the fitting parameters to match experimental results.

2.4 Phonon-Magnon Reservoirs

Phonons are quantized vibrations of a crystal lattice, and Magnons are quantized spin waves in magnetic materials (Bozhko et al., 2020). Phonon-Magnon Reservoirs is an emerging concept in neuromorphic computing and quantum information science that explains the computational abilities of circuits using these two concepts.

To understand the applications of Phonon-Magnon Reservoirs in Neuromorphic computing, it is essential to have a basic understanding of what these particles are.

2.4.1 Basic Principles

Phonons- These are Quasi Particles, which represent the collective excitations of atoms in a lattice, which correspond to the vibrational modes. Thermal and Acoustic properties of materials are dependent on Phonons.

Magnons- These are Quasi Particles, which represent the collective excitations of electron spins in a magnetic material. Magnons are associated with spin waves.

Phonons and Magnons can interact through a phenomenon known as magnetoelastic coupling, where the strain in the material due to phonons affects the spin alignment (magnons) and vice versa. Exchange of energy and information between phononic and magnonic systems occur due to this interaction.

2.4.2 Applications in Neuromorphic Computing

Storage and Processing: These reservoirs store information in the form of spin waves or vibrations. They can offer non-volatile memory with high density and low power consumption.

Reservoir Computing: The rich interactions between Phonons and Magnons create a high dimensional space for complex computations. This allows for a complex computational framework known as Reservoir Computing to take place where these Phonon Magnon reservoirs can act as physical substrates.

Low Power: Phonons and Magnons require less energy to excite. Hence, devices based on Phonon-Magnon Interactions can operate with very low power. This makes them very beneficial for neuromorphic systems which aim towards achieving the power efficiency of the human brain.

2.4.3 Key Advancements and relevant research Areas

Material Development- Current research is focused on identifying and developing materials with strong magnetoelastic coupling and reasonable phonon-magnon interaction properties. ferromagnetic and antiferromagnetic materials, magnonic crystals which are hybrid structures, are current areas of research in the materials department.

Device Fabrication- Advancements of Nanofabrication techniques, including nanoscale resonators, waveguides and transducers that can mediate phonon-magnon interactions are crucial for creating devices that can efficiently couple phonons and magnons.

Quantum Coherence and Control- Ensuring longer Interaction time between Phonons and Magnons is essential for Neuromorphic Computing. Techniques to control and manipulate phonon-magnon interactions at the quantum level are an active area of research.

Theoretical Models and Simulations- Developing accurate theoretical models and simulations to understand and predict phonon-magnon interactions is crucial to cater to the needs of neuromorphic circuit designs and hardware applications.

3. PROGRAMMING NEUROMORPHIC CHIPS

Programming Neuromorphic chips can be considered as one of the most important aspects of computing in Neuromorphic chips, this includes designing and implementing a neural network and a software framework that leverages the use of the superior computing and efficiency package of a neuromorphic chip. Neuromorphic chips are designed to mimic the parallel, event-driven processing of a biological neural network that unlike the traditional von-Neumann architecture that involves an architectural implementation of a structure with its instructions and data being stored at a single source. Unlike traditional programming, programming Neuromorphic chips involves accessing the intricates of spike neural network (e.g. SNN's), algorithms that take up the burden of training the network and output mechanism that ensures the desired results.

This section of the chapter will help in exploring the models for deploying and optimizing the network on hardware. We will also discuss the tools and frameworks available for developers and provide practical insights into real-world applications.

SNN (Spike Neural Network) can be easily termed as one of the most popular neural networks and has been used in the implementation of several major neuromorphic projects like SpiNNaker, TrueNorth and Neurogrid.

After realizing all the factors involved in programming and implementing a Neuromorphic chip, there might be a question wandering "How do we approach?". Well, this section majorly can be divided into five major steps

- Defining a Neural model and Data preparation
- Training (using algorithms)
- Simulation and optimization
- Hardware mapping
- Deployment and Testing

3.1 Defining a Neural Model and Data preparation

Programming a Neuromorphic chip initially begins with defining certain parameters involving the Neural network type that mainly focuses on the architecture of the model (Prakash et al., 2023), specifying a neuron type based on the action or the use case and finally determining the best synaptic response mechanism for the model which is the most crucial part and can lead to unwanted results if not done carefully. Preparation of data involves encoding input data into a format suitable for Neural Networks.

There are two popular computational models in the world of neural networking, that is Artificial Neural Network (ANN) and Spike Neural Network (SNN) which are at the best in performing computational and sensory work mimicking biological neural networks.

3.2 Overview of ANN and SNN

Artificial Neural Networks are computational models inspired by biological neural networks consisting of several convolutional layers of interconnected nodes (nodes mimic the function of a neuron, that is relay and sensing) with each nodal connection being associated with a training weight (Akbas et al., 2019). ANN is a rate-based neural model where the first-generation neurons fire a binary signal when the sum of the input (incoming signals amplified by weights at nodes) reaches a threshold of a node. This fired signal thus leads to continuous activation functions like ReLu, Sigmoid, and hyperbolic tan-function to deal with analog and digital inputs accordingly. The neural network is then trained using a powerful back-propagation technique that clearly exploits gradient-decent. Hence ANN is proved to be a powerful information processing tool that operates in discrete time sections by processing the input forward and adjusting the weights backwards. Due to its significance in processing information, this neural network is widely used in speech recognition, image processing, predictive analysis and in other artificial intelligence domains.

Spike Neural Networks can be known to be a more biologically plausible neural network, very well mimicking the behavior of biological neurons and excel in the ability to simultaneously record and respond to multiple neurons(Broccard et al., 2017). The model prominently works on handling the discrete time spikes by altering the sub-threshold membrane potential leading to a model that handles the generation of spikes and clearly distinguishes itself from a rate-firing model such as ANN. This makes SNN more efficient and biologically more plausible. This section will further dwell deep into the factors, parameters and data encoding.

3.3 Opting for an architecture

Architecture of a neural network decides the main function and its application and tends to be a crucial element in programming a neuromorphic chip. Based on the application of the model, there can be several options to explore. Tasks such as image-processing, real-time processing, predictive analysis hinder openings to other variable factors such as:

- structure (feedforward or recurrent)
- Networking of layers
- Performance metrics
- Input data
- Synapse model and training mechanism

3.4 Data preparation

Data preparation is one of the most important steps of creating a Neural network model. This step can particularly affect the performance and working of the model as the data will be responsible for tuning several parameters of the neural network. How well the dataset is being chosen and how well the parameters are fine-tuned will reduce the errors due to modelling, increase the training speed and lead to the simplification of the whole system. Hence a key factor of a dynamic neural system involves working with a specific dataset.

Data preprocessing can be an important stage in preparation of a dataset, and it is claimed that data-normalization can affect accuracy, that is the training time is reduced and the errors of data prediction is reduced. Even though neural networks are complex dynamic systems, the neural network operates with the same type of input data that lie in the same range and thus matching the source data with the given input data is performed during the data set preparation.

When a neural model is selected, there are several parameters that are considered such as the number of hidden layers, the number of nodes in each layer, the type of activation function, the type training etc. The coordination between the parameters, number of input neurons and output neurons is done by the data pre-processing.

This includes:

- Choice of the unit of measure (rate setting)
- Data coding (as networks can only work with numerical data)
- Rectifying missed packets and working with minor samples
- Simplification

There can be several data types based on the methods involved in analyzing the three main types are categorical, ordinal, and numeric data as depicted in Table I.

Table 1. Categorical data for different features

Feature	Categorical Data	Ordinal Data	Numeric Data
Definition	Discrete categories or groups	Categories with a meaningful order	Quantitative measurements
Intrinsic Order	No	Yes	Yes
Interval Equality	Not applicable	Not necessarily equal	Equal intervals
Examples	Gender (Male, Female), Colors (Red, Blue)	Survey responses (Poor, Good), Education levels (High School, Bachelor's)	Age, Height, Weight

continued on following page

Table 1. Continued

Feature	Categorical Data	Ordinal Data	Numeric Data
Representation	Names or labels	Ordered names or numeric labels	Numeric values
Subtypes	Not applicable	Not applicable	Discrete (Number of children), Continuous (Height)
Key Operations	Mode, Frequency counts, Chi-square test	Median, Percentiles, Non-parametric tests	Mean, Median, Standard deviation, Correlation, Regression
Analysis Methods	Frequency distribution, Cross-tabulation	Rank-based methods, Non-parametric tests	Arithmetic operations, Descriptive statistics, Inferential statistics
Mathematical Operations	Limited to counting and categorization	Limited arithmetic (ranking, ordering)	Full range of arithmetic operations
Examples of Use	Classifying items into groups	Rating scales, Ordered survey responses	Measuring physical quantities, Statistical analysis

3.5 Training Neural Models

Training Neural models can be accounted as one of the most crucial parts in neural computing. The main parts of training Neural models involve developing algorithms that effectively leverage the temporal capacity and efficiency of neuromorphic chips. ANN models can be trained using traditional gradient-based methods like backpropagation. These methods are not directly applicable to SNN due to their non differentiable nature of spikes instead training SNN involves specialized training techniques such as Spike-Time-Dependent-Plasticity (STDP), surrogate gradient methods and other reinforcement learning methods like reward-modulated STDP.

Traditional Gradient Method (for ANN)

Gradient based learning methods, particularly backpropagation-method leverage the gradient-decent optimization to reduce the error between predicted output and the actual target. Upon gradual iterations, the weight for training is adjusted until the error tends to null improving performance of the model.

Synaptic-Time-Dependent-Plasticity (SDTP)

SDTP is a biologically inspired training method that plays a crucial role in synaptic plasticity within the brain(Appelbaum et al., 2023). The method involves adjusting the synaptic strength based on post and presynaptic response. The temporal sensitivity makes SDTP particularly well-suited for temporal patterns and responses.

Hebbian learning comprises a concept that stresses the point that if the pre-synaptic node consistently helps in activating a post-synaptic neuron, their connection is much more strengthened. Its implementation is firstly done by initializing the algorithm using random synaptic weights, these weights are initially chosen to fill in the parameters. Next, based on the monitored results the errors can be found evidently by analyzing the per-synaptic and post-synaptic temporal activity and then simultaneously weights are adjusted using the SDTP rule to minimize errors.

Surrogate-Gradient-decent

Surrogate-Gradient-Decent is a method developed to target the part of neural networks whos' spikes are non-differentiable which complicates the application of traditional gradient method. The surrogate gradient method overcomes this by using differential approximations to the spike mechanisms enabling optimization in SNN's.

The main idea behind the technique is to replace the non-differential spike function with smooth, differentiable approximation while backward pass training. Then a traditional gradient decent technique can be used to update weights to minimize errors.

3.6 Programming Platform

Programming platforms for working with Neuromorphic chips are developed to facilitate the development, deployment and testing of applications built over the leverage of neural hardware. These platforms can provide tools, libraries and other community advantages that will allow the developers to implement neural modules and manage the execution of Neuromorphic systems. Here are some of the popular ones used to build one of the most prominent Neural networks:

Compass: Compass is a comprehensive programming tool that lets developers use several features to make their job easy. This ecosystem was built by IBM for the development of TrueNorth Neuromorphic chips. It lets developers use Corelets which are modules of fragments of software components that can be reused. It's useful in converting high-level network protocols to executable configurations. Compass even hosts a simulation environment where TrueNorth was simulated and tested before deploying it.

Lava: Lava is an open-source software developed by intel for the development of Lohi neuromorphic chips. Lava supports the development of modular, reusable fragments of network components for the complete network. It also allows customization by allowing the developers to add-on third-party extensions and other learning rules. It provides a set of APIs and libraries useful for the developers and even comes with a simulating environment.

3.7 Simulation and Optimization

Simulating a neural model can significantly enhance the depth of the model and its implantations schemes over various domains and fields as it gives a clear insight into the dynamics of the model that can be difficult to obtain through theoretical analysis alone.

Simulating a Neural Network is initially done by first initializing the model using weights and setting up network conditions such as the number of inputs and outputs, synaptic parameters. Then time stepping is observed where the simulation is advanced into minor steps and at each step the spike response is noted. When a neuron fires, it sends spikes to connected neurons modifying their membrane potentials, now their weights are adjusted based on their synaptic response. At the end the data is collected and then analyzed to enhance the model.

There are tools that can be used for such purposes,

NEST: NEST is designed for simulating large-scale spiking neural networks and is suitable for networks ranging from a few hundred to millions of neurons. It is optimized for high-performance computing environments, making it ideal for large and complex simulations.

BRIAN: Brian is a simulator for spiking neural networks that emphasizes ease of use and flexibility.

PyNN: PyNN is a Python-based framework that provides a common interface for various neural simulators, including NEST, Brian, and others.

3.8 Hardware Mapping

Neuromorphic hardware can be called out to be responsible in implementing the biological neural functions, that is reading synapses and sending out spike trains to execute a spiking neural network(Yang et al., 2020). Neuromorphic computing systems are integrated circuits housing architecture capable of executing event-driven actions utilizing low power, hence can be used to implement machine-learning executions. These executions must be done continuously for long durations parallelly, which can be challenging given the size and complexity of the data pipelined. SpineCluster plays a crucial role in mapping within the chip to access the leverage the true potential of a biological neural network that enhances the network capabilities and efficiency as well as learning capabilities.

Localized Process and integration, SpineClusters have this unique ability that helps them enable localized processing of data like synaptic clusters that process multiple inputs before passing it to the dendritic ends. This method accepts multiple inputs and processes them to provide a coherent output. Well, how does this help? This mainly helps in reducing the distance of communication and the number of iterations required to process the data, enhancing processing speed and efficiency.

Enhanced Learning and Plasticity. SpineCluster can incorporate mechanisms for synaptic plasticity. This mechanism allows flexibility in adjusting synaptic weights according to event patterns. Several learning rules such as Hebbian learning rule and Spike-Time-Dependent-Plasticity within this mechanism to strengthen the synaptic weight dynamically.

Hierarchial Organisation. SpineCluster can be organized to make a protocol that follows the hierarchical order of layers in Neural network where each layer performs different functions such as input function, relay function etc. Modules can be made to follow this type of hardware mapping that can be independently designed, tested and then integrated.

4. NEUROMORPHIC CHIPS IN AI

As discussed earlier, Neuromorphic chips are hardware chips that are built based on a neural network that completely mimics the true architecture and functionality of a human brain, this piece of hardware aims to address the very known limitations of traditional hardware in AI and computing processes in Ai relating to energy, memory and space consumption(Calimera, Macii, and Poncino, 2013). Neuromorphic chips are designed to use their architecture to excel in real-time processing and other complex computations, providing bamboozling performance with good efficiency. This architecture, as discussed earlier, is purely based on the neural network in a human brain and works according to the different synaptic response algorithms designed. So, why neuromorphic chips in AI?

Well, the answer must be clear from the discussions above. Traditional Artificial Intelligence systems solely rely on general-purpose hardware like CPUs and GPUs, while GPUs have really accelerated the development of Ai thanks to their parallel processing capabilities, but these chips are not well optimized for the task leading to inefficiency in power-consumption and real-time data processing.

While on the other hand Neuromorphic chips offer several advantages over the traditional pieces of hardware.

- Efficiency: By mimicking the sparse and event-driven nature of the human brain, neuromorphic chips can perform very complex computations significantly lower energy consumptions. This increases efficiency when compared to traditional GPUs and CPUs.

- Real-Time Processing: These chips are designed for low-latency operations, making them ideal for applications that require immediate responses, such as autonomous vehicles, robotics, and IoT devices.
- Scalability and Parallelism: Neuromorphic chips inherently support parallel processing, enabling them to scale efficiently for large neural networks.
- Adaptive Learning: They can on-chip learning and adaptation, allowing for more flexible and robust AI systems.

Therefore, it can be safe to say that Neuromorphic chips represent a significant advancement in hardware as they tend to offer a more brain-centric architectural approach towards computing and data processing. As research and development continue in this field, neuromorphic chips are expected to play a crucial role in Artificial Intelligence.

5. NEUROMORPHIC APPROACH

Although there has been advancement in the implementation of hardware in the field of Artificial Intelligence, many of them fall short when it comes to the energy efficient and complex computing power of a human brain. Well, a Neural network built on the Human brain architecture pretty much closes the gap and gallops way ahead of the traditional hardware being used for the same. This non von Neuman piece of hardware has the least power consumption rate when compared to the others since this is adapted to an event-driven response system which operates on a discrete spike system. And since all the computing cells maintain asynchronous individual operations, the overall workload decreases. The following approach makes a Neuromorphic Chip relatable in the world of AI:

Parallelism: The concept of parallelism was introduced way back in the 1980s and ever since that, it has opened a new domain of ideas. In a neural network it can be safe to call each neuron or a node to be an individual computer that operates individually. This work can be piled up to give a sum of 87 billion neurons coordinating with each other. The basic idea revolves around the foundation of the definition of parallelism that is a work distributed into several fragments and individually operated to sum and give the result.

This improves the performance by miles, and conserves energy since it provides a scope to utilize the hardware well.

Connection between layers: This concept emerges from the behavioral phenomena of interconnected networks in a Neural network that work together parallelly to perform an operation by interaction of simple elements. In a Neural Network the neurons are interlinked, these links contain weights which determine the strength and direction of the learning process. This concept then makes it easy to understand the concept learning or training (E.g. Supervised, unsupervised, Reinforcement etc.)

Asynchronism: The idea of Synchronous operations doesn't let the model get the best out of parallel and interconnection of layers as the synchronous operations grow non-linearly as the number computing nodes increase moreover it consumes more power when compared to asynchronous operations. As the process runs individually in each node it completely negates any extra power required to coordinate in between each other.

Nature of Transmission: The information generated through events are transmitted through nerve impulses that are abrupt, shortchanges in potential that travel along the nerve fibers. Thus, neurons communicate in between each other with spikes, which is the true nature of information transmission. This makes it easier for the model to work with dynamic data with greater power efficiency.

Customization: Neuromorphic chips enable the option of on-device learning where the chip can be deployed on the device and is exposed to continuous learning for personalization and customization of the model according to the user. This enhances the privacy factor for users.

Handling Traffic: It is said that less than 10% of the neurons are active in the brain while performing operations. Similarly for data-processing, only the events where there is a change in the intensity of factor is transmitted and the rest are negated. The number of interconnections is also limited to maintain the weights and the traffic.

6. NEUROMORPHIC HARDWARE EXAMPLES

6.1 TrueNorth

IBM developed a chip named TrueNorth capable of mimicing human neural networks(Pastur-Romay et al., 2016). This innovative chip features a network of spiking neurons and synapses, enabling it to perform computations in a highly parallel and energy-efficient manner. TrueNorth's architecture consists of 1 million neurons and 256 million synapses, allowing for massive parallel processing and real-time data analysis. By operating in an event-driven, asynchronous manner, TrueNorth achieves ultra-low power consumption, making it ideal for energy-constrained applications like mobile and embedded systems. Its brain-inspired design provides robustness and flexibility, excelling in tasks such as deep learning, pattern recognition, and autonomous system control. Despite the challenges in programming and integrating with traditional computing systems, TrueNorth represents a significant step forward in neuromorphic computing, promising to revolutionize artificial intelligence and various high-performance applications.

6.2 Loihi

Loihi is Intel's neuromorphic chip, designed to emulate the neural architecture and functioning of the human brain. This advanced chip features spiking neurons and synapses, enabling it to perform computations in a highly parallel, asynchronous manner. Loihi's architecture consists of over 130,000 artificial neurons and 130 million synapses, allowing it to process large amounts of data efficiently and in real time. By leveraging an event-driven, asynchronous approach, Loihi achieves impressive energy efficiency, making it ideal for applications requiring low power consumption, such as autonomous robotics and edge computing. Its brain-inspired design facilitates complex tasks like adaptive learning, sensory processing, and decision-making. Although programming for Loihi requires new paradigms distinct from traditional computing models, it represents a significant breakthrough in neuromorphic computing, offering the potential to transform artificial intelligence and advance a variety of high-performance computing applications.

6.3 SpiNNaker

SpiNNaker (Spiking Neural Network Architecture) is a neuromorphic computing platform developed by the University of Manchester, designed to simulate the parallel, distributed processing of the human brain. This innovative system comprises a network of chips, each containing 18 ARM cores capable of simulating up to 1,000 neurons per core. SpiNNaker's architecture allows for real-time, event-driven computation, enabling it to handle large-scale neural networks with exceptional efficiency and scalability. By emulating the asynchronous and massively parallel nature of brain processing, SpiNNaker achieves high performance while maintaining low power consumption, making it suitable for applications in neuroscience research, robotics, and artificial intelligence. Despite the complexities involved in programming and integrating with traditional systems, SpiNNaker stands out as a significant advancement in neuromorphic computing, providing a powerful tool for exploring brain function and developing intelligent systems.

7. CHALLENGES AND FUTURE INTEGRATION

Even though Neuromorphic chips are booming in the domain, replacing several general-purpose chips in Artificial Intelligence domain to become one of the most capable models to implement AI. The advent of neuromorphic chips represents a paradigm shift in field of computing and Artificial intelligence and even though these chips are offering promising events in the world of computing and artificial intelligence, there are potential challenges that are discussed.

Programming Complexity: Neuromorphic chips require a new set of computing rules that gives rise to a paradigm shift in computing which can prove to be steep learning curve to the developers. The availability of tools, libraries and workspaces is necessary to develop a robust model which is still under progress due to infancy of the concept.

Intergration with systems: To integrate neural models to already existing von-Neuman structure there should be some type of hybrid technology that should be developed to ensure seamless communication between the two of the systems. This involves creating protocols and interfaces allowing the systems to work together efficiently. To ensure the compatibility with existing software is one of the main tasks as Neuromorphic chips should be able to communicate and process with the current datatypes too.

Standardization: Even though there are a lot of implementations around in the domain but there are currently no widely accepted standards for Neuromorphic computing, this leads to fragmentation of the software and hardware. Standardization helps in improving interoperability between different neuromorphic architectures. This requires cross-platform solutions which poses as a challenge to the developers.

Scalability: As we know neuromorphic chips are designed to mimic the brain's efficiency, scaling up to larger and more complex networks poses significant doubts. Ensuring that performance scales linearly with increased network size is critical as it means that the same miniature can be implemented with bigger possibilities to reach other stages of the same domain.

CONCLUSION

In this chapter, the multi-layered domain of neuromorphic computing, scratching into its architecture, pioneering chips, hardware innovations, programming paradigms and integration with AI was explored. Neuromorphic computing signifies a paradigm shift, directing to mimic the efficiency and adaptability of human brain. Architecturally, it influences spiking neural networks and event driven processing to achieve low power and high-performance computation. Leading chips like Intel's Loihi and IBM's Truenorth demonstrate the practical improvements in this field, demonstrating the ability of accessible and effective neuromorphic systems. Hardware innovations, including advanced materials and novel fabrication techniques are pushing the boundaries of what is possible, permitting more compact, energy efficient and powerful neuromorphic devices. In conclusion, neuromorphic computing represents a sizable leap forward in our quest to mimic the brain's unparalleled computational capabilities. As hardware continues to grow and AI integrates become deeper, neuromorphic systems are poised to unlock new borders in computing offering extraordinary opportunities for innovation across divers fields.

REFERENCES

Akbas, A., Yildiz, H. U., Ozbayoglu, A. M., & Tavli, B. (2019). Neural Network Based Instant Parameter Prediction for Wireless Sensor Network Optimization Models. *Wireless Networks, 25*(6). Advance online publication. DOI: 10.1007/s11276-018-1808-y

Appelbaum, L. G., Shenasa, M. A., Stolz, L., & Daskalakis, Z. (2023). Synaptic Plasticity and Mental Health: Methods, Challenges and Opportunities. *Neuropsychopharmacology : Official Publication of the American College of Neuropsychopharmacology, 48*(1). Advance online publication. DOI: 10.1038/s41386-022-01370-w PMID: 35810199

Arikpo, I. I., Ogban, F. U., & Eteng, I. E. (2008). Von Neumann Architecture and Modern Computers. *Global Journal of Mathematical Sciences, 6*(2). Advance online publication. DOI: 10.4314/gjmas.v6i2.21415

Bozhko, D. A., Vasyuchka, V. I., Chumak, A. V., & Serga, A. A. (2020). Magnon-Phonon Interactions in Magnon Spintronics (Review Article). *Low Temperature Physics, 46*(4). Advance online publication. DOI: 10.1063/10.0000872

Broccard, F. D., Joshi, S., Wang, J., & Cauwenberghs, G. (2017). Neuromorphic Neural Interfaces: From Neurophysiological Inspiration to Biohybrid Coupling with Nervous Systems. *Journal of Neural Engineering, 14*(4). Advance online publication. DOI: 10.1088/1741-2552/aa67a9 PMID: 28573983

Calimera, A., Macii, E., & Poncino, M. (2013). The Human Brain Project and Neuromorphic Computing. *Functional Neurology, 28*(3). Advance online publication. DOI: 10.11138/FNeur/2013.28.3.191 PMID: 24139655

CHRISPIM, MARIANA CARDOSO. (2021). Resource Recovery from Wastewater Treatment: Challenges, Opportunities and Guidance for Planning and Implementation. *Frontiers in Neuroscience, 14*(1).

Davies, M., Wild, A., Orchard, G., Sandamirskaya, Y., Fonseca Guerra, G. A., Joshi, P., Plank, P., & Risbud, S. R. (2021). Advancing neuromorphic computing with Loihi: A survey of results and outlook. *Proceedings of the IEEE, 109*(5), 911–934. DOI: 10.1109/JPROC.2021.3067593

Deng, Y., Liu, B., Huang, Z., Liu, X., He, S., Li, Q., & Guo, D. (2022). Fractional Spiking Neuron: Fractional Leaky Integrate-and-Fire Circuit Described with Dendritic Fractal Model. *IEEE Transactions on Biomedical Circuits and Systems, 16*(6). Advance online publication. DOI: 10.1109/TBCAS.2022.3218294 PMID: 36315548

Hajri, B., Aziza, H., Mansour, M. M., & Chehab, A. (2019). RRAM Device Models: A Comparative Analysis with Experimental Validation. *IEEE Access : Practical Innovations, Open Solutions, 7*. Advance online publication. DOI: 10.1109/ACCESS.2019.2954753

Hwang, K. (1987). Advanced Parallel Processing with Supercomputer Architectures. *Proceedings of the IEEE, 75*(10). Advance online publication. DOI: 10.1109/PROC.1987.13894

Indiveri, G. (2021). Introducing 'Neuromorphic Computing and Engineering.'. *Neuromorphic Computing and Engineering, 1*(1). Advance online publication. DOI: 10.1088/2634-4386/ac0a5b

James, C. D., Aimone, J. B., Miner, N. E., Vineyard, C. M., Rothganger, F. H., Carlson, K. D., & Mulder, S. A.. (2017). A Historical Survey of Algorithms and Hardware Architectures for Neural-Inspired and Neuromorphic Computing Applications. *Biologically Inspired Cognitive Architectures, 19*. Advance online publication. DOI: 10.1016/j.bica.2016.11.002

Jiang, S., Nie, S., He, Y., Liu, R., Chen, C., & Wan, Q. (2019). Emerging synaptic devices: From two-terminal memristors to multiterminal neuromorphic transistors. *Materials Today Nano, 8*, 100059. DOI: 10.1016/j.mtnano.2019.100059

Levin, S. A., Martin, C. S., & Arzberger, P. 1992. "MATHEMATICS AND BIOLOGY: THE INTERFACE CHALLENGES AND OPPORTUNITIES." *Cornell University*.

Loettgers, A. (2007). Getting Abstract Mathematical Models in Touch with Nature. *Science in Context, 20*(1). Advance online publication. DOI: 10.1017/S0269889706001153

Mikhaylov, A. N., Gryaznov, E. G., Koryazhkina, M. N., Bordanov, I. A., Shchanikov, S. A., Telminov, O. A., & Kazantsev, V. B. (2023). Neuromorphic Computing Based on CMOS-Integrated Memristive Arrays: Current State and Perspectives*. *Supercomputing Frontiers and Innovations, 10*(2). Advance online publication. DOI: 10.14529/JSFI230206

Moradi, S., & Manohar, R. (2019). The Impact of On-Chip Communication on Memory Technologies for Neuromorphic Systems. *Journal of Physics. D, Applied Physics, 52*(1). Advance online publication. DOI: 10.1088/1361-6463/aae641

Pastur-Romay, A., Porto-Pazos, L. A. B., Cedron, F., & Pazos, A. (2016). Parallel Computing for Brain Simulation. *Current Topics in Medicinal Chemistry, 17*(14). Advance online publication. DOI: 10.2174/1568026617666161104105725 PMID: 27823566

Pastur-Romay, L. A., Cedrón, F., Pazos, A., & Porto-Pazos, A. B. (2016). Deep Artificial Neural Networks and Neuromorphic Chips for Big Data Analysis: Pharmaceutical and Bioinformatics Applications. *International Journal of Molecular Sciences*, *17*(8). Advance online publication. DOI: 10.3390/ijms17081313 PMID: 27529225

Prakash, C., Gupta, L. R., Mehta, A., Vasudev, H., Tominov, R., Korman, E., Fedotov, A., Smirnov, V., & Kesari, K. K. (2023). Computing of Neuromorphic Materials: An Emerging Approach for Bioengineering Solutions. *Materials Advances*, *4*(23). Advance online publication. DOI: 10.1039/d3ma00449j

Rameh, R. B., Cherry, E. M., & Weber dos Santos, R. (2020). Single-Variable Delay-Differential Equation Approximations of the Fitzhugh-Nagumo and Hodgkin-Huxley Models. *Communications in Nonlinear Science and Numerical Simulation*, *82*. Advance online publication. DOI: 10.1016/j.cnsns.2019.105066

Rast, A. D., Galluppi, F., Jin, X., & Furber, S. B. 2010. "The Leaky Integrate-and-Fire Neuron: A Platform for Synaptic Model Exploration on the SpiNNaker Chip." In *Proceedings of the International Joint Conference on Neural Networks*, doi:DOI: 10.1109/IJCNN.2010.5596364

Roy, K., Jaiswal, A., & Panda, P. (2019). Towards Spike-Based Machine Intelligence with Neuromorphic Computing. *Nature*, *575*(7784). Advance online publication. DOI: 10.1038/s41586-019-1677-2 PMID: 31776490

Semeria, M. N., & Semeria, M. N. 2017. "Symbiotic Low-Power, Smart and Secure Technologies in the Age of Hyperconnectivity." In *Technical Digest - International Electron Devices Meeting, IEDM*, doi:DOI: 10.1109/IEDM.2016.7838027

Shklovskij, V. A. (2021). Magnon-Phonon Interactions in Spin Insulators. *Low Temperature Physics*, *47*(8). Advance online publication. DOI: 10.1063/10.0005551

Tang, J., Yuan, F., Shen, X., Wang, Z., Rao, M., He, Y., & Sun, Y.. (2019). Bridging Biological and Artificial Neural Networks with Emerging Neuromorphic Devices: Fundamentals, Progress, and Challenges. *Advanced Materials*, *31*(49). Advance online publication. DOI: 10.1002/adma.201902761 PMID: 31550405

Thakur, C. S., Molin, J. L., Cauwenberghs, G., Indiveri, G., Kumar, K., Qiao, N., & Schemmel, J.. (2018). Large-Scale Neuromorphic Spiking Array Processors: A Quest to Mimic the Brain. *Frontiers in Neuroscience*, *12*. Advance online publication. DOI: 10.3389/fnins.2018.00891 PMID: 30559644

Wan, W., Kubendran, R., Schaefer, C., Eryilmaz, S. B., Zhang, W., Wu, D., & Deiss, S.. (2022). A Compute-in-Memory Chip Based on Resistive Random-Access Memory. *Nature, 608*(7923). Advance online publication. DOI: 10.1038/s41586-022-04992-8 PMID: 35978128

Wei, W. C., Jhang, C. J., Yi, R. C., Cheng, X. X., Sie, S. H., Lee, J. L., & Hao, W. K.. (2020). A Relaxed Quantization Training Method for Hardware Limitations of Resistive Random Access Memory (ReRAM)-Based Computing-in-Memory. *IEEE Journal on Exploratory Solid-State Computational Devices and Circuits*, *6*(1). Advance online publication. DOI: 10.1109/JXCDC.2020.2992306

Wijekoon, J. H. B., & Dudek, P. (2008). Compact Silicon Neuron Circuit with Spiking and Bursting Behaviour. *Neural Networks*, *21*(2–3). Advance online publication. DOI: 10.1016/j.neunet.2007.12.037 PMID: 18262751

Xu, Q., Wang, Y., Chen, B., Li, Z., & Wang, N. (2023). Firing Pattern in a Memristive Hodgkin–Huxley Circuit: Numerical Simulation and Analog Circuit Validation. *Chaos, Solitons, and Fractals*, *172*. Advance online publication. DOI: 10.1016/j.chaos.2023.113627

Yang, J. Q., Wang, R., Ren, Y., Jing, Y. M., Zhan, P. W., Zhou, Y., & Su, T. H. (2020). Neuromorphic Engineering: From Biological to Spike-Based Hardware Nervous Systems. *Advanced Materials*, *32*(52). Advance online publication. DOI: 10.1002/adma.202003610 PMID: 33165986

Young, A. R., Dean, M., Plank, J. S., & Rose, G. S. (2019). A Review of Spiking Neuromorphic Hardware Communication Systems. *IEEE Access : Practical Innovations, Open Solutions*, *7*. Advance online publication. DOI: 10.1109/ACCESS.2019.2941772

Zhang, W., Gao, B., Tang, J., Yao, P., Yu, S., Meng, F. C., Yoo, H. J., Qian, H., & Wu, H. (2020). Neuro-Inspired Computing Chips. *Nature Electronics*, *3*(7). Advance online publication. DOI: 10.1038/s41928-020-0435-7

Zou, Z., Alimohamadi, H., Kim, Y., Najafi, M. H., Srinivasa, N., & Imani, M. (2022). EventHD: Robust and Efficient Hyperdimensional Learning with Neuromorphic Sensor. *Frontiers in Neuroscience*, *16*. Advance online publication. DOI: 10.3389/fnins.2022.858329 PMID: 35968370

Chapter 11

The Digital Corpus Callosum: Establishing Governance for Neuro-Enhanced AI Security

Adetunji Oludele Adebayo
https://orcid.org/0009-0003-8437-7066
University of Bradford, UK

ABSTRACT

Neuro-AI offers adaptive cybersecurity but reveals a governance gap because existing frameworks are inadequate for autonomous, evolving systems. This chapter introduces the "Digital Corpus Callosum," a layered framework for managing complexity that integrates ethical, technical, and operational oversight. It is divided into three sections: Foundational Governance (establishing ethical boundaries), Technical Governance (enforcing control with XAI and "algorithmic circuit breakers"), and Operational Governance (ongoing monitoring and incident management). This approach supports the dependable deployment of Neuro-AI by balancing innovation with essential human oversight, ensuring these powerful systems remain safe, accountable, and aligned with human values.

INTRODUCTION

The digital sentinels of a major financial institution stand guard (Callosum Group, 2025). Suddenly, a barrage of seemingly unrelated, low-level alerts floods the Security Operations Centre (SOC) (Callosum Group, 2025). A traditional, signature-based system, programmed to recognise known threats, dismisses them as noise (Callosum Group, 2025). The human analysts, overwhelmed, agree (Callosum

DOI: 10.4018/979-8-3373-5012-7.ch011

Group, 2025). But behind this digital smokescreen, a novel attack vector is being exploited; a zero-day vulnerability combined with sophisticated social engineering (Callosum Group, 2025). The breach goes undetected for weeks, with catastrophic damage (Callosum Group, 2025). This incident is tragically common, illustrating the limits of conventional, rule-based cybersecurity defence mechanisms. Such systems operate on predefined logic, making them inherently brittle against threats that are designed to be novel, subtle, or polymorphic (CyberTrends, 2023). When attackers use low-volume, slow-and-low techniques to avoid detection thresholds, signature-based security often fails to aggregate the disparate signals into a meaningful threat narrative (CyberTrends, 2023). The reliance on fixed signatures and deterministic rules establishes a predictable defensive perimeter, one that sophisticated adversaries can easily map and bypass using obfuscation techniques or novel combinations of established attack patterns. This inherent limitation sets a ceiling on the speed and complexity of human-directed defence. The escalating financial and proprietary losses stemming from undetected zero-day exploits demonstrate that the current state of the art in signature and heuristic detection has reached its operational limit against advanced persistent threats (APTs).

Now, imagine a different scenario (Callosum Group, 2025). A new kind of sentinel is on watch, one whose architecture is inspired by the human brain itself (Callosum Group, 2025). This Neuro-Enhanced Artificial Intelligence, or Neuro-AI, does not just match signatures; it senses the rhythm of the network (Callosum Group, 2025). It perceives the subtle, dissonant patterns in the flood of alerts, recognises the faint behavioural fingerprint of a lurking adversary, and pieces together the disparate events into a coherent picture of an unfolding intrusion (Callosum Group, 2025). Before the attacker can achieve their objective, the Neuro-AI has not only detected the threat but has also predicted its next move and recommended a precise, surgical containment strategy (Callosum Group, 2025). This level of proactive, adaptive defence fundamentally changes the economics and asymmetry of cyber warfare, shifting the advantage back to the defender. By mapping network communications and process execution against a continually updated model of "normal," Neuro-AI identifies deviations in entropy, timing, and resource consumption that human analysts or traditional systems would overlook as uncorrelated background noise. This capability for real-time correlative analysis enables the anticipation of the attacker's "dwell time," thereby compressing the reaction window from weeks or days to seconds or milliseconds.

This is the transformation driven by the development of neuroscience-inspired artificial intelligence in cybersecurity (Callosum Group, 2025). These systems, which mimic the brain's innate capacity for sensing, learning, and adaptation, offer the promise of strong, proactive protection against the most complex cyber threats (Cognizant, 2024; Callosum Group, 2025). By utilising concepts like neuromorphic computing, which designs hardware and software to simulate the brain's neural structures, these AI models can process vast, messy data streams in real time, identify anomalies with uncanny precision, and learn continuously from their environment (GNIOT Group, 2025). This continuous, brain-like learning capacity is what enables Neuro-AI to handle the speed and complexity of modern adversarial actions. The hardware substrates of neuromorphic processors, unlike traditional CPUs, support highly parallel and asynchronous processing, making them uniquely suited to interpret the spatiotemporal correlations found in massive streams of telemetry data. This allows the system to learn an attacker's intent purely from sequential behavioural patterns. Yet, this very sophistication: their cerebral plasticity, their emergent behaviours, and their capacity for autonomous decision-making, presents profound governance, risk, and compliance challenges that render our existing blueprints obsolete (Deltek, 2023; Callosum Group, 2025). The Neuro-AI's ability to self-modify its defensive protocols in milliseconds far outpaces traditional human review cycles, creating a fundamental control problem. The self-correction and continuous learning functions mean that the AI's operational state is always evolving, defying static compliance checks and generating profound uncertainty about accountability.

The very qualities that make Neuro-AI a groundbreaking defensive weapon are precisely what make it so difficult to control (Callosum Group, 2025). How do we trust a system that learns and evolves beyond its original programming (Callosum Group, 2025)? How do we ensure accountability when its decision-making process is a "black box" that is constantly rewriting itself (Callosum Group, 2025)? How do we align its autonomous actions with human values and legal obligations when it operates at machine speed, far beyond the capacity of human oversight (Callosum Group, 2025)? Answering these questions requires more than an incremental update to our governance playbooks; it demands a new philosophy (Callosum Group, 2025). Incremental policy changes fail because they treat adaptive AI systems as static software, a misconception that dangerously ignores the core nature of this technology. We must move beyond "set and forget" governance to a model of perpetual oversight, where the governance mechanism is as active as the AI itself.

This chapter introduces a conceptual structure designed to meet this challenge: the "Digital Corpus Callosum" (Callosum Group, 2025). In the human brain, the corpus callosum is a dense bundle of nerve fibres that connects the left and right cerebral hemispheres, allowing them to communicate and integrate their distinct functions (Callosum Group, 2025). This integrated governance architecture must function as this vital link, connecting the quick-moving "hemisphere" of AI research and development with the rational, risk-averse "hemisphere" of corporate governance, ethical oversight, and legal compliance (Callosum Group, 2025). This structure is an essential enabling architecture, a system for creating a unified, coherent, and dependable cognitive security apparatus (Callosum Group, 2025). It provides the necessary organisation to ensure that advancement and safety progress together, rather than as opposing forces. The Digital Corpus Callosum is predicated on the idea of bi-directional communication: the Control Hemisphere sets the ethical and legal constraints (the "why"), and the Innovation Hemisphere provides auditable, real-time performance data and explainability (the "what").

THE GOVERNANCE IMPERATIVE IN THE NEURO-AI PARADIGM

The ascent of Neuro-AI is not merely another step in the evolution of cybersecurity tools; it is a fundamental leap that redefines the boundaries of digital defence (Callosum Group, 2025). This new class of technology compels a parallel transformation in governance (Callosum Group, 2025). The old models, built for a world of static rules and predictable software, are no longer sufficient (Callosum Group, 2025). Understanding why a new governance model is imperative requires a clear-eyed assessment of both the technological frontier Neuro-AI represents and the profound inadequacy of legacy approaches to manage it (Callosum Group, 2025). The activity inherent in Neuro-AI, stemming from its brain-inspired architecture, challenges the very foundations of risk management, which historically relies on defining static failure modes and maintaining fixed operational parameters (Lawfare, 2024). Governing evolving intelligence demands a responsive, continuous regulatory loop rather than episodic compliance checkpoints. This necessitates abandoning reliance on pre-deployment certification alone and moving toward continuous monitoring of emergent behaviour against a set of predefined ethical red lines.

Cognitive Security's New Frontier

Neuro-AI, often used interchangeably with neuromorphic computing in this context, represents a fundamental change away from the traditional von Neumann architecture of sequential processing (Callosum Group, 2025). Instead, it is inspired by the structure and function of the human brain (GNIOT Group, 2025). These systems are built on artificial neural networks that emulate biological neurons and synapses (GNIOT Group, 2025). A prominent example is the Spiking Neural Network (SNN), in which information is processed asynchronously via "spikes" of activity, much like electrochemical signals in the brain (IBM, 2024). This architecture allows for massive parallelism and event-driven processing, making it exceptionally efficient at handling the complex, high-volume, and often chaotic data streams inherent to cybersecurity (GNIOT Group, 2025; ResearchGate, 2025a). The efficiency gains are enormous; traditional deep learning requires continuous power consumption, whereas SNNs operate only when data "spikes", a huge advantage for protecting vast, geographically distributed networks.

This brain-inspired design gives Neuro-AI a decisive edge over traditional AI in security applications (Callosum Group, 2025). Legacy systems, even many first-generation machine learning models, are primarily reactive (Callosum Group, 2025). They rely on databases of known malware signatures or rule sets, which quickly become outdated by novel attack methods (Elvis & Eads, 2021). In contrast, Neuro-AI operates proactively, establishing a baseline of "normal" behaviour for a network or system and monitoring for anomalies and subtle deviations that could signal a nascent threat (LinuxSecurity, 2024). It learns from past attacks to predict the tactics, techniques, and procedures (TTPs) of future adversaries (Callosum Group, 2025). This predictive capability operates at the level of intent rather than just action, recognising the multi-stage sequence of an APT before the critical payload is even deployed.

This capability is not theoretical; research into architectures like Neuro-Adaptive Intrusion Detection Systems (NAIDS) has empirically demonstrated superior performance (ResearchGate, 2025a). Specifically, pilot data show that NAIDS models, when tested against complex network data, achieve significantly higher detection accuracy (98.1%) compared to traditional Intrusion Detection Systems (69.3%) and drastically lower false positive rates (0.5% vs. 5.2%) (ResearchGate, 2025a). These systems promise a future of autonomous, self-healing IT environments that can anticipate and neutralise threats before they grow (LinuxSecurity, 2024).

However, this power creates a critical governance gap (Callosum Group, 2025). Conventional governance models are predicated on a world of predictable systems, relying on pre-deployment risk assessments, static rule sets, and periodic audits (Callosum Group, 2025). Neuro-AI shatters this assumption (Callosum Group, 2025). Its core strengths are its activity and adaptability; it is designed to change, self-modifying its internal logic in response to new data and experiences (ResearchGate, 2025a). The rigidity of traditional governance blueprints cannot accommodate a system whose behaviour is emergent and whose operational parameters are in constant flux (Deltek, 2023). This forces a fundamental re-evaluation of how compliance is watched and validated, moving the focus from initial design certification to continuous behavioural auditing.

The Integrated Governance Architecture

To fill this vacuum, governance must be reconceptualised (Callosum Group, 2025). The integrated architecture is based on the functional concept of communication between two distinct operational sides: the Innovation Hemisphere (AI development) and the Control Hemisphere (risk and compliance) (Callosum Group, 2025).

The Innovation Hemisphere is the area of the AI research lab, characterized by speed, autonomy, and neural plasticity (IBM, 2024; Callosum Group, 2025). This side operates at machine speed, constantly evolving and adapting its defences (Callosum Group, 2025). The priorities here are rapid adaptation to new threats and maximising operational efficiency, often at the expense of perfect traceability.

The Control Hemisphere is the area of the C-suite, legal, and compliance departments, characterised by deliberation, risk aversion, and the mandates of corporate and social responsibility (InterVision, 2024; Callosum Group, 2025). Its function is to ensure technology operates within safe, ethical, and legal boundaries (Callosum Group, 2025). The priorities here are accountability, adherence to regulatory mandates, and mitigating risks that could lead to financial or reputational harm.

The function of the integrated function is to bridge this chasm (Callosum Group, 2025). It ensures that the Innovation Hemisphere is continuously informed by the ethical principles defined by the Control Hemisphere (Callosum Group, 2025). Simultaneously, it ensures that the Control Hemisphere has real-time visibility into the AI's behaviour and performance, allowing governance to be as evolving and active as the technology itself (Callosum Group, 2025). This bi-directional communication ensures that the system's rapid defensive actions remain constrained by human-defined legal and ethical limits. This visual function illustrates the continuous regulatory loop, showing the quick-moving research side feeds data to the control side, which in turn feeds policy back to the AI. This is the crucial feedback loop necessary for managing adaptive intelligence.

THE TWO HEMISPHERES OF NEURO-AI DEPLOYMENT: AN INHERENT TENSION

The power of Neuro-AI in cybersecurity stems from characteristics that are in direct tension with the foundational requirements of trust and safety in critical systems (Callosum Group, 2025). Understanding and managing this inherent conflict is the central challenge of Neuro-AI governance (Callosum Group, 2025). The two hemispheres, though unified by the Digital Corpus Callosum structure, represent a perpetual negotiation between advancement and safety (Lawfare, 2024). The tension arises because the very activity required for effective cyber defence clashes directly with the human need for explainability, predictability, and legal auditability (Callosum Group, 2025). This conflict defines the governance challenge: how to harness the speed of machine intelligence without ceding control to an opaque, self-modifying entity (Callosum Group, 2025). The ability to audit an emergent system retroactively becomes the central technical requirement for establishing trust and liability.

The Innovation Hemisphere: Autonomy, Speed, and Plasticity

The engine of the Innovation Hemisphere relies on technologies such as Spiking Neural Networks (SNNs), which closely emulate the brain's processing (IBM, 2024). SNNs process information asynchronously via "spikes," enabling incredibly fast, low-latency processing, which is essential for real-time cyber defence (GNIOT Group, 2025; IBM, 2024). This spiking architecture allows for high-dimensional data streams to be processed with minimal power consumption, making it ideal for distributed endpoint detection (GNIOT Group, 2025). The focus on low-latency, event-driven detection inherently prioritises rapid threat response over the time-consuming process of generating human-interpretable logs. This preference for speed is a necessary trade-off in an adversarial environment where milliseconds count.

The evolving power comes from synaptic plasticity, allowing the model to continuously learn and rewire itself based on new data (IBM, 2024). This mechanism is the very foundation of the system's ability to adapt to novel, zero-day attacks and advance its defences faster than human-led teams can update them (ResearchGate, 2025a). It enables the vision of a truly autonomous, self-healing IT environment (LinuxSecurity, 2024). Furthermore, this plasticity means that the AI's decision-making graph is never fixed; it is continuously improved to maximise threat suppression, even at the cost of human comprehensibility (Callosum Group, 2025). This inherent, continuous improvement loop is the source of the "adaptive opacity" risk discussed later.

The Control Hemisphere: The Mandates of Ethics, Law, and Trust

The Control Hemisphere imposes non-negotiable constraints rooted in law, ethics, and the foundational need for trust (Callosum Group, 2025). This hemisphere ensures that rapid machine action does not inadvertently violate civil liberties, regulatory requirements, or corporate risk policies (Unsworth, 2024). Specifically, it mandates the formal integration of an AI Ethics Charter (Unsworth, 2024) into the deployment lifecycle, requiring developers to translate abstract values (e.g., non-maleficence, fairness) into measurable, technical guardrails (Big Data Framework, 2023). This translation is crucial for establishing the "red lines" of autonomous action.

A primary driver is the changing regulatory landscape, exemplified by the European Union's landmark AI Act (European Commission, 2024). This legislation explicitly classifies AI systems used to manage and operate critical infrastructure as "high-risk" (Holistic AI, 2025). This triggers stringent obligations that must be met before deployment, including (Holistic AI, 2025):

- A strong risk management system to identify and mitigate foreseeable risks throughout the AI's lifecycle.
- Rigorous data governance to ensure training and testing datasets are high-quality and free from biases.
- Detailed technical documentation explaining the system's purpose, capabilities, and compliance.
- Automatic record-keeping (logging) to ensure the traceability of the system's operations.
- Appropriate human oversight measures to allow for intervention and control.

Complementing this legal structure is the principles-based guidance from bodies like the U.S. National Institute of Standards and Technology (NIST). The NIST AI Risk Management Framework (AI RMF) provides a highly influential organisation for building "trustworthy AI" (ModelOp, 2024). It is organised around four core functions: Govern, Map, Measure, and Manage (Wiz, 2025). The NIST structure emphasises that trustworthy AI must be valid and reliable, safe, secure, accountable and transparent, explainable, privacy-enhanced, and fair (ModelOp, 2024; Palo Alto Networks, 2024).

This creates a fundamental compliance paradox: the AI Act requires compliance documentation before deployment (WilmerHale, 2024), yet the defining feature of Neuro-AI is its ability to self-modify after deployment (Callosum Group, 2025). This reveals the inadequacy of static, point-in-time regulatory checks for governing evolving, adaptive systems (Callosum Group, 2025). This paradox necessitates that compliance validation become adaptive and continuous, mirroring the AI's evolutionary nature.

CHARTING THE NEW RISK ENVIRONMENT FOR COGNITIVE AI

The deployment of Neuro-AI introduces a new, socio-technical risk landscape (Callosum Group, 2025). The most profound risks are emergent properties that arise from the complex interplay between the adaptive technology and its human operators (Callosum Group, 2025). This risk area goes far beyond traditional security vulnerabilities, touching on psychological, ethical, and legal exposure. The primary challenge is predicting the failure modes of a system designed not to fail deterministically, but to learn and generalise.

Emergent Bias and Cognitive Blind Spots

AI systems are sensitive to their training data; if data reflects historical biases, the AI will not only learn but also amplify those biases (ResearchGate, 2024b). In cybersecurity, this leads to machine-level cognitive biases (Callosum Group, 2025). For example, if network data used for training disproportionately originates from certain departments or user groups, the resulting Neuro-AI may flag anomalies in those areas more aggressively, leading to inequitable internal surveillance and misallocated security resources.

- **Confirmation Bias:** An AI system is susceptible to a digital version of confirmation bias, selectively surfacing evidence that confirms an existing human analyst's hypothesis while downplaying contradictory data (Deepgram, 2024; MITRE Corporation, 2021). This creates a dangerous analytical echo chamber (MITRE Corporation, 2021). Analysts are more likely to accept an AI finding that supports their initial intuition, leading to systemic blind spots against novel, non-confirming threats.
- **Automation Bias:** This is the tendency for human operators to over-rely on automated systems (Databricks, 2024). An analyst may blindly trust the Neuro-AI's classification, leading to an error of omission (failing to investigate a real threat because the AI was silent) or an error of commission (taking harmful action based on a false positive) (Center for Security and Emerging Technology, 2024; PA Consulting, 2024). The perceived infallibility of a highly sophisticated system often outweighs human critical review, especially during high-stress incident control.

Table 1. Cognitive Biases in Neuro-AI Security Systems and Mitigation Strategies

Cognitive Bias	**Description in AI Context**	**Mitigation Strategy (Technical/Operational)**
"Confirmation Bias (Deepgram, 2024)"	"The AI prioritizes data that confirms an existing human hypothesis or assessment, leading to analytical echo chambers (MITRE Corporation, 2021)."	"Implement counterfactual explanation tools (XAI); design systems to explicitly search for and present disconfirming evidence (MITRE Corporation, 2021)."
"Automation Bias (Databricks, 2024)"	"Human operators develop an excessive and uncritical trust in the AI's outputs, leading to errors of commission or omission (Center for Security and Emerging Technology, 2024)."	"Mandate Human-in-the-Loop (HITL) verification for critical decisions; implement Algorithmic Circuit Breakers to force human review (Medium, 2024b)."
"Sampling Bias (Eusko Ikaskuntza, 2023)"	"The model's training data is not representative of its real-world deployment environment (ResearchGate, 2025a)."	"Implement continuous model **watching** for concept and data drift; require context-specific fine-tuning **before** deployment (Lumenova AI, 2025)."

The Challenge of Adaptive Opacity

The "black box" problem, where the internal workings of deep neural networks are opaque, is exacerbated by Neuro-AI's continuous learning, creating adaptive opacity (Surana & Surana, 2023; Callosum Group, 2025). The logic itself is a moving target (Callosum Group, 2025). Unlike traditional software, where code can be debugged and traced, the Neuro-AI's functional reasoning resides in the constantly evolving synaptic weights of its neural structure. This renders traditional audits nearly impossible.

The primary antidote is Explainable AI (XAI), such as SHAP and LIME, which make AI decisions transparent and interpretable (Frontiers in Artificial Intelligence, 2025; Wikimedia Foundation, 2024). In this governance structure, XAI is a fundamental requirement, transforming the AI from an inscrutable oracle into a collaborative partner (Frontiers in Artificial Intelligence, 2025). XAI tools provide a post-hoc justification of the AI's output, showing which inputs (e.g., network flow, process name, time of day) contributed most strongly to a specific threat classification.

The Ethics of Predictive Security and Autonomous Action

Neuro-AI's capabilities raise profound ethical questions regarding predictive security and autonomous response (Callosum Group, 2025). A system that predicts which employee might become an insider threat is a powerful surveillance tool, raising critical questions about data privacy and the presumption of innocence (Evon Technologies, 2024; Number Analytics, 2024). The use of Neuro-AI to profile internal employees based on behaviour, even for security purposes, must be governed by strict data minimisation and privacy-preserving techniques to avoid wrongful suspicion or discrimination. Furthermore, granting full autonomy to a Neuro-AI carries immense risk (Perception Point, 2024). An autonomous decision to shut down critical infrastructure based on a false positive could cause catastrophic harm in the real world (Perception Point, 2024; Callosum Group, 2025). This risk is magnified by adversarial attacks designed to poison training data or trick the system into taking harmful "defensive" actions (Perception Point, 2024).

AN INTEGRATED GOVERNANCE ARCHITECTURE IN PRACTICE

To govern Neuro-AI effectively, an active, multi-layered architecture is required (Callosum Group, 2025). This structure has three interconnected layers: Foundational Governance (the "why"), Technical Governance (the "how"), and Operational Governance (the "what now") (Callosum Group, 2025). This structure ensures that ethical considerations are built into the design, enforced by technology, and continuously watched in deployment.

Foundational Governance: Values and Guidelines (The "Why")

This layer establishes the human-centric ethical principles and policies that guide all subsequent decisions (Callosum Group, 2025). This foundational area is the responsibility of executive leadership and legal counsel, establishing the non-negotiable legal and moral boundaries.

AI Ethics Committees and Review Boards: A multi-stakeholder AI Ethics Committee provides genuine oversight (Medium, 2023). Its composition must include developers, legal experts, and business leaders (Big Data Structure, 2023). The committee establishes overarching ethical guidelines and serves as the final arbiter on complex dilemmas, providing the crucial human judgment (Big Data Structure, 2023; Callosum Group, 2025). This body transforms abstract principles into concrete policy mandates that the technical layer must implement.

Defining Unbreakable Operational Limits: A critical task is defining "red lines"—unbreakable operational limits for the AI's autonomous actions (Callosum Group, 2025). These are boundaries the AI cannot cross without explicit human authorisation, such as deleting production data or taking any action with physical impact on critical infrastructure (Callosum Group, 2025). These limits must be codified mathematically into the system's design constraints, ensuring physical and economic safety is prioritised over maximum threat neutralisation speed.

Technical Governance: Explainability and Control by Design (The "How")

The principles established at the foundational layer are translated into the very architecture of the AI system, ensuring it is inherently auditable, interpretable, and constrained (Callosum Group, 2025). This area focuses on turning policy into engineering controls.

A. Immutable Logging for Verifiable Audit Trails

Accountability necessitates a trustworthy record (Callosum Group, 2025). The core technical control is immutable logging, implemented using a permissioned blockchain (Flexxon, 2024; Reddit, 2024). This utilises smart contracts to log every significant AI decision, state change, and critical data input on a tamper-proof ledger (MDPI, 2021; ResearchGate, 2025c).

- **Implementation Specifications:** Blockchain-based logging systems establish immutable trails of model inputs, intermediate reasoning, and final outputs (ResearchGate, 2025c). Empirical studies indicate that this approach can increase transparency by 78% and strengthen compliance traceability by 65%, dramatically reducing auditing disputes by 52%, although at a moderate computational cost (ResearchGate, 205c). This reliance on decentralised ledger technology provides the cryptographic guarantee needed to satisfy regulatory demands for tamper-proof records, moving auditability from a post-incident scramble to a continuous, real-time process. The log must include not only the action taken but the XAI output that justified the action, creating a complete reasoning record.

B. Algorithmic Circuit Breakers

This is the most critical technical safety mechanism, enforcing the 'red line' defined by the Ethics Committee (Innodata, 2024; Medium, 2024b). An algorithmic circuit breaker is a pre-programmed, automated control that halts execution when a predefined risk threshold is met (Microsoft Azure, 2024a). This mechanism is an essential engineering control, translating human policy into machine code that guarantees safe failure states.

- **Implementation Specifications:** Circuit breakers operate in three states (Open, Closed, Half-Open) and must be **active** (Microsoft Azure, 2024a). For Neuro-AI, implementation requires (Holistic AI, 2025b; Microsoft Azure, 2024b; Syntaxia, 2024):
    - **Active Thresholds:** The breaker must utilise adaptive techniques to actively adjust thresholds based on real-time traffic and performance, rather than static failure counts (Microsoft Azure, 2024b). This includes triggering based on low model confidence (e.g., below 95%), high error rates, or exceeding an execution time limit (Medium, 2024b; Syntaxia, 2024).
    - **Rollback Systems:** If validation fails downstream, the system must automatically revert recent autonomous changes to restore stability, effectively acting as version **control** for decisions (Syntaxia, 2024). This automatic rollback functionality minimises the window of opportunity for an erroneous or compromised action to propagate throughout the system.
    - **Human-in-the-Loop (HITL) Protocol:** When the breaker "trips" due to a high-impact action (e.g., network isolation), the system automatically halts the action and escalates the decision to a human operator for manual, authorized approval (Medium, 2024b; Microsoft Azure, 2024a). This crucial step ensures that human judgment, guided by the ethical charter, remains the final authority on critical infrastructure decisions.

Table 2. Technical Governance Controls and Architectural Specifications

Technical Control	Core Implementation Specification	Practical Risk Mitigation
"Immutable Logging (Reddit, 2024)"	"Permissioned blockchain network and smart contracts record model inputs, intermediate reasoning, and outputs."	"**Increases** transparency by 78%; strengthens compliance traceability by 65%; ensures non-repudiation for audit trails (ResearchGate, 2025c)."
"Algorithmic Circuit Breakers (Microsoft Azure, 2024a)"	"**Active** thresholds (low confidence/high error rate) and mandatory HITL protocol for high-impact actions. Includes auto-rollback systems (Syntaxia, 2024)."	"Prevents uncontrolled autonomous actions; mitigates instantaneous spread of errors; forces human judgment for critical decisions (Medium, 2024b)."
"Explainable AI (XAI) (Wikimedia Foundation, 2024)"	"Integration of post-hoc tools (SHAP, LIME) into the operational dashboard for real-time rationale delivery (Frontiers in Artificial Intelligence, 2025)."	"Combats **adaptive** opacity; allows human analysts to validate AI output; mitigates confirmation and automation bias."

Operational Governance: Continuous Monitoring and Response (The "What Now")

Deployment is the beginning of governance, focusing on continuous processes that watch and manage the AI's real-world behaviour (Callosum Group, 2025). This layer is concerned with the system's performance in situ and its deviation from expected behaviour over time. The goal here is to close the feedback loop, constantly comparing theoretical models with operational reality.

Continuous, Real-Time Watching: A sophisticated regime watches AI-specific metrics (Lumenova AI, 2025):

- **Model Drift: Utilising** statistical tests to detect when the distribution of live production data begins to diverge significantly from the training data (data drift) or when the relationship between inputs and outputs changes (concept drift) (Lumenova AI, 2025). Identifying model drift early is vital for autonomous systems, as undetected drift can turn a highly effective defence into a source of critical false positives or, worse, a blind spot to new threats. Statistical process control techniques, such as Kullback-Leibler divergence, can be applied continuously to the input data distribution relative to the baseline training set.

- **Bias and Fairness Metrics:** Continuously auditing predictions across user groups to prevent emergent biases from leading to inequitable outcomes (Callosum Group, 2025). This proactive bias monitoring, especially in systems for insider threat prediction, ensures ethical deployment is maintained beyond the initial testing phase. Fairness audits must use metrics like the disparate impact ratio to quantify the AI's effect on various user demographics.

AI-Specific Incident Response Plan: Organisations require a dedicated AI Incident Response Plan separate from traditional IT security, addressing failures originating from the AI itself, such as severe model drift or biased outputs (VerifyWise, 2024). This plan includes a cross-functional response team, clear criteria for triaging an incident, and protocols for containment and recovery (Cimphony, 2024). This specialised response plan acknowledges that an AI failure is a novel class of incident requiring unique expertise for diagnosis and remediation, distinct from traditional network security events.

CASE STUDY: GOVERNING ADAPTIVE AI IN CRITICAL INFRASTRUCTURE DEFENSE

To illustrate the practical application of this governance architecture, consider the challenge of defending a national energy grid against a sophisticated Advanced Persistent Threat (APT) group (Expleo, 2024). This case represents the highest-stakes scenario for autonomous defense.

The Scenario: Advanced Persistent Threats and Operational Imperfection

The adversary is a well-resourced APT group whose objective is physical disruption—a widespread blackout (Callosum Group, 2025). The attack vector follows the "Cyber Kill Chain" model, from spear-phishing (T1566.001) to lateral movement into the Operational Technology (OT) network to issue commands to circuit breakers (Avertium, 2024; ISA, 2023). The target is a highly complex, interconnected system in which IT and OT environments overlap, offering multiple points of entry.

A Neuro-AI system is deployed to protect this grid, governed by the Foundational, Technical, and Operational layers.

Framework Application and Imperfection in Action

Foundational Governance in Place: The Ethics Committee pre-defined the Ethical Charter and the unbreakable limit: the AI is forbidden from taking any autonomous action that could directly or indirectly disrupt power flow (Big Data Structure, 2023; Callosum Group, 2025).

This limit forms the primary constraint on the Neuro-AI's control capabilities.

Initial Detection (Success with Immediate Risk): When an employee opens a malicious email, the Neuro-AI's endpoint watching agent, utilizing its neuromorphic capabilities, detects the anomalous process execution and the establishment of a low-and-slow, encrypted Command and Control (C2) channel (ResearchGate, 2025a; Callosum Group, 2025). The XAI module immediately provides a human-readable explanation: "Alert: Unusual network traffic consistent with C2 communication (T1071). Model confidence: 99.1%" (ResearchGate, 2025b). Every step of this detection is logged instantly onto the immutable blockchain ledger (Reddit, 2024).

Critical Event 1: The False Positive (Operational Limitation): Following the initial intrusion, the AI detects a subsequent surge of legitimate network traffic—a planned, routine software update—but the timing and volume closely mimic a Distributed Denial of Service (DDoS) preparatory phase. Due to sampling bias (the training data lacked this specific maintenance profile), the AI assigns a high confidence score of 97% to a DDoS threat and recommends a pre-emptive throttle of network bandwidth to the OT environment (Callosum Group, 2025).

Control in Action (Circuit Breaker Activation): Although throttling is a low-impact action, its high-confidence recommendation on a high-risk system automatically triggers the algorithmic circuit breaker (Microsoft Azure, 2024a). The action is halted, and the decision is escalated to the human operator (Medium, 2024b). The SOC analyst, seeing the AI's high confidence but also the XAI rationale, which cites a high data-flow deviation, manually verifies the traffic against the maintenance schedule. The analyst identifies the AI's mistake—a false positive—and overrides the recommendation, preventing disruption to the legitimate software update. This forced human intervention, facilitated by the circuit breaker, prevents an error of commission and illustrates the structure's resilience against automation bias (Center for Security and Emerging Technology, 2024).

Critical Event 2: Lateral Movement and Escalation: The attacker attempts lateral movement from the compromised IT workstation to the OT network (ResearchGate, 2024a). The AI detects this cross-domain access attempt as a critical threat indicator and analyses the situation (Callosum Group, 2025). The AI determines that the optimal response is to isolate the compromised IT workstation (Callosum Group, 2025). Immutable Logging

Control in Action (HITL Enforcement): Because this action involves severing a network connection, it is categorised as a high-impact operation. The AI's recommendation triggers a critical circuit breaker, enforcing the Foundational layer's unbreakable limit (Callosum Group, 2025). The autonomous action is halted and escalated (Microsoft Azure, 2024a). The SOC analyst, armed with the clear evidence log, quickly validates the threat and manually authorises the containment action. The attack is stopped before the adversary accesses the industrial controls (Callosum Group, 2025). The blackout is averted.

This case study demonstrates that the integrated Governance Architecture functions not only to ensure compliance but to actively manage the inevitable imperfections of adaptive AI, ensuring that decision speed is balanced with human judgment and safety mandates.

FUTURE DIRECTIONS AND EMERGING CHALLENGES

As we stand on the cusp of this new era of cognitive security, the integrated governance structure provides a necessary model for governance in the present day (Callosum Group, 2025). Looking ahead, three key areas will shape the future of Neuro-AI governance (Callosum Group, 2025).

The Evolving Regulatory Landscape

The future of AI regulation is defined by fragmentation, not harmony (Dentons, 2025). The European Union has established its comprehensive, risk-based AI Act (European Commission, 2024; Smith Law, 2024). In contrast, the United States appears to be heading toward a more sector-specific, advancement-focused approach (Dentons, 2025). This global divergence necessitates a governance structure capable of adaptive, context-aware compliance (Dentons, 2025). The patchwork of global regulations, where one jurisdiction demands pre-certification (EU) and others rely on voluntary industry standards (US), creates a difficult compliance burden for multinational organisations deploying Neuro-AI defences (Dentons, 2025). The long-term challenge is creating mechanisms for cross-jurisdictional compliance that honour local laws without stifling the AI's global, adaptive defensive capabilities. Standardization efforts, such as those by the International Organization for Standardization (ISO), will be paramount in providing common technical specifications that can satisfy diverse legal requirements.

Governing Evolving Cognitive Architectures

The technology is rapidly evolving beyond initial neuromorphic computing concepts (Callosum Group, 2025). The next wave of Neuro-AI systems promises to bridge the current gap between perception and reasoning.

- **Neuro-Symbolic AI:** This approach combines the data-driven, pattern-matching strengths of neural networks with the explicit, rule-based reasoning of symbolic AI (Gartner, 2024; Piplai et al., 2023). By encoding ethical rules and legal constraints directly into the AI's symbolic knowledge base, systems may become inherently more explainable and auditable (Innova Solutions, 2024; ResearchGate, 2023). This offers the possibility of generating logical, step-by-step explanations for decisions, which could significantly alleviate the black box problem (Callosum Group, 2025). The governance implications here are highly positive, as the symbolic component can serve as a built-in compliance layer, self-checking the neural network's recommendations against hard-coded legal boundaries. This technical control may finally satisfy the "right to explanation" mandated by regulations like the European Union's General Data Protection Regulation (GDPR).
- **Collective (Swarm) AI:** This involves a decentralised collective of many smaller, interacting AI agents (Medium, 2024). Governance for such a system shifts from controlling a central "brain" to designing and auditing the simple interaction rules of the individual agents to ensure that their emergent collective behaviour is safe and aligned with organisational goals (Royal Society Publishing, 2024). This raises new questions about accountability when emergent group behaviour leads to error (Callosum Group, 2025). Tracking responsibility in a swarm environment is complex, requiring a shift from centralised audits to decentralised ledger technology (DLT) or blockchain to track the minute interactions between agents that collectively lead to an outcome (Royal Society Publishing, 2024). The governance focus must move from individual agent intent to the thermodynamics of the collective system's stability and emergent behaviour.

Long-Term Ethical Implications of Adaptive Security

We must grapple with profound, long-term ethical questions that arise from deploying intelligent, perpetually adapting systems (Callosum Group, 2025). These questions require societal debate, not just technical solutions.

- **The Diffusion of Responsibility:** If an AI security system evolves and self-modifies over years, it becomes distinct from the system its original developers created (Callosum Group, 2025). If a catastrophic error occurs, the "responsibility gap" makes assigning accountability a deep ethical and legal problem (ResearchGate, 2024c). Determining whether the fault lies with the original programmers, the data curators, or the autonomous adaptation mechanism will become a major area of legal contention (ResearchGate, 2024c). Future liability frameworks may need to recognise the AI itself as an organisational entity capable of causing harm, necessitating new forms of cyber insurance.
- **The Atrophy of Human Expertise:** Over-reliance on highly effective autonomous systems can lead to the erosion of human skill (Callosum Group, 2025). If SOC analysts rely solely on the AI's perfect recommendations, their own expertise may atrophy, leaving the organisation dangerously vulnerable if the AI system fails or is specifically targeted by an adaptive adversarial AI (Callosum Group, 2025). Mitigation strategies must include mandatory Human-in-the-Loop (HITL) scenarios designed not only for error prevention but also for continuous maintenance of human skills and critical analysis (Medium, 2024b). These training environments must simulate AI failure to prevent human complacency and dependency.

CONCLUSION

Neuro-Enhanced Artificial Intelligence offers a future of strong, proactive cybersecurity, but its power necessitates a commensurate transformation in governance (Callosum Group, 2025). This chapter introduced an integrated governance architecture, framed by the Digital Corpus Callosum concept, built to bridge the divide between technological advancement and ethical control (Callosum Group, 2025).

The structure is an active, continuous feedback loop of Foundational, Technical, and Operational layers (Callosum Group, 2025). Its practical managerial significance lies in its mandated technical controls: the use of immutable logging on a permissioned ledger to ensure a tamper-proof audit trail (ResearchGate, 2025c), and the deployment of algorithmic circuit breakers and Explainable AI (XAI) to enforce human oversight and accountability for critical decisions (Frontiers in Artificial Intelligence, 2025; Medium, 2024b). As the realistic case study illustrated, this architecture is designed to manage operational imperfections and inevitable false positives, ensuring decision speed is balanced with human judgment and safety mandates.

The challenges are increasing amid global regulatory fragmentation and the emergence of more complex architectures such as Neuro-Symbolic and Swarm AI (Dentons, 2025; Medium, 2024). The integrated governance structure is not a final answer, but a necessary, living architecture that must evolve alongside the cognitive technology it governs (Callosum Group, 2025). By integrating human values and technical controls, we forge a path toward trustworthy autonomy.

REFERENCES

Avertium. (2024). The top 5 cyber threats in the energy sector. Retrieved from https://www.avertium.com/resources/threat-reports/top-5-cyber-threats-in-energy-sector

Big Data Framework. (2023). *The role of AI ethics boards: Navigating the ethical landscape of artificial intelligence*. Retrieved from https://www.bigdataframework.org/knowledge/the-role-of-ai-ethics-boards-navigating-the-ethical-landscape-of-artificial-intelligence/

Callosum Group. (2025). *The digital corpus callosum: Establishing governance for neuro-enhanced AI security*. (User-provided document).

Center for Security and Emerging Technology. (2024). *AI safety and automation bias*. Georgetown University. Retrieved from https://cset.georgetown.edu/wp-content/uploads/CSET-AI-Safety-and-Automation-Bias.pdf

Cimphony. (2024). *AI incident response plans: Checklist and best practices*. Retrieved from https://www.cimphony.ai/insights/ai-incident-response-plans-checklist-and-best-practices

Cognizant. (2024). *Amplify cybersecurity resilience with neuro cybersecurity*. Retrieved from https://www.cognizant.com/us/en/services/neuro-intelligent-automation/ai-cybersecurity

Consulting, P. A. (2024). *What is automation bias and how can you prevent it?* Retrieved from https://www.paconsulting.com/insights/what-is-automation-bias-how-to-prevent

CyberTrends. (2023). *Advanced persistent threat case studies*. Retrieved from https://www.cybertrends.it/wp-content/uploads/pubblicazioni/APTcasestudies.pdf

Databricks. (2024). *What is automation bias?* Databricks Glossary. Retrieved from https://www.databricks.com/glossary/automation-bias

Deepgram. (2024). *Confirmation bias in machine learning*. AI Glossary. Retrieved from https://deepgram.com/ai-glossary/confirmation-bias

Deltek. (2023). *Traditional AI vs. generative AI: What's the difference?* Deltek Innovation. Retrieved from https://www.deltek.com/en/innovation/ai/traditional-ai-vs-generative-ai

Dentons. (2025). *AI trends for 2025: AI regulation, governance, and ethics*. Retrieved from https://www.dentons.com/en/insights/articles/2025/january/10/ai-trends-for-2025-ai-regulation-governance-and-ethics

Elvis, M., & Eads, B. (2021). Will the improved use of AI in cybersecurity make it harder for attackers to exploit vulnerabilities? *Quora*. Retrieved from https://www.quora.com/Will-the-improved-use-of-AI-in-cybersecurity-make-it-harder-for-attackers-to-exploit-vulnerabilities

European Commission. (2024). *Regulatory framework proposal on artificial intelligence*. Retrieved from https://digital-strategy.ec.europa.eu/en/policies/regulatory-framework-ai

Eusko Ikaskuntza. (2023). *Human cognitive biases present in artificial intelligence*. Retrieved from https://www.eusko-ikaskuntza.eus/en/riev/human-cognitive-biases-present-in-artificial-intelligence/rart-24782/

Evon Technologies. (2024). Ethical considerations in predictive analytics: Ensuring fairness and accountability. Retrieved from https://evontech.com/component/easyblog/ethical-considerations-in-predictive-analytics-ensuring-fairness-and-accountability-1-1.html?Itemid=159

Expleo. (2024). *Guarding the grid: Essential cybersecurity measures for smart grids*. Retrieved from https://expleo.com/global/en/insights/blog/guarding-grid-cybersecurity-smart-grids/

Flexxon. (2024). *Securing generative AI workflows with immutable data*. Retrieved from https://estore.flexxon.com/blogs/immutable-storage/securing-generative-ai-workflows-with-immutable-data

Frontiers in Artificial Intelligence. (2025). Explainable artificial intelligence (XAI) for enhanced transparency in intrusion detection systems. *Frontiers in Artificial Intelligence*. Retrieved from https://www.frontiersin.org/journals/artificial-intelligence/articles/10.3389/frai.2025.1526221/full

Gartner. (2024). *Neuro-symbolic AI*. Gartner Glossary. Retrieved from https://www.gartner.com/en/information-technology/glossary/neuro-symbolic-ai

GNIOT Group of Institutions. (2025). *Neuromorphic computing for AI-powered cyber defense*. GNIOT Blog. Retrieved from https://www.gniotgroup.edu.in/blog/index.php/2025/03/20/neuromorphic-computing-for-ai-powered-cyber-defense/

Holistic, A. I. (2025). *How to identify high-risk AI systems according to the EU AI act*. Retrieved from https://www.holisticai.com/blog/identify-high-risk-ai-systems-according-to-eu-ai-act

Holistic, A. I. (205b). *Implementing the circuit breaker pattern in a microservices based application*. Retrieved from https://blog.bitsrc.io/implementing-circuit-breaker-pattern-in-a-microservices-based-application-5d759021d09a

IBM. (2024). *Neuromorphic computing*. IBM Think. Retrieved from https://www.ibm.com/think/topics/neuromorphic-computing

Innodata. (2024). *How to design plan–act–observe–adjust architectures for agentic AI*. Retrieved from https://innodata.com/how-to-design-architectures-for-agentic-ai/

Innova Solutions. (2024). *From petabytes to peace of mind: LLM & graphs for neuro-symbolic AI security on GCP*. Retrieved from https://innovasolutions.com/blog/from-petabytes-to-peace-of-mind-llm-graphs-for-neuro-symbolic-ai-security-on-gcp/

InterVision. (2024). *AI and data governance: The new competitive advantage for IT leaders*. Retrieved from https://intervision.com/blog-ai-and-data-governance/

ISA. (2023). *Lessons learned from a forensic analysis of the Ukrainian power grid cyberattack malware*. ISA Blog. Retrieved from https://blog.isa.org/lessons-learned-forensic-analysis-ukrainian-power-grid-cyberattack-malware

Lawfare. (2024). *A dynamic governance model for AI*. Retrieved from https://www.lawfaremedia.org/article/a-dynamic-governance-model-for-ai

LinuxSecurity. (2024). *Embracing neuroscience-inspired AI for proactive linux security*. Retrieved from https://linuxsecurity.com/news/security-trends/embracing-neuroscience-inspired-ai

Lumenova, A. I. (2025). *Does your AI monitoring system follow these best practices?* Retrieved from https://www.lumenova.ai/blog/ai-monitoring-system-best-practices/

MDPI. (2021). An approach based on signal processing and artificial intelligence to identify PIR and main contact instants. Retrieved from https://www.mdpi.com/1996-1073/18/2/377

Medium. (2023). *Role of ethics committees and review boards, and governance structures for responsible AI*. Retrieved from https://medium.com/tech-ai-made-easy/role-of-ethics-committees-and-review-boards-and-governance-structures-for-responsible-ai-61da34203553

Medium. (2024). Generative AI "agile swarm intelligence" (part 1): Autonomous agent swarms foundations, theory, and advanced applications. Retrieved from https://medium.com/@armankamran/generative-ai-agile-swarm-intelligence-part-1-autonomous-agent-swarms-foundations-theory-and-9038e3bc6c37

Medium. (2024b). *Stop the AI drift: Governing autonomous decisions*. Retrieved from https://medium.com/@SophiaNellon/stop-the-ai-drift-governing-autonomous-decisions-ccb96a5dfc2d

Microsoft Azure. (2024a). *Circuit breaker pattern*. Azure Architecture Center. Retrieved from https://learn.microsoft.com/en-us/azure/architecture/patterns/circuit-breaker

Microsoft Azure. (2024b). *Adaptive techniques for circuit breakers*. Retrieved from https://learn.microsoft.com/en-us/azure/architecture/patterns/circuit-breaker

MITRE Corporation. (2021). *Intelligence after next: Breaking past AI's confirmation bias*. Retrieved from https://www.mitre.org/sites/default/files/2021-08/pr-21-0090-intelligence-after-next-breaking-past-ai-confirmation-bias.pdf

ModelOp. (2024). *NIST AI RMF*. Retrieved from https://www.modelop.com/ai-governance/ai-regulations-standards/nist-ai-rmf

Number Analytics. (2024). *The ethics of AI surveillance*.

Palo Alto Networks. (2024). *NIST AI risk management* ***structure*** *(AI RMF)*. Cyberpedia. Retrieved from https://www.paloaltonetworks.com/cyberpedia/nist-ai-risk-management-framework

Perception Point. (2024). *Top 6 AI security risks and how to defend your organization*. Retrieved from https://perception-point.io/guides/ai-security/top-6-ai-security-risks-and-how-to-defend-your-organization/

Piplai, A., Ramezani, N., & Sun, H. (2023). *Knowledge-enhanced neuro-symbolic AI for cybersecurity and privacy*. arXiv. Retrieved from https://arxiv.org/abs/2308.02031

Reddit. (2024). Ħ WiseID and AI agents - "Blockchain-based immutable logs". *r/Hedera*. Retrieved from https://www.reddit.com/r/Hedera/comments/1itbwi3/%C4%A7_wiseid_and_ai_agents_blockchainbased_immutable/

ResearchGate. (2023). *Neurosymbolic AI in cybersecurity: Bridging pattern recognition and symbolic reasoning*. Retrieved from https://www.researchgate.net/publication/376827715_Neurosymbolic_AI_in_Cybersecurity_Bridging_Pattern_Recognition_and_Symbolic_Reasoning

ResearchGate. (2024a). *Analysing recent APT incidents: Case studies and lessons learned*. Retrieved from https://www.researchgate.net/publication/387298480_Analysing_Recent_APT_Incidents_Case_Studies_and_Lessons_Learned

ResearchGate. (2024b). *Cognitive bias in AI development: Understanding the psychological and societal influences that shape AI model design and outcomes*. Retrieved from https://www.researchgate.net/publication/387382926_Cognitive_Bias_in_AI_Development_Understanding_the_Psychological_and_Societal_Influences_that_Shape_AI_Model_Design_and_Outcomes

ResearchGate. (2024c). *Reviewing the ethical implications of AI in decision making processes*. Retrieved from https://www.researchgate.net/publication/378295986_REVIEWING_THE_ETHICAL_IMPLICATIONS_OF_AI_IN_DECISION_MAKING_PROCESSES

ResearchGate. (2025a). *Neuro-adaptive intrusion detection systems: A brain-inspired ML architecture for autonomous threat hunting*. Retrieved from https://www.researchgate.net/publication/390945241_Neuro-Adaptive_Intrusion_Detection_Systems_A_Brain-Inspired_ML_Architecture_for_Autonomous_Threat_Hunting

ResearchGate. (2025b). *Explainable AI (XAI) techniques for cybersecurity in zero-trust architectures*. Retrieved from https://www.researchgate.net/publication/392064017_Explainable_AI_XAI_Techniques_for_Cybersecurity_in_Zero-Trust_Architectures

ResearchGate. (205c). *Blockchain-based logging for auditing AI decisions*. Retrieved from https://www.researchgate.net/publication/396889319_Blockchain-Based_Logging_for_Auditing_AI_Decisions

Royal Society Publishing. (2024). On the ethical governance of swarm robotic systems in the real world. *Philosophical Transactions. Series A, Mathematical, Physical, and Engineering Sciences*, *382*(2282). https://royalsocietypublishing.org/doi/10.1098/rsta.2024.0142

Smith Law. (2024). *The EU AI Act and its implications for US companies*. Retrieved from https://www.google.com/search?q=https://www.smithlaw.com/resources-insights/the-eu-ai-act-and-its-implications-for-us-companies

Surana & Surana. (2023). *AI-black box phenomenon*. Retrieved from https://suranaandsurana.com/ai-black-box-phenomenon/

Syntaxia. (2024). *AI agent safety: Circuit breakers for autonomous systems*. Retrieved from https://www.syntaxia.com/post/ai-agent-safety-circuit-breakers-for-autonomous-systems

Unsworth, C. (2024). *An ethical charter for artificial intelligence*. Retrieved from https://www.craigunsworth.com/articles/an-ethical-charter-for-artificial-intelligence

VerifyWise. (2024). *AI incident response plan*. Retrieved from https://verifywise.ai/lexicon/ai-incident-response-plan/

Wikimedia Foundation. (2024). *Explainable artificial intelligence*. Retrieved from https://en.wikipedia.org/wiki/Explainable_artificial_intelligence

WilmerHale. (2024). What are high-risk AI systems within the meaning of the EU's AI Act, and what requirements apply to them? *WilmerHale Privacy and Cybersecurity Law Blog*. Retrieved from https://www.wilmerhale.com/en/insights/blogs/wilmerhale-privacy-and-cybersecurity-law/20240717-what-are-highrisk-ai-systems-within-the-meaning-of-the-eus-ai-act-and-what-requirements-apply-to-them

Wiz. (2025). *NIST AI risk management* ***structure****: A tl;dr*. Retrieved from https://www.wiz.io/academy/nist-ai-risk-management-framework

Compilation of References

. Ahmadi, S. (2025). *Adaptive Cybersecurity: Dynamically Retrainable Firewalls for Real-Time Network Protection.*

. Balisane, H., Egho-Promise, E. I., Lyada, E., & Aina, F. (2024). TOWARDS IMPROVED THREAT MITIGATION IN DIGITAL ENVIRONMENTS: A COMPREHENSIVE FRAMEWORK FOR CYBERSECURITY ENHANCEMENT. *International Journal of Research -GRANTHAALAYAH, 12*(5). https://doi.org/DOI: 10.29121/granthaalayah.v12.i5.2024.5655

. Deleon, J., Hatherleigh, C., Cumberbatch, A., Ashworth, J., & Heathcote, L. (2024). *Predictive Profiling Framework for Ransomware Detection Using Contextual Signature Extraction.*

. Grootswagers, T., & Robinson, A. K. (n.d.). *OVERFITTING THE LITERATURE TO ONE SET OF STIMULI AND DATA.*

. Hatt, A., Blackwood, C., Lockhart, B., Ravenscroft, J., & Wainwright, N. (2024). *Dynamic Ransomware Detection through Adaptive Anomaly Partitioning Framework.*

. Koutsoutos, S., Christou, T., & Efremidis, S. (2006). *An Intrusion Detection System for Network-Initiated Attaclcs Using a Hybrid Neural Network.*

. Kurupathi, S. R., & Maass, W. (2020). *Survey on Federated Learning Towards Privacy Preserving AI.* 235–253. https://doi.org/DOI: 10.5121/csit.2020.101120

. Lekota, N. F. (2024). *Governance Considerations of Adversarial Attacks on AI Systems.*

. Lloyd Booz, K., & Hamilton, A. (2018). *Bias Amplification in Artificial Intelligence Systems.*

. Moore, B. E., & Col, L. (2013). *THE BRAIN COMPUTER INTERFACE FUTURE: TIME FOR A STRATEGY.*

. Moradi, S., Qiao, N., Stefanini, F., & Indiveri, G. (2017). *A scalable multi-core architecture with heterogeneous memory structures for Dynamic Neuromorphic Asynchronous Processors (DYNAPs).* https://doi.org/DOI: 10.1109/TBCAS.2017.2759700

. Navarro, M., Herrero, Á., Corchado, E., & Julián, V. (2010). *Approaching Real-Time Intrusion Detection through MOVICAB-IDS.*

. Rishad, S. M. S. I. (2025). LEVERAGING AI AND MACHINE LEARNING FOR PREDICTING, DETECTING, AND MITIGATING CYBERSECURITY THREATS: A COMPARATIVE STUDY OF ADVANCED MODELS. *International Journal of Computer Science & Information System, 10*(01), 06–25. https://doi.org/DOI: 10.55640/ijcsis/Volume10Issue01-02

. Rizvi, M. (2023). Enhancing cybersecurity: The power of artificial intelligence in threat detection and prevention. *International Journal of Advanced Engineering Research and Science, 10*(5), 055–060. https://doi.org/DOI: 10.22161/ijaers.105.8

. Rjoub, G., Bentahar, J., Wahab, O. A., Mizouni, R., Song, A., Cohen, R., Otrok, H., & Mourad, A. (2023). *A Survey on Explainable Artificial Intelligence for Cybersecurity.* https://doi.org/DOI: 10.1109/TNSM.2023.3282740

. Rodríguez-Barroso, N., Stipcich, G., Jiménez-López, D., Ruiz-Millán, J. A., Martínez-Cámara, E., González-Seco, G., Luzón, M. V., Veganzones, M. Á., & Herrera, F. (2020). *Federated Learning and Differential Privacy: Software tools analysis, the Sherpa.ai FL framework and methodological guidelines for preserving data privacy.* https://doi.org/DOI: 10.1016/j.inffus.2020.07.009

. Vasdani, T. V. (2020). Robot Justice: China's use of Internet Courts, The Lawyer's Daily, LexisNexis, Canada. lasted visited: 28/April/2025

. Zhu, T., Ye, D., Wang, W., Zhou, W., & Yu, P. S. (2020). *More Than Privacy: Applying Differential Privacy in Key Areas of Artificial Intelligence.* https://doi.org/DOI: 10.1109/TKDE.2020.3014246

Aarland, M. (2024). Cybersecurity in digital supply chains in the procurement process: Introducing the digital supply chain management framework. *Information and Computer Security.*

Abdelkader, S., Amissah, J., Kinga, S., Mugerwa, G., Emmanuel, E., Mansour, D. E. A., & Prokop, L. (2024). Securing modern power systems: Implementing comprehensive strategies to enhance resilience and reliability against cyber-attacks. *Results in Engineering, 102647.* Advance online publication. DOI: 10.1016/j.rineng.2024.102647

Abdullahi, M., Baashar, Y., Alhussian, H., Alwadain, A., Aziz, N., Capretz, L. F., & Abdulkadir, S. J. (2022). Detecting Cybersecurity Attacks in Internet of Things Using Artificial Intelligence Methods: A Systematic Literature Review. In *Electronics (Switzerland)* (Vol. 11, Issue 2). MDPI. https://doi.org/DOI: 10.3390/electronics11020198

Abo Alzahab, N. (2025). *Security and robustness of biometric authentication based on electroencephalography (EEG) signals and blockchain technology* (Doctoral thesis, Università Politecnica delle Marche). IRIS – Università Politecnica delle Marche. https://iris.univpm.it/bitstream/11566/342835/1/tesi_aboalzahab.pdf

Abuabid, A. A. (2025). A data-driven approach to cybersecurity situational awareness: Insights from machine learning. *Journal of Innovative Digital Transformation*, *2*, 131–155. DOI: 10.1108/jidt-03-2025-0013

Adabara, I., Olaniyi Sadiq, B., Nuhu Shuaibu, A., Ibarahim Danjuma, Y., & Venkateswarlu, M. (2025). A Review of Agentic AI in Cybersecurity: Cognitive Autonomy, Ethical Governance and Quantum-Resilient Defense. *F1000 Research*. PMID: 41169871

Aderu, N. (2025). AI-Driven Autonomous Middleware: Revolutionizing Enterprise IT Systems Management. *European Journal of Computer Science and Information Technology*.

Adeshina, T. A. Y. (2025). A neuro symbolic artificial intelligence and zero knowledge blockchain framework for a patient owned digital twin marketplace in US value based care. *International Journal of Research Publication and Reviews*, *6*(6).

Aggarwal, N. K., & Ford, E. (2013). The Neuroethics and Neurolaw of Brain Injury. *Behavioral Sciences & the Law*, *31*(6), 789–802. DOI: 10.1002/BSL.2086;C-TYPE:STRING:JOURNAL

Aharoni, E., Vincent, G. M., Harenski, C. L., Calhoun, V. D., Sinnott-Armstrong, W., Gazzaniga, M. S., & Kiehl, K. A. (2013). Neuroprediction of future rearrest. *Proceedings of the National Academy of Sciences of the United States of America*, *110*, 6223–6228. DOI: 10.1073/pnas.1219302110

Ajayi, A. M., Omokanye, A. O., Olowu, O., Adeleye, A. O., Omole, O. M., & Wada, I. U. (2024). Detecting insider threats in banking using AI-driven anomaly detection with a data science approach to cybersecurity. *International Journal of Cybersecurity Research*.

Ajibuwa, O., Hamdaoui, B., & Yavuz, A. A. (2023). *A Survey on AI/ML-Driven Intrusion and Misbehavior Detection in Networked Autonomous Systems: Techniques, Challenges and Opportunities*. https://arxiv.org/abs/2305.05040

Akbas, A., Yildiz, H. U., Ozbayoglu, A. M., & Tavli, B. (2019). Neural Network Based Instant Parameter Prediction for Wireless Sensor Network Optimization Models. *Wireless Networks, 25*(6). Advance online publication. DOI: 10.1007/s11276-018-1808-y

Akopyan, F. (2016)... *Design and Tool Flow of IBM's TrueNorth, 59–60*. Advance online publication. DOI: 10.1145/2872334.2878629

Al Siam, A., Hassan, M. M., & Bhuiyan, T. (2025, February). Artificial Intelligence for Cybersecurity: A State of the Art. In *2025 IEEE 4th International Conference on AI in Cybersecurity (ICAIC)* (pp. 1-7). IEEE.

Alam, A. (2023a). Media multitasking with M-learning technology in real-time classroom learning: Analysing the dynamics in formal educational settings for the future of E-learning in India. In *2023 2nd International Conference on Smart Technologies and Systems for Next Generation Computing (ICSTSN)* (pp. 1-6). IEEE.

Alam, A. (2023b). The secret sauce of student success: Cracking the code by navigating the path to personalized learning with educational data mining. In *2023 2nd International Conference on Smart Technologies and Systems for Next Generation Computing (ICSTSN)* (pp. 1-8). IEEE.

Alam, A., & Mohanty, A. (2022, December). Facial analytics or virtual avatars: competencies and design considerations for student-teacher interaction in AI-powered online education for effective classroom engagement. In *International Conference on Communication, Networks and Computing* (pp. 252-265). Cham: Springer Nature Switzerland.

Alam, A., & Mohanty, A. (2023, January). Learning on the move: a pedagogical framework for state-of-the-art mobile learning. In *International Conference on Data Management, Analytics & Innovation* (pp. 735-748). Singapore: Springer Nature Singapore.

Alam, A. (2022). Impact of university's human resources practices on professors' occupational performance: Empirical evidence from India's higher education sector. In Rajagopal, R., & Behl, R. (Eds.), *Inclusive businesses in developing economies: Converging people, profit, and corporate citizenship* (pp. 107–131). Springer International Publishing., DOI: 10.1007/978-3-031-12217-0_6

Alam, A. (2023c). Intelligence unleashed: An argument for AI-enabled learning ecologies with real world examples of today and a peek into the future. In *International Conference on Innovations in Computer Science, Electronics & Electrical Engineering*-2022 (Vol. 2717, No. 1, p. 030001). AIP Publishing LLC.

Alam, A., & Mohanty, A. (2024). Integrated constructive robotics in education (ICRE) model: A paradigmatic framework for transformative learning in educational ecosystem. *Cogent Education, 11*(1), 2324487.

Albladi, S. M., & Weir, G. R. S. (2018). User characteristics that influence judgment of social engineering attacks in social networks. Hum.-Centric Comput. Inf. Sci., 8(1).

Al-Faliti, S. A. (2024). *The Impact of Using Artificial Intelligence on the Litigation System in the Courts of the Sultanate of Oman and the Arab Republic of Egypt: Between Reality and Hope*. Scientific Research, Al-Zahraa College for Girls.

Ali, A. (2024). AI-Powered Shield: Transforming Cybersecurity with Neural Network Innovations *(Preprint)*. https://doi.org/DOI: 10.2196/preprints.69000

Ali, A., Septyanto, A. W., Chaudhary, I., Al Hamadi, H., Alzoubi, H. M., & Khan, Z. F. (2022, February). Applied artificial intelligence as event horizon of cyber security. In *2022 International Conference on Business Analytics for Technology and Security (ICBATS)* (pp. 1-7). IEEE.

Alkhatri, M., Deab, D. U., & Alzitawi, M. (2024). The role of artificial intelligence in addressing cybersecurity challenges. *International Journal of Academic Research in Business & Social Sciences, 14*(4).

Al-Marzouqi, A. A. (2021). *Electronic Litigation (Smart Litigation) and Electronic Litigation (Smart Judiciary): A Comparative Study of the Legislation of the United Arab Emirates with Some Arab and Foreign Systems*. University of Sharjah Journal of Legal Sciences.

Almojel, F., & Mishra, S. (2024). Advancing Hospital Cybersecurity Through IoT-Enabled Neural Network for Human Behavior Analysis and Anomaly Detection. In *IJACSA)* [). www.ijacsa.thesai.org]. *International Journal of Advanced Computer Science and Applications, 15*(5), •••.

Almousa, M., & Zhang, T., & Sarrafzadeh Abdolhossein and Anwar, M. (2022). Phishing website detection: How effective are deep learning-based models and hyperparameter optimization? *Security and Privacy, 5*(6).

AlOmar, B., & Trabelsi, Z. (2025). Integrating Generative AI into Cybersecurity Curricula. *2025 IEEE Global Engineering Education Conference (EDUCON)*, (39),1-15, 2025

Alserhani, F. M. (2025). Intrusion Detection and Real-Time Adaptive Security in Medical Internet of Things Using a Cyber-Physical System Design. *Sensors (Basel)*, •••, 25.

Al-Shar'ah, H. A. (2020). *Electronic Litigation and Electronic Courts*. Dar Al-Thaqafa for Publishing and Distribution.

Al-Taleb, N., & Saqib, N. A. (2022). Towards a hybrid machine learning model for intelligent cyber threat identification in smart city environments. *Applied Sciences (Basel, Switzerland)*, *12*(4), 1863.

Al-Turjman, F. (2024). Deep reinforcement learning applications in cybersecurity: Trends and future directions. *Future Generation Computer Systems*, *152*, 541–554. DOI: 10.1016/j.future.2023.11.009

Alwakeel, M. (2025). Neuro-Driven Agent-Based Security for Quantum-Safe 6G Networks. *Mathematics*, *13*(13), 2074. DOI: 10.3390/math13132074

Alzaabi, F. R., & Mehmood, A. (2024). A review of recent advances, challenges, and opportunities in malicious insider threat detection using machine learning methods. *IEEE Access : Practical Innovations, Open Solutions*, *12*, 30907–30927.

Alzahrani, A. A. (2023). Using Artificial Intelligence and Cybersecurity in Medical and Healthcare Applications. *Alzahrani, AA*.

Aminu, M. A., Hussain, A., & See, S. (2024). Spiking neural networks for efficient cybersecurity intrusion detection. *IEEE Access : Practical Innovations, Open Solutions*, *12*, 15632–15647. DOI: 10.1109/ACCESS.2024.3358912

Anda, R. F., Felitti, V. J., Bremner, J. D., Walker, J. D., Whitfield, C., Perry, B. D., Dube, S. R., & Giles, W. H. (2005). The enduring effects of abuse and related adverse experiences in childhood: A convergence of evidence from neurobiology and epidemiology. *European Archives of Psychiatry and Clinical Neuroscience*, *256*(3), 174. DOI: 10.1007/S00406-005-0624-4

Anderson, N. E., Allen, C. H., & Kiehl, K. A. (2024). A neurocriminological perspective on violence. In *Handbook of Gun Violence* (pp. 423–441). Elsevier., DOI: 10.1016/B978-0-323-95272-9.00019-X

Andrade, R. O., Fuertes, W., Cazares, M., Ortiz-Garcés, I., & Navas, G. (2022). An exploratory study of cognitive sciences applied to cybersecurity. *Electronics (Basel)*, *11*(11), 1692.

Ani, U. D., He, H., & Tiwari, A. (2019). Human factor security: Evaluating the cybersecurity capacity of the industrial workforce. *Journal of Systems and Information Technology*, *21*(1), 2–35.

Appelbaum, L. G., Shenasa, M. A., Stolz, L., & Daskalakis, Z. (2023). Synaptic Plasticity and Mental Health: Methods, Challenges and Opportunities. *Neuropsychopharmacology : Official Publication of the American College of Neuropsychopharmacology*, *48*(1). Advance online publication. DOI: 10.1038/s41386-022-01370-w PMID: 35810199

Aragonés Lozano, M., Pérez Llopis, I., & Esteve Domingo, M. (2023). Threat hunting architecture using a machine learning approach for critical infrastructures protection. *Big Data and Cognitive Computing*, *7*(2), 65.

Arikpo, I. I., Ogban, F. U., & Eteng, I. E. (2008). Von Neumann Architecture and Modern Computers. *Global Journal of Mathematical Sciences*, *6*(2). Advance online publication. DOI: 10.4314/gjmas.v6i2.21415

Artzt, M., & Dung, T. V. (2022). Artificial Intelligence and Data Protection: How to Reconcile Both Areas from the European Law Perspective. *Vietnamese Journal of Legal Sciences*, *7*(2), 39–58. DOI: 10.2478/vjls-2022-0007

Ashraf, M., Patterson, G., Kilhoffer, Z., Han, X., Brady, N., Rahn, A., & Yeh, T. (2023, June). Using fNIRS To Understand Adults' Empathy for Children in AI and Cybersecurity Scenarios. In *Proceedings of the 22nd Annual ACM Interaction Design and Children Conference* (pp. 630-634).

Avertium. (2024). The top 5 cyber threats in the energy sector. Retrieved from https://www.avertium.com/resources/threat-reports/top-5-cyber-threats-in-energy-sector

Baki, S., Umit, A., & Gonen, B. (2017). Phishing detection using cognitive and machine learning approaches. *International Journal of Information Security Science*, *6*(4), 70–81. http://www.ijiss.org/ijiss/index.php/ijiss/article/view/250

Balasubramanian, P., Nazari, S., Kholgh, D.K., Mahmoodi, A.B., Seby, J., & Kostakos, P. (2024). TSTEM: A Cognitive Platform for Collecting Cyber Threat Intelligence in the Wild. *ArXiv, abs/2402.09973*.

Barsallo Yi, E. A., Majors, J. D., Padala, A. V., Wu, D., Machiry, A., & Bagchi, S. (2024, June). Multi-Device Context-Sensitive Attacks Against Privacy. In *Proceedings of the Fifteenth ACM Conference on Data and Application Security and Privacy* (pp. 209-220).

Basit, A., Zafar, S., Liu, J., & Javed, A. (2020). A comprehensive survey of AI for phishing detection. *IEEE Access : Practical Innovations, Open Solutions, 8*, 116–125. DOI: 10.1109/ACCESS.2020.2979038 PMID: 33110340

Bechara, A. (2005). Decision making, impulse control and loss of willpower to resist drugs: A neurocognitive perspective. *Nature Neuroscience, 8*(11), 1458–1463. DOI: 10.1038/NN1584

Berryessa, C. M., & Raine, A. (2017). Neurocriminology. In *The Routledge Companion to Criminological Theory and Concepts* (pp. 78–82). Taylor and Francis., DOI: 10.4324/9781315744902-18

Bhardwaj, T., Upadhyay, H., Sharma, T. K., & Fernandes, S. L. (Eds.). (2023). *Artificial Intelligence in Cyber Security: Theories and Applications*. Springer.

Bhaware, A., Varshney, G., Kour, J., Bishnoi, T., Jain, M., & Sharma, D. (2024, May). A Privacy Preserving Context Sensitive Kernel. In *Proceedings of the 2024 ACM Workshop on Wireless Security and Machine Learning* (pp. 20-25).

Big Data Framework. (2023). *The role of AI ethics boards: Navigating the ethical landscape of artificial intelligence*. Retrieved from https://www.bigdataframework.org/knowledge/the-role-of-ai-ethics-boards-navigating-the-ethical-landscape-of-artificial-intelligence/

Bilal, F. B. (2023). The Role of Artificial Intelligence in Promoting Effective Justice Before the Judiciary. A Comparative Study with the Legal and Judicial Systems in the State of Qatar. Master's Thesis, Qatar University.

Bilal, F. B. (2023). *Smart Litigation in Qatari Courts: Between Reality and Hope. A Comparative Study*. Supreme Judicial Council.

Bizzarri, A., Yu, C.-E., Jalaian, B., Riguzzi, F., & Bastian, N. D. (2024a). A synergistic approach in network intrusion detection by neurosymbolic AI [Preprint]. *arXiv*. https://arxiv.org/abs/2406.00938

Bizzarri, A., Yu, C.-E., Jalaian, B., Riguzzi, F., & Bastian, N. D. (2024b). *A neurosymbolic artificial intelligence network intrusion detection system*. In *Proceedings of the 33rd International Conference on Computer Communications and Networks (ICCCN)* (pp. 1–8). IEEE. https://doi.org/DOI: 10.1109/ICCCN61486.2024.10637618

Blair, R. J. R. (2005). Applying a cognitive neuroscience perspective to the disorder of psychopathy. *Development and Psychopathology, 17*(3), 865–891. DOI: 10.1017/S0954579405050418

Blitz, M. J. (2017). *The Fifth Amendment: Self-Incrimination and the Brain*. 59–79. https://doi.org/DOI: 10.1007/978-3-319-50004-1_4

Boccardi, V., Tagliafico, L., Persia, A., Page, E., Ottaviani, S., Cremonini, A. L., Borgarelli, C., Pisciotta, L., Mecocci, P., Nencioni, A., & Monacelli, F. (2024). The Potential Effects of Red Wine and Its Components on Neurocognitive Disorders: A Narrative Review. In *Nutrients* (Vol. 16, Issue 20). Multidisciplinary Digital Publishing Institute (MDPI). https://doi.org/DOI: 10.3390/nu16203431

Boi, F., Moraitis, T., De Feo, V., Diotalevi, F., Bartolozzi, C., Indiveri, G., & Vato, A. (2016). A bidirectional brain-machine interface featuring a neuromorphic hardware decoder. *Frontiers in Neuroscience*, *10*. Advance online publication. DOI: 10.3389/fnins.2016.00563 PMID: 28018162

Bormpotsis, C., Nanos, M., & Patel, A. (2025). A Neuroscience-Informed AI Framework to Decode the Complexities of Neurofinance. *IEEE Transactions on Technology and Society*.

Boskovic, I., Perera, N., & Otgaar, H. (2025). Cross-Cultural Perspectives on Psychological Research Practices and Opportunities: Do We All Have the (Same) Chance? *Psychological Research on Urban Society*, *8*(2), 4.

Bozhko, D. A., Vasyuchka, V. I., Chumak, A. V., & Serga, A. A. (2020). Magnon-Phonon Interactions in Magnon Spintronics (Review Article). *Low Temperature Physics*, *46*(4). Advance online publication. DOI: 10.1063/10.0000872

Broccard, F. D., Joshi, S., Wang, J., & Cauwenberghs, G. (2017). Neuromorphic Neural Interfaces: From Neurophysiological Inspiration to Biohybrid Coupling with Nervous Systems. *Journal of Neural Engineering*, *14*(4). Advance online publication. DOI: 10.1088/1741-2552/aa67a9 PMID: 28573983

Brundage, M., Avin, S., Clark, J., Toner, H., Eckersley, P., Garfinkel, B., Dafoe, A., Scharre, P., Zeitzoff, T., Filar, B., Anderson, H., Roff, H., Allen, G. C., Steinhardt, J., Flynn, C., Héigeartaigh, S. Ó., Beard, S., Belfield, H., Farquhar, S., . . . Amodei, D. (2018). The malicious use of artificial intelligence: Forecasting, prevention, and mitigation. *arXiv*. https://doi.org//arxiv.1802.07228DOI: 10.48550

Cai, Y., Llorca, J., Tulino, A. M., & Molisch, A. F. (2021, June 1). Optimal Cloud Network Control with Strict Latency Constraints. *IEEE International Conference on Communications*. https://doi.org/DOI: 10.1109/ICC42927.2021.9500573

Calimera, A., Macii, E., & Poncino, M. (2013). The Human Brain Project and Neuromorphic Computing. *Functional Neurology*, *28*(3). Advance online publication. DOI: 10.11138/FNeur/2013.28.3.191 PMID: 24139655

Callosum Group. (2025). *The digital corpus callosum: Establishing governance for neuro-enhanced AI security*. (User-provided document).

Campbell, C. C. (2019). Solutions for counteracting human deception in social engineering attacks. *Information Technology & People*, *32*(5), 1130–1152.

Carré, J. M., & Olmstead, N. A. (2015). Social neuroendocrinology of human aggression: Examining the role of competition-induced testosterone dynamics. *Neuroscience*, *286*, 171–186. DOI: 10.1016/j.neuroscience.2014.11.029

Center for Security and Emerging Technology. (2024). *AI safety and automation bias*. Georgetown University. Retrieved from https://cset.georgetown.edu/wp-content/uploads/CSET-AI-Safety-and-Automation-Bias.pdf

Chamberlain, S. R., & Sahakian, B. J. (2007). The neuropsychiatry of impulsivity. *Current Opinion in Psychiatry*, *20*(3), 255–261. DOI: 10.1097/YCO.0B013E-3280BA4989

Chandra, P., Sharma, H., & Sachan, N. (2025). Explainable and Responsible AI in Neuroscience: Cognitive Neurostimulation. *Explainable and Responsible Artificial Intelligence in Healthcare*, 27-63.

Chapagain, D., Kshetri, N., & Pokharel, B. P. (2025). AISCliteracy: Assessing Artificial Intelligence and Cybersecurity Literacy Levels and Learning Needs of Students. *arXiv preprint arXiv:2506.23321*.

Charmet, F., Tanuwidjaja, H. C., Ayoubi, S., Gimenez, P.-F., Han, Y., Jmila, H., Blanc, G., Takahashi, T., & Zhang, Z. (2022). Explainable artificial intelligence for cybersecurity: A literature survey. *Annales des Télécommunications*, *77*(11–12), 789–812.

Chen, C., Liu, J., Tan, H., Li, X., Wang, K. I.-K., Li, P., Sakurai, K., & Dou, D. (2024). *Trustworthy Federated Learning: Privacy, Security, and Beyond*. https://arxiv.org/abs/2411.01583

Chio, C., & Freeman, D. (2018). *Machine learning and security: Protecting systems with data and algorithms*. O'Reilly Media.

Chisty, N. M. A., Baddam, P. R., & Amin, R. (2022). Strategic approaches to safe-guarding the digital future: Insights into next-generation cybersecurity. *Engineering International*, *10*(2), 69–84.

Choudhury, O., Gkoulalas-Divanis, A., Salonidis, T., Sylla, I., Park, Y., Hsu, G., & Das, A. (2020). *Anonymizing Data for Privacy-Preserving Federated Learning*. https://arxiv.org/abs/2002.09096

Chowdhury, R. H., Prince, N. U., Abdullah, S. M., & Mim, L. A. (2024). The role of predictive analytics in cybersecurity: Detecting and preventing threats. *World Journal of Advanced Research and Reviews, 23*(2), 1615–1623.

CHRISPIM, MARIANA CARDOSO. (2021). Resource Recovery from Wastewater Treatment: Challenges, Opportunities and Guidance for Planning and Implementation. *Frontiers in Neuroscience, 14*(1).

Cimphony. (2024). *AI incident response plans: Checklist and best practices.* Retrieved from https://www.cimphony.ai/insights/ai-incident-response-plans-checklist-and-best-practices

Cognizant. (2024). *Amplify cybersecurity resilience with neuro cybersecurity.* Retrieved from https://www.cognizant.com/us/en/services/neuro-intelligent-automation/ai-cybersecurity

Consulting, P. A. (2024). *What is automation bias and how can you prevent it?* Retrieved from https://www.paconsulting.com/insights/what-is-automation-bias-how-to-prevent

Corradini, I. (2020). Redefining the approach to cybersecurity. In Studies in Systems, Decision and Control (pp. 49–62). Springer International Publishing.

CyberTrends. (2023). *Advanced persistent threat case studies.* Retrieved from https://www.cybertrends.it/wp-content/uploads/pubblicazioni/APTcasestudies.pdf

Dal Verne, T. D. M. C. (2023). Artificial Intelligence, Neuroscience and Emotional Data. What Role for Private Autonomy in the Digital Market? *Erasmus L. Rev., 16*, 83.

Dalal, A. (2018). Cybersecurity And Artificial Intelligence: How AI Is Being Used in Cybersecurity To Improve Detection And Response To Cyber Threats. *Turkish Journal of Computer and Mathemafics Educafion, 9*(3), 1704–1709.

Dangi, A. K., Pant, K., Alanya-Beltran, J., Chakraborty, N., Akram, S. V., & Balakrishna, K. (2023, January). A review of use of artificial intelligence on cyber security and the fifth-generation cyber-attacks and its analysis. In *2023 International Conference on Artificial Intelligence and Smart Communication (AISC)* (pp. 553–557). IEEE. https://doi.org/DOI: 10.1109/AISC56872.2023.10092161

Dang, Y., Huang, K., Huo, J., Yan, Y., Huang, S., Liu, D., Gao, M., Zhang, J., Qian, C., Wang, K., Liu, Y., Shao, J., Xiong, H., & Hu, X. (2024). *Explainable and Interpretable Multimodal Large Language Models: A Comprehensive Survey.* https://arxiv.org/abs/2412.02104

Dapel, M. E., Asante, M., Uba, C. D., & Agyeman, M. O. (2023). Artificial Intelligence Techniques in Cybersecurity Management. In Advanced Sciences and Technologies for Security Applications (pp. 241–255). Springer International Publishing.

Darktrace. (2022). *Darktrace AI stops sophisticated ransomware attack at South African financial services provider.* PR Newswire. https://www.prnewswire.com/news-releases/darktrace-ai-stops-sophisticated-ransomware-attack-at-south-african-financial-services-provider-301517557.html

Darktrace. (2023). *Under the radar: Insider threats detected by Darktrace.* https://darktrace.com/news/under-the-radar-insider-threats-detected-by-darktrace

Dasso, A., Funes, A., Montejano, G., Riesco, D., Uzal, R., & Debnath, N. (2016, March). Model-based evaluation of cybersecurity implementations. In *Information Technology: New Generations: 13th International Conference on Information Technology* (pp. 303–313). Springer International Publishing.

Databricks. (2024). *What is automation bias?* Databricks Glossary. Retrieved from https://www.databricks.com/glossary/automation-bias

Davies, M., Wild, A., Orchard, G., Sandamirskaya, Y., Guerra, G. A. F., Joshi, P., Plank, P., & Risbud, S. R. (2021). Advancing neuromorphic computing with Loihi: A survey of results and outlook. *Proceedings of the IEEE, 109*(5), 911–934. DOI: 10.1109/jproc.2021.3067593

De Dreu, C. K. W. (2012). Oxytocin modulates cooperation within and competition between groups: An integrative review and research agenda. *Hormones and Behavior, 61*(3), 419–428. DOI: 10.1016/J.YHBEH.2011.12.009

Decety, J., & Jackson, P. L. (2004). The functional architecture of human empathy. *Behavioral and Cognitive Neuroscience Reviews, 3*(2), 71–100. DOI: 10.1177/1534582304267187

Deepgram. (2024). *Confirmation bias in machine learning.* AI Glossary. Retrieved from https://deepgram.com/ai-glossary/confirmation-bias

Delfin, C., Krona, H., Andiné, P., Ryding, E., Wallinius, M., & Hofvander, B. (2019). Prediction of recidivism in a long-term follow-up of forensic psychiatric patients: Incremental effects of neuroimaging data. *PLoS One, 14*(5), e0217127. DOI: 10.1371/JOURNAL.PONE.0217127

Deltek. (2023). *Traditional AI vs. generative AI: What's the difference?* Deltek Innovation. Retrieved from https://www.deltek.com/en/innovation/ai/traditional-ai-vs-generative-ai

Deng, Y., Liu, B., Huang, Z., Liu, X., He, S., Li, Q., & Guo, D. (2022). Fractional Spiking Neuron: Fractional Leaky Integrate-and-Fire Circuit Described with Dendritic Fractal Model. *IEEE Transactions on Biomedical Circuits and Systems, 16*(6). Advance online publication. DOI: 10.1109/TBCAS.2022.3218294 PMID: 36315548

Dentons. (2025). *AI trends for 2025: AI regulation, governance, and ethics*. Retrieved from https://www.dentons.com/en/insights/articles/2025/january/10/ai-trends-for-2025-ai-regulation-governance-and-ethics

Dhirani, L. L., Mukhtiar, N., Chowdhry, B. S., & Newe, T. (2023). Ethical dilemmas and privacy issues in emerging technologies: A review. *Sensors (Basel), 23*(3), 1151. PMID: 36772190

Di Salvo, M. (2025). The Protection of Neural Rights in the Age of Neurotechnologies and AI. The Ethical Challenge for Law and Neuroscience. *Russ. J. Econ. & L., 19*, 202.

Dom, G., Schouler-Ocak, M., Bhui, K., Demunter, H., Kuey, L., Raballo, A., Frydecka, D., Misiak, B., Gorwood, P., & Samochowiec, J. (2018). Mass violence, radicalization and terrorism: A role for psychiatric profession? *European Psychiatry : the Journal of the Association of European Psychiatrists, 49*, 78–80. DOI: 10.1016/J.EURPSY.2018.01.001

Duary, S., Choudhury, P., Mishra, S., Sharma, V., Rao, D. D., & Aderemi, A. P. (2024, February). Cybersecurity threats detection in intelligent networks using predictive analytics approaches. In *2024 4th International Conference on Innovative Practices in Technology and Management (ICIPTM)* (pp. 1–5). IEEE.

Ejeofobiri, C. K., Victor-Igun, O. O., & Okoye, C. (2024). AI-Driven Secure Intrusion Detection for Internet of Things (IOT) Networks. *Asian Journal of Mathematics and Computer Research, 31*(4), 40–55. DOI: 10.56557/ajomcor/2024/v31i48971

El-Din, R. E. (2024). *Artificial Intelligence and the Judicial System: Global Experiences. Scientific Research*. Mansoura University.

Elvis, M., & Eads, B. (2021). Will the improved use of AI in cybersecurity make it harder for attackers to exploit vulnerabilities? *Quora*. Retrieved from https://www.quora.com/Will-the-improved-use-of-AI-in-cybersecurity-make-it-harder-for-attackers-to-exploit-vulnerabilities

European Commission. (2024). *Regulatory framework proposal on artificial intelligence*. Retrieved from https://digital-strategy.ec.europa.eu/en/policies/regulatory-framework-ai

Europol. (2025, March 18). *Criminals use AI in 'proxy' attacks for hostile powers, warns Europol. Financial Times.* https://www.ft.com/content/755593c8-8614-4953-a4b2-09a0d2794684

Eusko Ikaskuntza. (2023). *Human cognitive biases present in artificial intelligence.* Retrieved from https://www.eusko-ikaskuntza.eus/en/riev/human-cognitive-biases-present-in-artificial-intelligence/rart-24782/

Evon Technologies. (2024). Ethical considerations in predictive analytics: Ensuring fairness and accountability. Retrieved from https://evontech.com/component/easyblog/ethical-considerations-in-predictive-analytics-ensuring-fairness-and-accountability-1-1.html?Itemid=159

Expleo. (2024). *Guarding the grid: Essential cybersecurity measures for smart grids.* Retrieved from https://expleo.com/global/en/insights/blog/guarding-grid-cybersecurity-smart-grids/

Familoni, B. T. (2024). Cybersecurity challenges in the age of Ai: Theoretical approaches and practical solutions. Comput. Sci. IT Res. j., 5(3), 703–724.

Farah, M. J. (2012). Neuroethics: The ethical, legal, and societal impact of neuroscience. *Annual Review of Psychology, 63*(Volume 63, 2012), 571–591. https://doi.org/DOI: 10.1146/ANNUREV.PSYCH.093008.100438/CITE/REFWORKS

Faraji, M. R., Shikder, F., Hasan, M. H., Islam, M. M., & Akter, U. K. (2024). Examining the role of artificial intelligence in cyber security (CS): A systematic review for preventing prospective solutions in financial transactions. *International Journal (Toronto, Ont.), 5*(10), 4766–4782.

Farrington, D. P. (2005). Childhood origins of antisocial behavior. *Clinical Psychology & Psychotherapy, 12*(3), 177–190. DOI: 10.1002/CPP.448;WGROUP:STRING:-PUBLICATION

Fernández-García, C. E., Marín, D. V., & Velásquez, H. S. (2023). Neurohacking and Artificial Intelligence in the Vulnerability of the Human Brain: Are We Facing a Threat? In *Artificial Intelligence in Higher Education and Scientific Research: Future Development* (pp. 117–128). Springer Nature Singapore.

Ferrag, M. A., Maglaras, L., Moschoyiannis, S., & Janicke, H. (2020). Deep learning for cyber security intrusion detection: Approaches, datasets, and comparative studies. *Journal of Information Security and Applications, 50*, 102419. DOI: 10.1016/j.jisa.2019.102419

Fetaji, B., & Samanta, D. (2025). Artificial Intelligence in cybersecurity: A comprehensive analysis of machine learning applications on phishing URLs and malware API calls for devising cyber defense strategies. In *Research Square*.

Firasta, S., Srivastava, Y. R., & Rao, V. (2024). Cognitive Detection of Anomalies in Autonomous In-Vehicle Network Communication. *2024 International Conference on Advancements in Power, Communication and Intelligent Systems (APCI)*, 1-6.

Fisher, H., Shahar, M., & Resheff, Y. S. (2024). *Neural Fingerprints for Adversarial Attack Detection*. https://arxiv.org/abs/2411.04533

Flexxon. (2024). *Securing generative AI workflows with immutable data*. Retrieved from https://estore.flexxon.com/blogs/immutable-storage/securing-generative-ai-workflows-with-immutable-data

Frontiers in Artificial Intelligence. (2025). Explainable artificial intelligence (XAI) for enhanced transparency in intrusion detection systems. *Frontiers in Artificial Intelligence*. Retrieved from https://www.frontiersin.org/journals/artificial-intelligence/articles/10.3389/frai.2025.1526221/full

Gadicha, V. B., Gadicha, A. B., Zuhair, M., Khan, Z. I., & Burange, M. S. (2025). Revolutionizing Security Information and Event Management (SIEM) Systems: Harnessing Deep Learning for Advanced Threat Detection. In *Project Management Information Systems: Empowering Decision Making and Execution* (pp. 233-262). IGI Global Scientific Publishing.

Galinec, D. (2023). Cyber Security and Cyber Defense: Challenges and Building of Cyber Resilience Conceptual Model. *International Journal of Applied Sciences & Development*, *1*, 83–88. DOI: 10.37394/232029.2022.1.10

Gartner. (2024). *Neuro-symbolic AI*. Gartner Glossary. Retrieved from https://www.gartner.com/en/information-technology/glossary/neuro-symbolic-ai

Gatla, T. R. (2022). A critical examination of shielding the cyberspace: A review on the role of Ai in cyber security. Int. j. *Innov. Eng. Res. Technol.*, *9*(9), 55–60.

Gavazzi, S. M., Yarcheck, C. M., Sullivan, J. M., Jones, S. C., & Khurana, A. (2008). Global risk factors and the prediction of recidivism rates in a sample of first-time misdemeanant offenders. *International Journal of Offender Therapy and Comparative Criminology*, *52*(3), 330–345. DOI: 10.1177/0306624X07305481;PAGE:STRING:ARTICLE/CHAPTER

George, A. S. (2024). Emerging trends in AI-driven cybersecurity: An in-depth analysis. *Partners Universal Innovative Research Publication*, *2*(4), 15–28.

Georgiadou, A., Mouzakitis, S., Bounas, K., & Askounis, D. (2022). A cyber-security culture framework for assessing organization readiness. *Journal of Computer Information Systems*, *62*(3), 452–462.

Gkintoni, E., Antonopoulou, H., Sortwell, A., & Halkiopoulos, C. (2025). Challenging cognitive load theory: The role of educational neuroscience and artificial intelligence in redefining learning efficacy. *Brain Sciences*, *15*(2), 203. PMID: 40002535

Glenn, A. L., & Raine, A. (2014a). Neurocriminology: Implications for the punishment, prediction and prevention of criminal behaviour. In *Nature Reviews Neuroscience* (Vol. 15, pp. 54–63). https://doi.org/DOI: 10.1038/nrn3640

GNIOT Group of Institutions. (2025). *Neuromorphic computing for AI-powered cyber defense*. GNIOT Blog. Retrieved from https://www.gniotgroup.edu.in/blog/index.php/2025/03/20/neuromorphic-computing-for-ai-powered-cyber-defense/

Goodfellow, I., Bengio, Y., & Courville, A. (2016). *Deep learning*. MIT Press.

Goodfellow, I., Shlens, J., & Szegedy, C. (2015). Explaining and harnessing adversarial examples. *International Conference on Learning Representations (ICLR)*.

Goodkind, M., Eickhoff, S. B., Oathes, D. J., Jiang, Y., Chang, A., Jones-Hagata, L. B., Ortega, B. N., Zaiko, Y. V., Roach, E. L., Korgaonkar, M. S., Grieve, S. M., Galatzer-Levy, I., Fox, P. T., & Etkin, A. (2015). Identification of a common neurobiological substrate for mental Illness. *JAMA Psychiatry*, *72*(4), 305–315. DOI: 10.1001/JAMAPSYCHIATRY.2014.2206

Goswami, M. (2024). AI-based anomaly detection for real-time cybersecurity. International journal of research and review techniques, 3(1), 45-53.

Guan, Y., & Chen, Q. (2021). Research on Intelligent Perception and Cognitive Computing of Information Security System Based on Computer Big Data. *Wireless Communications and Mobile Computing*, *3281825*. Advance online publication. DOI: 10.1155/2021/3281825

Gundu, T. (2024). Learn, Unlearn and Relearn: Adaptive Cybersecurity Culture Model. *Iccws*, *19*(1), 95–102.

Guo, Y., Huo, P., Huang, S., Gou, G., & Li, Q. (2025). Multi-Receptor Skin with Highly Sensitive Tele-Perception Somatosensory Flexible Electronics in Healthcare: Multimodal Sensing and AI-Powered Diagnostics. *Advanced Healthcare Materials*, •••, 2502901. PMID: 40619754

Gururaj, H. L., Janhavi, V., & Ambika, V. (Eds.). (2024). *Social Engineering in Cybersecurity: Threats and Defenses*. CRC Press.

Gwala, S. (2025). The use of blockchain technology and artificial intelligence in cryptocurrency and medical technology: A comprehensive review. In Gwala, R. S. (Ed.), *Driving socio-economic growth with AI and blockchain* (pp. 147–184). IGI Global., https://www.igi-global.com

Habeeb, M. S. (2024). Predictive analytics and cybersecurity. In *Intelligent techniques for predictive data analytics* (pp. 151–169). Wiley., DOI: 10.1002/9781394227990.ch8

Hajri, B., Aziza, H., Mansour, M. M., & Chehab, A. (2019). RRAM Device Models: A Comparative Analysis with Experimental Validation. *IEEE Access : Practical Innovations, Open Solutions, 7.* Advance online publication. DOI: 10.1109/ACCESS.2019.2954753

Hakim, S. B., Adil, M., Velasquez, A., Xu, S., & Song, H. H. (2025). Neuro-Symbolic AI for Cybersecurity: State of the Art, Challenges, and Opportunities. *arXiv preprint arXiv:2509.06921.*

Harju, H., Tuisku, J., & Nummenmaa, L. (2025). *Shared brain basis of aggression in clinical, forensic, and healthy samples: A meta-analysis.* https://doi.org/DOI: 10.1101/2025.02.17.638609

Harms, M. B., Birn, R., Provencal, N., Wiechmann, T., Binder, E. B., Giakas, S. W., Roeber, B. J., & Pollak, S. D. (2017). Early life stress, FK506 binding protein 5 gene (FKBP5) methylation, and inhibition-related prefrontal function: A prospective longitudinal study. *Development and Psychopathology, 29*(5), 1895–1903. DOI: 10.1017/S095457941700147X

Hashikawa, Y., Hashikawa, K., Falkner, A. L., & Lin, D. (2017). Ventromedial hypothalamus and the generation of aggression. *Frontiers in Systems Neuroscience, 11*, 94. Advance online publication. DOI: 10.3389/fnsys.2017.00094

Hassabis, D., Kumaran, D., Summerfield, C., & Botvinick, M. (2017). Neuroscience-inspired artificial intelligence. *Neuron, 95*(2), 245–258. DOI: 10.1016/j.neuron.2017.06.011 PMID: 28728020

Heartfield, R., & Loukas, G. (2018). Detecting semantic social engineering attacks with the weakest link: Implementation and empirical evaluation of a human-as-a-security-sensor framework. *Computers & Security, 76*, 101–127.

Hinrichs, R., Subramanian, L., Ayala, A., Endicott-Popovsky, B., & Stoll, S. (2024, November). AI-Enhanced Cybersecurity Training: Integrating Ethical Reasoning and Personalized Learning Pathways. In *Proceedings of the Future Technologies Conference* (pp. 606-622). Cham: Springer Nature Switzerland.

Hinrichs, R., Subramanian, L., Ayala, A., Endicott-Popovsky, B., & Stoll, S. (2024, November). *AI-enhanced cybersecurity training: Integrating ethical reasoning and personalized learning pathways.* In *Proceedings of the Future Technologies Conference* (pp. 606–622). Springer Nature Switzerland. https://doi.org/DOI: 10.1007/978-3-031-49514-4_40

Hirstein, W. (2022). Neuroscience and Normativity: How Knowledge of the Brain Offers a Deeper Understanding of Moral and Legal Responsibility. *Criminal Law and Philosophy*, *16*(2), 327–351. DOI: 10.1007/S11572-021-09600-W/METRICS

Hitzler, P., Eberhart, A., Ebrahimi, M., Sarker, M. K., & Zhou, L. (2022). Neuro-symbolic approaches in artificial intelligence. *National Science Review*, *9*(6), nwac035. PMID: 35673530

Hogea, E., & Onchis, D. (2024). *Sisteme Hibride de Invatare Automata si Aplicatii*. https://arxiv.org/abs/2406.11870

Holistic, A. I. (2025). *How to identify high-risk AI systems according to the EU AI act*. Retrieved from https://www.holisticai.com/blog/identify-high-risk-ai-systems-according-to-eu-ai-act

Holistic, A. I. (205b). *Implementing the circuit breaker pattern in a microservices based application*. Retrieved from https://blog.bitsrc.io/implementing-circuit-breaker-pattern-in-a-microservices-based-application-5d759021d09a

Hramov, A. E., Ghosh, D., Pisarchik, A. N., Pavlov, A., Stoyanov, D., Zaikin, A., & Sanjuan, M. (2025). Artificial intelligence and complex networks meet natural sciences. *The European Physical Journal. Special Topics*, •••, 1–16.

Huda, M., Awaludin, A., & Siregar, H. K. (2024). Legal Challenges in Regulating Artificial Intelligence: A Comparative Study of Privacy and Data Protection Laws. In *IJSH* (Vol. 01, Issue 2). https://dejournals.org/index.php/ijsh

Husak, M., Bartoš, V., Sokol, P., & Gajdoš, A. (2021). Predictive methods in cyber defense: Current experience and research challenges. *Future Generation Computer Systems*, *115*, 517–530.

Hwang, K. (1987). Advanced Parallel Processing with Supercomputer Architectures. *Proceedings of the IEEE*, *75*(10). Advance online publication. DOI: 10.1109/PROC.1987.13894

IBM. (2024). *Neuromorphic computing*. IBM Think. Retrieved from https://www.ibm.com/think/topics/neuromorphic-computing

Ilieva, R., & Stoilova, G. (2024, September). Challenges of AI-driven cybersecurity. In *2024 XXXIII International Scientific Conference Electronics (ET)* (pp. 1–4). IEEE.

Indiveri, G. (2021). Introducing 'Neuromorphic Computing and Engineering.'. *Neuromorphic Computing and Engineering, 1*(1). Advance online publication. DOI: 10.1088/2634-4386/ac0a5b

Inkster, B. (2021). Cybersecurity: A critical priority for digital mental health. In *PsyArXiv*.

Innodata. (2024). *How to design plan–act–observe–adjust architectures for agentic AI*. Retrieved from https://innodata.com/how-to-design-architectures-for-agentic-ai/

Innova Solutions. (2024). *From petabytes to peace of mind: LLM & graphs for neuro-symbolic AI security on GCP*. Retrieved from https://innovasolutions.com/blog/from-petabytes-to-peace-of-mind-llm-graphs-for-neuro-symbolic-ai-security-on-gcp/

InterVision. (2024). *AI and data governance: The new competitive advantage for IT leaders*. Retrieved from https://intervision.com/blog-ai-and-data-governance/

Irwandy, I., & Mangilep, A. U. A. Anggraeni Rini and Noor, N. B., Niartiningsih, A., & Latifah, N. (2024). Cybersecurity culture among healthcare workers in Indonesia: Knowledge gaps, demographic influences, and strategic policy solutions. In Research Square.

ISA. (2023). *Lessons learned from a forensic analysis of the Ukrainian power grid cyberattack malware*. ISA Blog. Retrieved from https://blog.isa.org/lessons-learned-forensic-analysis-ukrainian-power-grid-cyberattack-malware

Islam, S. A. M., Bari, M. S., Sarkar, A., Khan, A. J. M. O. R., & Paul, R. (2024). AI-powered threat intelligence: Revolutionizing cybersecurity with proactive risk management for critical sectors. [JAIGS]. *Journal of Artificial Intelligence General Science, 7*(1), 1–8. DOI: 10.60087/jaigs.v7i01.291

James, C. D., Aimone, J. B., Miner, N. E., Vineyard, C. M., Rothganger, F. H., Carlson, K. D., & Mulder, S. A.. (2017). A Historical Survey of Algorithms and Hardware Architectures for Neural-Inspired and Neuromorphic Computing Applications. *Biologically Inspired Cognitive Architectures, 19*. Advance online publication. DOI: 10.1016/j.bica.2016.11.002

Jiang, S., Nie, S., He, Y., Liu, R., Chen, C., & Wan, Q. (2019). Emerging synaptic devices: From two-terminal memristors to multiterminal neuromorphic transistors. *Materials Today Nano, 8*, 100059. DOI: 10.1016/j.mtnano.2019.100059

Jones, O. D., & Shen, F. X. (2012). Law and Neuroscience in the United States. *International Neurolaw: A Comparative Analysis*, 349–380. https://doi.org/DOI: 10.1007/978-3-642-21541-4_19

Juarez, D., Arteaga, I., Cortes, H., Vazquez-Roque, R., Lopez-Lopez, G., Flores, G., Treviño, S., Guevara, J., & Diaz, A. (2023). Chronic resveratrol administration reduces oxidative stress and brain cell loss and improves memory of recognition in old rats. *Synapse (New York, N.Y.)*, *77*(4). Advance online publication. DOI: 10.1002/syn.22271 PMID: 37130656

Jumagaliyeva, A., Abdykerimova, E., Turkmenbayev, A., Serimbetov, B., Muratova, G., Yersultanova, Z., & Zhiyembayev, Z. (2024). IDENTIFYING PATTERNS AND MECHANISMS OF AI INTEGRATION IN BLOCKCHAIN FOR E-VOTING NETWORK SECURITY. *Eastern-European Journal of Enterprise Technologies*, *4*(2(130)), 6–18. DOI: 10.15587/1729-4061.2024.305696

Kabanda, G. (2023). Bayesian Models in Cognitive Neuroscience. In *Artificial Intelligence and Knowledge Processing* (pp. 157–185). CRC Press.

Karpatou, P. A. (2025). *The evolution of cybersecurity threats & the rise of artificial intelligence* (Bachelor's thesis, University of Piraeus). Dione: Institutional Repository of the University of Piraeus. https://dione.lib.unipi.gr/xmlui/handle/unipi/17786

Karunamurthy, A., Kiruthivasan, R., & Gauthamkrishna, S. (2023). Human-in-the-loop intelligence: Advancing AI-centric cybersecurity for the future. *Qijmsrd*, *2*(3), 20–43.

Karunamurthy, A., Kiruthivasan, R., & Gauthamkrishna, S. (2023). Human-in-the-loop intelligence: Advancing ai-centric cybersecurity for the future. Quing. *International Journal of Multidisciplinary Scientific Research and Development*, *2*(3), 20–43.

Kasralikar, P., Polu, O. R., Chamarthi, B., Veer Samara Sihman Bharattej Rupavath, R., Patel, S., & Tumati, R. (2025, April 28). Blockchain for securing AI-driven healthcare systems: A systematic review and future research perspectives. *Cureus*, *17*(4), e83136. Advance online publication. DOI: 10.7759/cureus.83136 PMID: 40438823

Kaushik, K., Khan, A., Kumari, A., Sharma, I., & Dubey, R. (2024). Ethical considerations in AI-based cybersecurity. In *Next-generation cybersecurity: AI, ML, and blockchain* (pp. 437–470). Springer Nature Singapore.

Kayode, B., Adebola, N. T., & Akerele, S. (2025). The state of AI-driven cybersecurity: Trends, challenges, and opportunities. *Journal of Artificial Intelligence. Machine Learning & Data Science, 3*(2), 2731–2739.

Khalaf, N. Z., Al Barazanchi, I. I., Radhi, A. D., Parihar, S., Shah, P., & Sekhar, R. (2025). Development of real-time threat detection systems with AI-driven cybersecurity in critical infrastructure. *Mesopotamian Journal of CyberSecurity, 5*(2), 501–513.

Khan, O. U., Abdullah, S. M., Olajide, A. O., Sani, A. I., Faisal, S. M. W., Ogunola, A. A., & Lee, M. D. (2024). The future of cybersecurity: Leveraging artificial intelligence to combat evolving threats and enhance digital defense strategies. *Journal of Computational Analysis and Applications, 33*(8).

Kicho, Yu. (2022). *Khanh Nguyen, & Younghee Park*. Flexible and Robust Real-time Intrusion Detection Systems to Network Dynamics., DOI: 10.1109/ACCESS.2017. DOI

Kim, J., Park, M., & Kim, H., & Cho Suhyoun and Kang, P. (2019). Insider threat detection based on user behavior modeling and anomaly detection algorithms. *Applied Sciences (Basel, Switzerland), 9*(19), 4018.

Kolicic, B., Caron, A., Hicks, C., & Mavroudis, V. (2024). *Inherently Interpretable and Uncertainty-Aware Models for Online Learning in Cyber-Security Problems.* https://arxiv.org/abs/2411.09393

Kolosnjaji, B., Zarras, A., Webster, G., & Eckert, C. (2016). Deep learning for classification of malware system call sequences. In *Australasian Joint Conference on Artificial Intelligence* (pp. 137–149). Springer. https://doi.org/DOI: 10.1007/978-3-319-50127-7_11

Kraft, C. J., & Giordano, J. (2017). Integrating brain science and law: Neuroscientific evidence and legal perspectives on protecting individual liberties. *Frontiers in Neuroscience, 11*(NOV). Advance online publication. DOI: 10.3389/FNINS.2017.00621

Kritika, E. (2025). A neuroscience perspective on AI and cybersecurity. ISACA Journal, (1).

Kritika, E. (2025c). Brainjacking: The cybersecurity nightmare of the future. https://www.researchgate.net/profile/Er-Kritika/publication/391858141_Brainjacking_The_Cybersecurity_Nightmare_of_the_Future/links/682ac6438a76251f22e2b799/Brainjacking-The-Cybersecurity-Nightmare-of-the-Future.pdf

Kritika, E. (2025a). A comprehensive study on navigating the integration of neuropsychology and cybersecurity. *International Journal of Advanced Networking and Applications*, *17*(1), 6788–6798.

Kritika, E. (2025b). Ethical frontiers: Navigating the intersection of neurotechnology and cybersecurity. *Journal of Experimental Neurology*, *6*(1), 21–25.

Kritika, M. (2024). Neuro-driven cybersecurity: Strengthening digital defense. *London Journal of Research in Computer Science and Technology*, *24*(1), 17–26.

Kritika, M. (2025d). A comprehensive study on navigating neuroethics in cyberspace. *AI and Ethics*, *5*(1), 93–100.

Kumar, A., Rathore, P. S., Ahuja, S., & Lilhore, U. K. (Eds.). (2025). *Integrating Neurocomputing with Artificial Intelligence*. John Wiley & Sons.

La Tona, G., Terranova, M. C., Vernuccio, F., Lo Re, G., Salerno, S., Zerbo, S., & Argo, A. (2020). Lie Detection: fMRI. *Radiology in Forensic Medicine: From Identification to Post-Mortem Imaging*, 197–202. https://doi.org/DOI: 10.1007/978-3-319-96737-0_18

Lara, F. (2023). Neurorehabilitation of Offenders, Consent and Consequentialist Ethics. *Neuroethics*, *16*(1), 1–15. DOI: 10.1007/S12152-022-09510-1/METRICS

Lawfare. (2024). *A dynamic governance model for AI*. Retrieved from https://www.lawfaremedia.org/article/a-dynamic-governance-model-for-ai

Lee, J., Kim, J., Kim, I., & Han, K. (2019). Cyber threat detection based on artificial neural networks using event profiles. *IEEE Access : Practical Innovations, Open Solutions*, *7*, 165607–165626.

Leider, A., & Li, S. (2025, February). Brain-Computer Interactions in Extended Reality with Artificial Intelligence and Cloud Computing. In *2025 Conference on Artificial Intelligence x Multimedia (AIxMM)* (pp. 51-54). IEEE.

Lepri, B., Oliver, N., & Pentland, A. (2021). Ethical machines: The human-centric use of artificial intelligence. *iScience*, *24*(3), 102249. PMID: 33763636

Levin, S. A., Martin, C. S., & Arzberger, P. 1992. "MATHEMATICS AND BIOLOGY: THE INTERFACE CHALLENGES AND OPPORTUNITIES." *Cornell University*.

Li, M., Laiu, P., Nichols, J. A., Huettel, M., Sikkema, I., Mathur, M., Hollifield, S., & Hankins, M. (2025). Cognitive IoT and Edge Computing for Intrusion Detection with Federated TinyML. *2025 IEEE World AI IoT Congress (AIIoT)*, 0677-0684.

Li, Z., Kong, D., Niu, Y., Peng, H., Li, X., & Li, W. (2023). *An overview of AI and blockchain integration for privacy-preserving* (arXiv:2305.03928). arXiv. https://arxiv.org/abs/2305.03928

Li, J., Li, X., & Zhang, C. (2022). Analysis on Security and Privacy-preserving in Federated Learning. In *Highlights in Science* (Vol. 2022). Engineering and Technology SDPIT.

LinuxSecurity. (2024). *Embracing neuroscience-inspired AI for proactive linux security*. Retrieved from https://linuxsecurity.com/news/security-trends/embracing-neuroscience-inspired-ai

Liu, H., Wang, W., & Li, H. (2024). *Interpretable Multimodal Misinformation Detection with Logic Reasoning*. https://arxiv.org/abs/2305.05964

Liu, L., Chen, C., Zhang, J., De Vel, O., & Xiang, Y. (2019). Insider threat identification using the simultaneous neural learning of multi-source logs. *IEEE Access : Practical Innovations, Open Solutions*, *7*, 183162–183176.

Liu, R., Shi, J., Chen, X., & Lu, C. (2024). Network anomaly detection and security defense technology based on machine learning: A review. *Computers & Electrical Engineering*, *119*, 109581.

Liv, N., & Greenbaum, D. (2023). Cyberneurosecurity. In *Policy, identity, and neurotechnology: The neuroethics of brain-computer interfaces* (pp. 233–251). Springer International Publishing.

Li, W., Meng, W., Kwok, L., & Ip, H. H. (2017). Developing advanced fingerprint attacks on challenge-based collaborative intrusion detection networks. *Cluster Computing*, *21*, 299–310.

Lo, D. L. (2021). Can AI replace a judge in the courtroom? UNSW. Sydney. https://www.unsw.edu.au/newsroom/news/2021/10/can-ai-replace-judge-courtroom

Loaiza, F. L., Birdwell, J. D., Kennedy, G. L., & Visser, D. (2022). *Utility of artificial intelligence and machine learning in cybersecurity*. Institute for Defense Analyses.

Loettgers, A. (2007). Getting Abstract Mathematical Models in Touch with Nature. *Science in Context*, *20*(1). Advance online publication. DOI: 10.1017/S0269889706001153

Lumenova, A. I. (2025). *Does your AI monitoring system follow these best practices?* Retrieved from https://www.lumenova.ai/blog/ai-monitoring-system-best-practices/

Luo, Z., Tessler, C., Lin, T., Yuan, Y., He, T., Xiao, W., Guo, Y., ... (2025). “Emergent Active Perception and Dexterity of Simulated Humanoids from Visual Reinforcement Learning.” *arXiv preprint arXiv:2505.12278*

Maennel, K., & Maennel, O. M. (2024, December). Human-AI collaboration and cyber security training: Learning analytics opportunities and challenges. In *2024 17th International Conference on Security of Information and Networks (SIN)* (pp. 1–8). IEEE.

Mahajan, S., Khurana, M., & Estrela, V. V. (Eds.). (2024). *Applying Artificial Intelligence in Cybersecurity Analytics and Cyber Threat Detection*. John Wiley & Sons.

Malik, W., & Gul, S. (2024). Bridging the Gap: Exploring the Intersection of Cybersecurity and Human Security in the Digital Age. *Competitive Research Journal Archive*, *2*(04), 195–202.

Mannes, A. (2020). *Successful Research in AI Governance*. Risk, and Artificial Intelligence.

Margetts, H. (2022). Rethinking AI for Good Governance. *Daedalus*, *151*(2), 360–371. DOI: 10.1162/DAED_a_01922

Margolin, G., & Gordis, E. B. (2000). The effects of family and community violence on children. *Annual Review of Psychology*, *51*, 445–479. DOI: 10.1146/ANNUREV.PSYCH.51.1.445

Marsh, T. (2023). Deepfakes and the challenge to evidentiary integrity in modern courts. *International Review of Digital Forensics*, *11*(3), 120–138.

Martiri, E., Vajjhala, N. R., & Dalipi, F. (Eds.). (2025). *AI-enabled threat intelligence and cyber risk assessment* (1st ed.). CRC Press., DOI: 10.1201/9781003504979

Mathov, Y., Levy, E., Katzir, Z., Shabtai, A., & Elovici, Y. (2021). *Not All Datasets Are Born Equal: On Heterogeneous Data and Adversarial Examples*. https://arxiv.org/abs/2010.03180

McCullum, T., & Mancera, L. C. C. (2025). Neurotechnology Combined with Artificial Intelligence and Neurorights: A Legal Discussion. *Rev. Prop. Inmaterial*, *39*, 145.

MDPI. (2021). An approach based on signal processing and artificial intelligence to identify PIR and main contact instants. Retrieved from https://www.mdpi.com/1996-1073/18/2/377

Medium. (2023). *Role of ethics committees and review boards, and governance structures for responsible AI.* Retrieved from https://medium.com/tech-ai-made-easy/role-of-ethics-committees-and-review-boards-and-governance-structures-for-responsible-ai-61da34203553

Medium. (2024). Generative AI "agile swarm intelligence" (part 1): Autonomous agent swarms foundations, theory, and advanced applications. Retrieved from https://medium.com/@armankamran/generative-ai-agile-swarm-intelligence-part-1-autonomous-agent-swarms-foundations-theory-and-9038e3bc6c37

Medium. (2024b). *Stop the AI drift: Governing autonomous decisions.* Retrieved from https://medium.com/@SophiaNellon/stop-the-ai-drift-governing-autonomous-decisions-ccb96a5dfc2d

Meghraoui, L., & Belkhamza, Z. (2025, March). Cognitive Warfare and Cybersecurity: Strategic Implications for Global Security. In *Proceedings of the 19th International Conference on Cyber Warfare and Security*. Academic Conferences and publishing limited.

Merat, S., & Almuhtadi, W. (2024, January). Innovative Application of a Sleepwalking-Based Artificial Neural Model for Cybersecurity Risk Assessment. In *2024 IEEE International Conference on Consumer Electronics (ICCE)* (pp. 1-8). IEEE.

Microsoft Azure. (2024a). *Circuit breaker pattern.* Azure Architecture Center. Retrieved from https://learn.microsoft.com/en-us/azure/architecture/patterns/circuit-breaker

Microsoft Azure. (2024b). *Adaptive techniques for circuit breakers.* Retrieved from https://learn.microsoft.com/en-us/azure/architecture/patterns/circuit-breaker

Mikhaylov, A. N., Gryaznov, E. G., Koryazhkina, M. N., Bordanov, I. A., Shchanikov, S. A., Telminov, O. A., & Kazantsev, V. B. (2023). Neuromorphic Computing Based on CMOS-Integrated Memristive Arrays: Current State and Perspectives*. *Supercomputing Frontiers and Innovations*, *10*(2). Advance online publication. DOI: 10.14529/JSFI230206

Minssen, T., Seitz, C., Aboy, M., & Compagnucci, M. C. (2020). The EU-US Privacy Shield Regime for CrossBorder Transfers of Personal Data under the GDPR What are the legal challenges and how might these affect cloudbased technologies, big data, and AI in the medical sector? *European Pharmaceutical Law Review*, *4*(1), 34–50. DOI: 10.21552/eplr/2020/1/6

Mitchell, A., Potter, L., Palmer, X. L., & Barnett, M. (2025, March). Exploring the Intersection of Cybersecurity, Neurocapitalism, and Biodesign. In *Proceedings of the 19th International Conference on Cyber Warfare and Security*. Academic Conferences and publishing limited.

MITRE Corporation. (2021). *Intelligence after next: Breaking past AI's confirmation bias*. Retrieved from https://www.mitre.org/sites/default/files/2021-08/pr-21-0090-intelligence-after-next-breaking-past-ai-confirmation-bias.pdf

ModelOp. (2024). *NIST AI RMF*. Retrieved from https://www.modelop.com/ai-governance/ai-regulations-standards/nist-ai-rmf

Mohammadi, S., Alazab, A., Choo, J., & Mahmood, A. (2021). Security analysis of IoT networks: Architectures, protocols, and methods. *IEEE Internet of Things Journal*, *8*(5), 3536–3554.

Monteith, S., Glenn, T., Geddes, J. R., Achtyes, E. D., Whybrow, P. C., & Bauer, M. (2024). Artificial intelligence and cybercrime: Implications for individuals and the healthcare sector. *The British Journal of Psychiatry*, *225*(4), 421–423. PMID: 39308261

Moradi, S., & Manohar, R. (2019). The Impact of On-Chip Communication on Memory Technologies for Neuromorphic Systems. *Journal of Physics. D, Applied Physics*, *52*(1). Advance online publication. DOI: 10.1088/1361-6463/aae641

Morgan, S. (2020, November 13). *Cybercrime to cost the world $10.5 trillion annually by 2025*. Cybersecurity Ventures. https://cybersecurityventures.com/hackerpocalypse-cybercrime-report-2016/

Morgan, S. (2024, November 18). *Cybercrime to cost the world $10.5 trillion annually by 2025*. Cybercrime Magazine. https://cybersecurityventures.com/hackerpocalypse-cybercrime-report-2016/

Moustafa, A. (Ed.). (2022). *Cybersecurity and cognitive science*. Academic Press.

Müller, E., Arnold, E., Breitwieser, O., Czierlinski, M., Emmel, A., Kaiser, J., Mauch, C., Schmitt, S., Spilger, P., Stock, R., Stradmann, Y., Weis, J., Baumbach, A., Billaudelle, S., Cramer, B., Ebert, F., Göltz, J., Ilmberger, J., Karasenko, V., & Schemmel, J. (2022). A Scalable Approach to Modeling on Accelerated Neuromorphic Hardware. *Frontiers in Neuroscience*, *16*. Advance online publication. DOI: 10.3389/fnins.2022.884128 PMID: 35663548

Mulyadi, M., Fernando, Z. J., Putra, P. S., & Anditya, A. W. (2024). Unleashing Justice's Future: The Dawn of Neuro-Cognitive Risk Assessments (NCRA) in Transforming Rehabilitation. [Indonesian Journal of Criminal Law Studies]. *IJCLS, 9*(1), 61–86. DOI: 10.15294/IJCLS.V9I1.50152

Naeem, M. R., Amin, R., Farhan, M., Alotaibi, F. A., Alnfiai, M. M., Sampedro, G. A., & Karovič, V. (2024). Harnessing AI and analytics to enhance cybersecurity and privacy for collective intelligence systems. *PeerJ. Computer Science, 10*, e2264. PMID: 39314701

Nagar, A., Kumar, T., Bhamidipati, P., & Sandhia, G. K. (2022). Cybersecurity: The Part Played By Artificial Intelligence. *NeuroQuantology : An Interdisciplinary Journal of Neuroscience and Quantum Physics, 20*(15), 1629–1642.

Nalluri, S., Malyala, M. M., Kandagiri, H., & Kandagiri, K. K. (2025, June). Nscti: A hybrid neuro-symbolic framework for ai-driven predictive cyber threat intelligence. In *2025 4th International Conference on Computational Modelling, Simulation and Optimization (ICCMSO)* (pp. 14-21). IEEE.

Nasir, R., Afzal, M., Latif, R., & Iqbal, W. (2021). Behavioral based insider threat detection using deep learning. *IEEE Access : Practical Innovations, Open Solutions, 9*, 143266–143274.

Nasser Al-mhiqani, M., Ahmad, R., Zainal Abidin, Z., Yassin, W., Hassan, A., & Natasha Mohammad, A. (2020). New insider threat detection method based on recurrent neural networks. *Indonesian Journal of Electrical Engineering and Computer Science, 17*(3), 1474.

Nazir, A., & Khan, R.A. (2019). Combinatorial Optimization based Feature Selection Method: A study on Network Intrusion Detection. *ArXiv, abs/1906.04494.*

Nazir, I., & Tiwari, S. (2023). Impact of Machine Learning in Cybersecurity Augmentation. In Social Development and Governance Innovations in Education, Technology and Management (pp. 147–154). QTanalytics India.

Neelaveni, R., Sridevi, B., & Sivasankari, J. (2022). Securing Privacy Using Optimization and Statistical Models in Cognitive Radio Networks. *Computer Systems Science and Engineering, 42*(2).

Neupane, S., Ables, J., Anderson, W., Mittal, S., Rahimi, S., Banicescu, I., & Seale, M. (2022). *Explainable Intrusion Detection Systems (X-IDS): A Survey of Current Methods, Challenges, and Opportunities*. https://arxiv.org/abs/2207.06236

Nguyen, T. T., & Reddi, V. J. (2021). Deep reinforcement learning for cyber security. *IEEE Transactions on Neural Networks and Learning Systems, 34*(8), 3779–3795. DOI: 10.1109/tnnls.2021.3121870 PMID: 34723814

Nilawati, S., Amri, S., Hasanah, N., Saodah, S., Juliati, J., & Sapnita, S. (2024). Unraveling emotional regulation through multimodal neuroimaging techniques. *BrainBridge: Neuroscience and Biomedical Engineering, 1*(1), 1–26. DOI: 10.35335/A0CFDA08

NIST. (2021). *Digital Identity Guidelines (NIST Special Publication 800-63-3).* U.S. Department of Commerce, National Institute of Standards and Technology.

Noonan, C. (2018). *Spy the lie: Detecting malicious insiders. Office of Scientific and Technical Information.* OSTI.

Novelli, C., Taddeo, M., & Floridi, L. (2024). *Accountability in Artificial Intelligence: What It Is and How It Works.* https://ec.europa.eu/digital-inglemarket/en/news/definition-artificial-intelligence-main-capabilities-

Number Analytics. (2024). *The ethics of AI surveillance.*

Obi, O. C., Akagha, O. V., Dawodu, S. O., Anyanwu, A. C., Onwusinkwue, S., & Ahmad, I. A. I. (2024). Comprehensive review on cybersecurity: Modern threats and advanced defense strategies. Comput. Sci. IT Res. j., 5(2), 293–310.

OECD. (2019). *OECD Principles on Artificial Intelligence.* Organisation for Economic Co-operation and Development.

Oh, S. H., Jeong, M. K., Kim, H. C., & Park, J. (2023). Applying Reinforcement Learning for Enhanced Cybersecurity against Adversarial Simulation. *Sensors (Basel), 23*(6). Advance online publication. DOI: 10.3390/s23063000 PMID: 36991711

Okika, N., Okoh, O. F., & Etuk, E. E. (2025). Mitigating Insider Threats and Social Engineering Tactics in Advanced Persistent Threat Operations through Behavioral Analytics and Cybersecurity Training. *International Journal of Advance Research Publication and Reviews, 2*(3), 11–27.

Onchis, D. M., Gillich, G. R., Hogea, E., & Tufisi, C. (2023). Neuro-symbolic model for cantilever beams damage detection. *Computers in Industry, 151*, 103991.

Ortega Giménez, A. (n.d.). TUTELA JURISDICCIONAL ANTE UN TRATAMIENTO ILÍCITO INTERNACIONAL DE DATOS PERSONALES Y EL NUEVO REGLAMENTO GENERAL DE PROTECCIÓN DE DATOS DE LA UNIÓN EUROPEA Jurisdictional protection against an illicit international treatment of personal data and the new general regulations for data protection of the European Union. *Revista Acta Judicial*, (6), 2–23.

Palo Alto Networks. (2024). *NIST AI risk management **structure** (AI RMF)*. Cyberpedia. Retrieved from https://www.paloaltonetworks.com/cyberpedia/nist-ai-risk-management-framework

Panda, S. P. (2025). The Evolution and Defense Against Social Engineering and Phishing Attacks. [IJSR]. *International Journal of Scientific Research.*

Parisa, S. K., & Banerjee, S. (2024). AI-Enabled Cloud Security Solutions: A Comparative Review of Traditional vs. Next-Generation Approaches. *International Journal of Statistical Computation and Simulation, 16*(1).

Pastur-Romay, A., Porto-Pazos, L. A. B., Cedron, F., & Pazos, A. (2016). Parallel Computing for Brain Simulation. *Current Topics in Medicinal Chemistry, 17*(14). Advance online publication. DOI: 10.2174/1568026617666161104105725 PMID: 27823566

Pastur-Romay, L. A., Cedrón, F., Pazos, A., & Porto-Pazos, A. B. (2016). Deep Artificial Neural Networks and Neuromorphic Chips for Big Data Analysis: Pharmaceutical and Bioinformatics Applications. *International Journal of Molecular Sciences, 17*(8). Advance online publication. DOI: 10.3390/ijms17081313 PMID: 27529225

Pasupathieswaran, M., & Kapilan Bharathi, G. (2024). *Digital Battlefronts: Rethinking Legal Frontiers in Cyberwarfare and AI Conflicts*. www.ijfmr.com

Patel, J., & Shah, H. (2021). Creating Safe and Secure AI-From Computer Design to Cloud Technology. *International Research. Journal of Engineering and Applied Sciences (Asian Research Publishing Network), 9*(4), 10–55083.

Pazouki, S., Golilarz, N. A., Kazemi-Razi, S. M., & Aydeger, A. (2022, July). A self-healing cybersecurity mechanism for cyberattacks targeting artificial neural network-based human brain implants controlling smart homes. In *2022 International Conference on Electrical, Computer and Energy Technologies (ICECET)* (pp. 1-6). IEEE.

Pehle, C., Billaudelle, S., Cramer, B., Kaiser, J., Schreiber, K., Stradmann, Y., Weis, J., Leibfried, A., Müller, E., & Schemmel, J. (2022). *The BrainScaleS-2 accelerated neuromorphic system with hybrid plasticity*. https://arxiv.org/abs/2201.11063

Perception Point. (2024). *Top 6 AI security risks and how to defend your organization*. Retrieved from https://perception-point.io/guides/ai-security/top-6-ai-security-risks-and-how-to-defend-your-organization/

Perez, C. L., Orozco, C. M. V., & Rodríguez, I. H. (2026). General Overview Cybersecurity and Artificial Intelligence. *Reshaping Criminology with AI*, 63-90.

Phoenix Children's Hospital. (2019). *Case study: Phoenix Children's Hospital takes on cybersecurity*. BlackBerry Cylance. https://blogs.blackberry.com/en/2019/07/case-study-phoenix-childrens-hospital-takes-on-cybersecurity

Piplai, A., Ramezani, N., & Sun, H. (2023). *Knowledge-enhanced neuro-symbolic AI for cybersecurity and privacy*. arXiv. Retrieved from https://arxiv.org/abs/2308.02031

Poldrack, R. A., Huckins, G., & Varoquaux, G. (2020). Establishment of Best Practices for Evidence for Prediction: A Review. In *JAMA Psychiatry* (Vol. 77, pp. 534–540). American Medical Association., DOI: 10.1001/jamapsychiatry.2019.3671

Prakash, C., Gupta, L. R., Mehta, A., Vasudev, H., Tominov, R., Korman, E., Fedotov, A., Smirnov, V., & Kesari, K. K. (2023). Computing of Neuromorphic Materials: An Emerging Approach for Bioengineering Solutions. *Materials Advances*, *4*(23). Advance online publication. DOI: 10.1039/d3ma00449j

Priyanshu, A., Maurya, Y., & Hong, Z. (2024). *AI Governance and Accountability: An Analysis of Anthropic's Claude*. https://arxiv.org/abs/2407.01557

Prokopowicz, D., Gołębiowska, A., & Such-Pyrgiel, M. (2023). The role of big data and data science in the context of information security and cybersecurity. *Journal of Modern Science*, *53*(4), 9–42. DOI: 10.13166/jms/177036

Pustilnik, A. C. (2013). Neurotechnologies at the Intersection of Criminal Procedure and Constitutional Law. *The Constitution and the Future of Criminal Justice in America*, 109–134. https://doi.org/DOI: 10.1017/CBO9781139108034.011

Raine, A., & Marek, W. K. (2013). The anatomy of violence: The biological roots of crime. In *American Journal of Forensic Psychology* (Vol. 31, pp. 67–71). https://doi.org/DOI: 10.1080/10511253.2018.1445334

Raine, A. (2008). From Genes to Brain to Antisocial Behavior. *Current Directions in Psychological Science*, *17*(5), 323–328. DOI: 10.1111/J.1467-8721.2008.00599.X

Raine, A., Buchsbaum, M. S., Stanley, J., Lottenberg, S., Abel, L., & Stoddard, J. (1994). Selective reductions in prefrontal glucose metabolism in murderers. *Biological Psychiatry, 36*(6), 365–373. DOI: 10.1016/0006-3223(94)91211-4

Raine, A., Lencz, T., Bihrle, S., LaCasse, L., & Colletti, P. (2000). Reduced prefrontal gray matter volume and reduced autonomic activity in antisocial personality disorder. *Archives of General Psychiatry, 57*(2), 119–127. DOI: 10.1001/ARCHPSYC.57.2.119

Ramakrishnan, S., & Chittibala, D. R. (2024). Enhancing Cyber Resilience: Convergence of SIEM, SOAR, and AI in 2024. In *International Journal of Computing and Engineering* (Vol. 5, Issue 2). www.carijournals.orgwww.carijournals.orgwww.carijournals.org

Ramalingam, R., Arthi, K., Bhavani, M. M., & Sunitha, T. (2025). AI-Enhanced Security Information and Event Management (SIEM) System. In *Deep Learning Innovations for Securing Critical Infrastructures* (pp. 75-94). IGI Global Scientific Publishing.

Rameh, R. B., Cherry, E. M., & Weber dos Santos, R. (2020). Single-Variable Delay-Differential Equation Approximations of the Fitzhugh-Nagumo and Hodgkin-Huxley Models. *Communications in Nonlinear Science and Numerical Simulation, 82*. Advance online publication. DOI: 10.1016/j.cnsns.2019.105066

Rast, A. D., Galluppi, F., Jin, X., & Furber, S. B. 2010. "The Leaky Integrate-and-Fire Neuron: A Platform for Synaptic Model Exploration on the SpiNNaker Chip." In *Proceedings of the International Joint Conference on Neural Networks*, doi:DOI: 10.1109/IJCNN.2010.5596364

Ravi Kumar, M., Jain, U., Francis, F., Senthil Kumar, S., Adhvaryu, R., & Natrayan, L. (2024). Cognitive Digital Twin Systems for Predictive Security in AI-Enhanced IoT Environments. *2024 First International Conference on Software, Systems and Information Technology (SSITCON)*, 1-6.

Rayhan, A. (2024, April). Cybersecurity in the digital age: Assessing threats and strengthening defenses. In *Conference* (pp. 1–26). Cybersecurity Awareness.

Raza, A., Ali, A. K. S., & Hussain, A. A. (2024). AI-driven approaches to cyber and information security: Machine learning algorithms for threat prediction and anomaly detection. *Spectrum of Engineering Sciences*, 2(4), 565–573.

Reddit. (2024). Ħ WiseID and AI agents - "Blockchain-based immutable logs". *r/Hedera*. Retrieved from https://www.reddit.com/r/Hedera/comments/1itbwi3/%C4%A7_wiseid_and_ai_agents_blockchainbased_immutable/

ResearchGate. (2023). *Neurosymbolic AI in cybersecurity: Bridging pattern recognition and symbolic reasoning*. Retrieved from https://www.researchgate.net/publication/376827715_Neurosymbolic_AI_in_Cybersecurity_Bridging_Pattern_Recognition_and_Symbolic_Reasoning

ResearchGate. (2024a). *Analysing recent APT incidents: Case studies and lessons learned*. Retrieved from https://www.researchgate.net/publication/387298480_Analysing_Recent_APT_Incidents_Case_Studies_and_Lessons_Learned

ResearchGate. (2024b). *Cognitive bias in AI development: Understanding the psychological and societal influences that shape AI model design and outcomes*. Retrieved from https://www.researchgate.net/publication/387382926_Cognitive_Bias_in_AI_Development_Understanding_the_Psychological_and_Societal_Influences_that_Shape_AI_Model_Design_and_Outcomes

ResearchGate. (2024c). *Reviewing the ethical implications of AI in decision making processes*. Retrieved from https://www.researchgate.net/publication/378295986_REVIEWING_THE_ETHICAL_IMPLICATIONS_OF_AI_IN_DECISION_MAKING_PROCESSES

ResearchGate. (2025a). *Neuro-adaptive intrusion detection systems: A brain-inspired ML architecture for autonomous threat hunting*. Retrieved from https://www.researchgate.net/publication/390945241_Neuro-Adaptive_Intrusion_Detection_Systems_A_Brain-Inspired_ML_Architecture_for_Autonomous_Threat_Hunting

ResearchGate. (2025b). *Explainable AI (XAI) techniques for cybersecurity in zero-trust architectures*. Retrieved from https://www.researchgate.net/publication/392064017_Explainable_AI_XAI_Techniques_for_Cybersecurity_in_Zero-Trust_Architectures

ResearchGate. (205c). *Blockchain-based logging for auditing AI decisions*. Retrieved from https://www.researchgate.net/publication/396889319_Blockchain-Based_Logging_for_Auditing_AI_Decisions

Reyes, A. C., & Amador, A. A. (2009). Qualitative and quantitative EEG abnormalities in violent offenders with antisocial personality disorder. *Journal of Forensic and Legal Medicine*, *16*(2), 59–63. DOI: 10.1016/J.JFLM.2008.08.001

Rezaee, K., Rezakhani, S. M., Khosravi, M. R., & Moghimi, M. K. (2024). A survey on deep learning-based real-time crowd anomaly detection for secure distributed video surveillance. *Personal and Ubiquitous Computing*, *28*(1), 135–151.

Rigoni, D., Pellegrini, S., Mariotti, V., Cozza, A., Mechelli, A., Ferrara, S. D., Pietrini, P., & Sartori, G. (2010). How Neuroscience and Behavioural Genetics Improve Psychiatric Assessment: Report on a Violent Murder Case. *Frontiers in Behavioral Neuroscience, 4*, 160. DOI: 10.3389/FNBEH.2010.00160

Ring, M., Wunderlich, S., Scheuring, D., Landes, D., & Hotho, A. (2019). A survey of network-based intrusion detection data sets. *Computers & Security, 86*, 147–167. DOI: 10.1016/j.cose.2019.06.005

Rios-Campos, C., Paz, S. C. V., & Vilema, G. O., D\'\iaz, L. M. R., Zambrano, D. P. F., Zambrano, G. M. M., Viteri, J. D. C. L., Vara, F. E. O., Vallejos, P. A. A., Llontop, R. F. G., & Anchundia-Gómez, O. (2024). Cybersecurity and artificial intelligence (AI). *S. F. J. of Dev., 5*(8), e4276.

Rios-Campos, C., Paz, S. C. V., Vilema, G. O., Díaz, L. M. R., Zambrano, D. P. F., Zambrano, G. M. M., & Anchundia-Gómez, O. (2024). Cybersecurity and artificial intelligence (AI). *South Florida Journal of Development, 5*(8), e4276–e4276.

Rivas, A., Collarana, D., Torrente, M., & Vidal, M.-E. (2024). A neuro-symbolic system over knowledge graphs for link prediction. *Semantic Web, 15*(4), 1307–1331.

Royal Society Publishing. (2024). On the ethical governance of swarm robotic systems in the real world. *Philosophical Transactions. Series A, Mathematical, Physical, and Engineering Sciences, 382*(2282). https://royalsocietypublishing.org/doi/10.1098/rsta.2024.0142

Roy, K., Jaiswal, A., & Panda, P. (2019). Towards spike-based machine intelligence with neuromorphic computing. *Nature, 575*(7784), 607–617. DOI: 10.1038/s41586-019-1677-2 PMID: 31776490

Ryngaert, C., & Taylor, M. (2020). Symposium on the GDPR and international law. The GDPR as global data protection regulation? *AJIL Unbound, 114*, 5–9. https://doi.org/DOI: 10.1017/aju.2019.80

Saeed, S., Suayyid, S. A., Al-Ghamdi, M. S., Al-Muhaisen, H., & Almuhaideb, A. M. (2023). A systematic literature review on cyber threat intelligence for organizational cybersecurity resilience. *Sensors (Basel), 23*(16). PMID: 37631808

Saikia, S., Athilingam, V. P., & Ahmed, F. (2023). Cybersecurity and Intraoperative Artificial Intelligence Decision Support: Challenges and Solutions Related to Ethical Issues. In *Ethical Issues in AI for Bioinformatics and Chemoinformatics* (pp. 107-118). CRC Press.

Sander, J., Cohen, A., Dasari, V. R., Venable, B., & Jalaian, B. (2025). *On Accelerating Edge AI: Optimizing Resource-Constrained Environments*. https://arxiv.org/abs/2501.15014

Saputra, A. R. (2023). Aspects of Personal Data Protection According to International Law. [FJSS]. *Formosa Journal of Social Sciences*, *2*(3), 417–424. DOI: 10.55927/fjss.v2i3.6192

Sarker, I. H. (2023). Multi-aspects AI -based modeling and adversarial learning for cybersecurity intelligence and robustness: A comprehensive overview. *Security and Privacy*, *6*(5). Advance online publication. DOI: 10.1002/spy2.295

Sarker, I. H. (2024). *AI-driven cybersecurity and threat intelligence: Cyber automation, intelligent decision-making, and explainability*. Springer Nature., DOI: 10.1007/978-3-031-42906-4

Sarker, I. H., Furhad, M. H., & Nowrozy, R. (2021). Ai-driven cybersecurity: An overview, security intelligence modeling and research directions. *SN Computer Science*, *2*(3), 173. PMID: 33778771

Sashwin, K., Nithika, K. S., Priyadharshini, S., & Maduvant, S. P. (2024, March). Analysis, Trends, and Utilization of Security Information and Event Management (SIEM) in Critical Infrastructures. In *2024 10th International Conference on Advanced Computing and Communication Systems (ICACCS)* (Vol. 1, pp. 1980-1984). IEEE.

Savopoulos, P., & Lindell, A. K. (2018). Born criminal? Differences in structural, functional and behavioural lateralization between criminals and noncriminals. In *Laterality* (Vol. 23, pp. 738–760). Routledge., DOI: 10.1080/1357650X.2018.1432631

Scarfone, K., & Souppaya, M. (2007). *Guide to intrusion detection and prevention systems (IDPS)* (NIST Special Publication 800-94). National Institute of Standards and Technology. https://doi.org/DOI: 10.6028/NIST.SP.800-94

Schauer, F. (2010). Neuroscience, lie-detection, and the law: Contrary to the prevailing view, the suitability of brain-based lie-detection for courtroom or forensic use should be determined according to legal and not scientific standards. *Trends in Cognitive Sciences*, *14*(3), 101–103. DOI: 10.1016/j.tics.2009.12.004

Scholarship@western, S., & Loganathan, G. (2018). *Real-time Intrusion Detection using Multidimensional Sequence-Real-time Intrusion Detection using Multidimensional Sequence-to-Sequence Machine Learning and Adaptive Stream Processing to-Sequence Machine Learning and Adaptive Stream Processing Part of the Digital Communications and Networking Commons, and the Systems and Communications Commons*. https://ir.lib.uwo.ca/etdhttps://ir.lib.uwo.ca/etd/5523

Sekhar Bhusal, C. (2021). Systematic review on social engineering: Hacking by manipulating humans. *J. Inf. Secur.*, *12*(01), 104–114.

Semeria, M. N., & Semeria, M. N. 2017. "Symbiotic Low-Power, Smart and Secure Technologies in the Age of Hyperconnectivity." In *Technical Digest - International Electron Devices Meeting, IEDM*, doi:DOI: 10.1109/IEDM.2016.7838027

Sendjaja, T., Irwandi, E. P., Suryani, Y., & Fatmawati, E. (2024). Cybersecurity in the digital age: Developing robust strategies to protect against evolving global digital threats and cyber attacks. *The International Journal of Science in Society*, *6*(1), 1008–1019.

Seng, K. P., & Ang, L. M. (2022). Embedded intelligence: State-of-the-art and research challenges. *IEEE Access : Practical Innovations, Open Solutions*, *10*, 59236–59258.

Sententia, W. (2004). Neuroethical Considerations: Cognitive Liberty and Converging Technologies for Improving Human Cognition. *Annals of the New York Academy of Sciences*, *1013*(1), 221–228. DOI: 10.1196/ANNALS.1305.014

Seo, D., Patrick, C. J., & Kennealy, P. J. (2008). Role of serotonin and dopamine system interactions in the neurobiology of impulsive aggression and its comorbidity with other clinical disorders. *Aggression and Violent Behavior*, *13*(5), 383–395. DOI: 10.1016/J.AVB.2008.06.003

Shafique, M. (2024). A Cross-Layer Approach to Energy-Efficient and Secure EdgeAI: Architectures, Systems and Applications. *2024 5th CPSSI International Symposium on Cyber-Physical Systems (Applications and Theory) (CPSAT)*, 1-1.

Shahana, A., Hasan, R., Farabi, S. F., Akter, J., Al Mahmud, M. A., Johora, F. T., & Suzer, G. (2024). AI-driven cybersecurity: Balancing advancements and safeguards. *Journal of Computer Science and Technology Studies*, *6*(2), 76–85.

Shah, S., & Issac, B. (2018). Performance comparison of next-generation antivirus tools. *Journal of Information Security Research*, *9*(3), 130–140. DOI: 10.6025/jisr/2018/9/3/130-140

Shamay-Tsoory, S. G., Harari, H., Aharon-Peretz, J., & Levkovitz, Y. (2010). The role of the orbitofrontal cortex in affective theory of mind deficits in criminal offenders with psychopathic tendencies. *Cortex*, *46*(5), 668–677. DOI: 10.1016/j.cortex.2009.04.008

Shappie, A. T., Dawson, C. A., & Debb, S. M. (2020). Personality as a predictor of cybersecurity behavior. *Psychol. Pop. Media*, *9*(4), 475–480.

Sheikhbahei, E., & Ari, A. A. (2024). Harnessing the power of emerging digital technologies for improved sustainability and productivity in biomedical engineering and neuroscience. *Scientific Hypotheses*, *1*, 47–52.

Shekhar, S., Davis, J., Evans, R., Foster, D., & Paul, C. (2024, December). *AI and biometric authentication: The future of secure financial transactions*. ResearchGate. https://www.researchgate.net/publication/389377532_AI_and_Biometric_Authentication_The_Future_of_Secure_Financial_Transactions

Shendkar, B. D. (2024). Explainable machine learning models for real-time threat detection in cybersecurity. *Panamer. Math. J.*, *35*(1s), 264–275.

Shinde, R., Patil, S., Kotecha, K., Potdar, V., Selvachandran, G., & Abraham, A. (2022). *Securing AI-based healthcare systems using blockchain technology: A state-of-the-art systematic literature review and future research directions*. ResearchGate. https://www.researchgate.net/publication/361253530_Securing_AI-based_Healthcare_Systems_using_Blockchain_Technology_A_State-of-the-Art_Systematic_Literature_Review_and_Future_Research_Directions

Shiwlani, A., Hasan, S. U., & Kumar, S. (2024). Artificial Intelligence in Neuro-education: A Systematic Review of AI Applications Aligned with Neuroscience Principles for Optimizing Learning Strategies. *Journal of Development and Social Sciences*, *5*(4), 578–593.

Shklovskij, V. A. (2021). Magnon-Phonon Interactions in Spin Insulators. *Low Temperature Physics*, *47*(8). Advance online publication. DOI: 10.1063/10.0005551

Shone, N., Ngoc, T. N., Phai, V. D., & Shi, Q. (2018). A deep learning approach to network intrusion detection. *IEEE Transactions on Emerging Topics in Computational Intelligence*, *2*(1), 41–50. DOI: 10.1109/TETCI.2017.2772792

Siddique, R. A., & Jahankhani, H. (2024). An Investigation of Artificial Intelligence (AI) and Cybersecurity: Case of AI Integration in German Cybersecurity Strategy. In *Navigating the Intersection of Artificial Intelligence, Security, and Ethical Governance: Sentinels of Cyberspace* (pp. 123–146). Springer Nature Switzerland.

Singh, A. (2024). Toward Robust and Scalable Wireless Ad Hoc Networks: An Approach to Adaptive Routing and Security. *2024 12th International Conference on Intelligent Systems and Embedded Design (ISED)*, 1-6.

Singh, T. (2025). Neuroscience, Sociology, and Anthropology. In *Cybersecurity, Psychology and People Hacking* (pp. 73–94). Springer Nature Switzerland.

Smith Law. (2024). *The EU AI Act and its implications for US companies*. Retrieved from https://www.google.com/search?q=https://www.smithlaw.com/resources-insights/the-eu-ai-act-and-its-implications-for-us-companies

Smith, J. (2023). Cybersecurity implications of AI adoption in judicial institutions. *Journal of Law. Technology & Ethics*, *5*(2), 66–89.

Sommer, R., & Paxson, V. (2010). Outside the closed world: On using machine learning for network intrusion detection. In *Proceedings of the 2010 IEEE Symposium on Security and Privacy* (pp. 305–316). IEEE. https://doi.org/DOI: 10.1109/SP.2010.25

Song, Y., Zhang, L., Liu, Y., & Pan, Y. (2024). Spiking neural P systems for malware and phishing detection: A review. *IEEE Transactions on Neural Networks and Learning Systems*, *35*(2), 555–568. DOI: 10.1109/TNNLS.2023.3241829 PMID: 35877793

Surana & Surana. (2023). *AI-black box phenomenon*. Retrieved from https://suranaandsurana.com/ai-black-box-phenomenon/

Sutaria, K., Rajan, D. K., Pathak, G. P., & Dange, P. (2025, April). Context-Sensitive Graph Reduction and Partitioning for Enhanced Cyber Attack Investigation. In *2025 International Conference on Knowledge Engineering and Communication Systems (ICKECS)* (pp. 1-6). IEEE.

Syntaxia. (2024). *AI agent safety: Circuit breakers for autonomous systems*. Retrieved from https://www.syntaxia.com/post/ai-agent-safety-circuit-breakers-for-autonomous-systems

Talanov, M., Vallverdu, J., Adamatzky, A., Toschev, A., Suleimanova, A., Leukhin, A., Posdeeva, A., Mikhailova, Y., Rodionova, A., Mikhaylov, A., Serb, A., Shchanikov, S., Gerasimova, S., Dehshibi, M. M., Hramov, A., Kazantsev, V., Tsoy, T., Magid, E., Lavrov, I., & Warwick, K. (2022). *Neuropunk Revolution. Hacking Cognitive Systems towards Cyborgs 3.0.* https://arxiv.org/abs/2205.06538

Tang, J., Yuan, F., Shen, X., Wang, Z., Rao, M., He, Y., & Sun, Y.. (2019). Bridging Biological and Artificial Neural Networks with Emerging Neuromorphic Devices: Fundamentals, Progress, and Challenges. *Advanced Materials*, *31*(49). Advance online publication. DOI: 10.1002/adma.201902761 PMID: 31550405

Tariq, M. (Ed.). (2025c). *Emerging multisector applications of AI and IoT*. IGI Global., DOI: 10.4018/979-8-3373-4332-7

Tekin, U., & Dener, M. (2025). A bibliometric analysis of studies on artificial intelligence in neuroscience. *Frontiers in Neurology*, *16*, 1474484. PMID: 40040909

Temara, S. (2024). Harnessing the power of artificial intelligence to enhance next-generation cybersecurity. In *Preprints*.

Tesink, V., Douglas, T., Forsberg, L., Ligthart, S., & Meynen, G. (2023). Neurointerventions in Criminal Justice: On the Scope of the Moral Right to Bodily Integrity. *Neuroethics*, *16*(3), 1–11. DOI: 10.1007/S12152-023-09526-1/METRICS

Thakur, C. S., Molin, J. L., Cauwenberghs, G., Indiveri, G., Kumar, K., Qiao, N., & Schemmel, J.. (2018). Large-Scale Neuromorphic Spiking Array Processors: A Quest to Mimic the Brain. *Frontiers in Neuroscience*, *12*. Advance online publication. DOI: 10.3389/fnins.2018.00891 PMID: 30559644

Thapaliya, S., & Bokani, A. (2024). Leveraging artificial intelligence for enhanced cybersecurity: Insights and innovations. *SADGAMAYA*, *1*(1), 46–52. DOI: 10.3126/sadgamaya.v1i1.66888

Thapliyal, V., & Thapliyal, P. (2024). Machine learning for cybersecurity: Threat detection, prevention, and response. *Darpan International Research Analysis*, *12*(1), 1–7.

Timmers, P. (2019). Ethics of AI and Cybersecurity When Sovereignty is at Stake. In *Minds and Machines* (Vol. 29, Issue 4, pp. 635–645). Springer. https://doi.org/DOI: 10.1007/s11023-019-09508-4

Tortora, L., Meynen, G., Bijlsma, J., Tronci, E., & Ferracuti, S. (2020). Neuroprediction and A.I. in Forensic Psychiatry and Criminal Justice: A Neurolaw Perspective. *Frontiers in Psychology*, *11*, 493506. DOI: 10.3389/FPSYG.2020.00220/BIBTEX

Truong, N., Sun, K., Wang, S., Guitton, F., & Guo, Y. (2021). *Privacy Preservation in Federated Learning: An insightful survey from the GDPR Perspective*. https://arxiv.org/abs/2011.05411

Udeh, E. O., Amajuoyi, P., Adeusi, K. B., & Scott, A. O. (2024). The integration of artificial intelligence in cybersecurity measures for sustainable finance platforms: An analysis. Comput. Sci. IT Res. j., 5(6), 1221–1246.

UNESCO. (2021). *Recommendation on the Ethics of Artificial Intelligence*. United Nations Educational, Scientific and Cultural Organization.

University of Southampton. (2025). *The growing demand for AI skills in criminal justice*. Southampton Online. https://www.online.southampton.ac.uk/blog/growing-demand-ai-skills-criminal-justice [Accessed 10 Dec 2025].

Unsworth, C. (2024). *An ethical charter for artificial intelligence*. Retrieved from https://www.craigunsworth.com/articles/an-ethical-charter-for-artificial-intelligence

Urbaniok, F., Hardegger, J., Rossegger, A., & Endrass, J. (2006). Neurobiologischer determinismus: Fragwürdige schlussfolgerungen über menschliche entscheidungsmöglichkeiten und forensische schuldfähigkeit. *Fortschritte der Neurologie-Psychiatrie*, *74*(8), 431–441. DOI: 10.1055/S-2006-944237

Usman, H., Tariq, I., & Nawaz, B. (2023a). IN THE REALM OF THE MACHINES: AI'S INFLUENCE UPON INTERNATIONAL LAW AND POLICY. *Journal of Social Research Development*, *4*(2), 383–399. DOI: 10.53664/jsrd/04-02-2023-13-383-399

van Haastrecht, M., Yigit Ozkan, B., Brinkhuis, M., & Spruit, M. (2021). Respite for SMEs: A systematic review of Socio-technical cybersecurity metrics. *Applied Sciences (Basel, Switzerland)*, *11*(15), 6909.

Van Veen, V., Cohen, J. D., Botvinick, M. M., Stenger, V. A., & Carter, C. S. (2001). Anterior Cingulate Cortex, Conflict Monitoring, and Levels of Processing. *NeuroImage*, *14*(6), 1302–1308. DOI: 10.1006/NIMG.2001.0923

Verhoeven, F. E. A., Booij, L., Kruijt, A. W., Cerit, H., Antypa, N., & Van der Does, W. (2012). The effects of MAOA genotype, childhood trauma, and sex on trait and state-dependent aggression. *Brain and Behavior*, *2*(6), 806–813. DOI: 10.1002/BRB3.96

VerifyWise. (2024). *AI incident response plan*. Retrieved from https://verifywise.ai/lexicon/ai-incident-response-plan/

Vijaya, G., & Ramesh, K. (2025). IAS and Its Impact in Neuroscience. *Handbook of Intelligent Automation Systems Using Computer Vision and Artificial Intelligence*, 407-421.

Volkow, N. D., Fowler, J. S., & Wang, G. J. (2003). The addicted human brain: Insights from imaging studies. *The Journal of Clinical Investigation*, *111*(10), 1444–1451. DOI: 10.1172/JCI18533

Wang, H., Deng, Y., Yoo, S., & Lin, Y. (2023). *Exploring Robust Features for Improving Adversarial Robustness*. https://arxiv.org/abs/2309.04650

Wang, H., Tangirala, G. K., Naidu, G. P., Mayville, C., Roy, A., Sun, J., & Mandava, R. B. (2024). *Anomaly Detection for Incident Response at Scale*. https://arxiv.org/abs/2404.16887

Wang, J., Chen, H., Issa, M., Huang, S., & Imani, M. (2023). *Late Breaking Results: Scalable and Efficient Hyperdimensional Computing for Network Intrusion Detection*. https://arxiv.org/abs/2304.06728

Wang, J., Sun, Q., & Zhou, C. (2023). Insider threat detection based on deep clustering of multi-source behavioral events. *Applied Sciences (Basel, Switzerland), 13*(24), 13021.

Wang, M. (2024). Generative AI: A New Challenge for Cybersecurity. *Journal of Computer Science and Technology Studies*, *6*(2), 13–18.

Wan, W., Kubendran, R., Schaefer, C., Eryilmaz, S. B., Zhang, W., Wu, D., & Deiss, S.. (2022). A Compute-in-Memory Chip Based on Resistive Random-Access Memory. *Nature*, *608*(7923). Advance online publication. DOI: 10.1038/s41586-022-04992-8 PMID: 35978128

Waxman, M. C. (2017). *Cyber Strategy & Policy: International Law Dimensions.* https://scholarship.law.columbia.edu/faculty_scholarshiphttps://scholarship.law.columbia.edu/faculty_scholarship/2025

Wei, W. C., Jhang, C. J., Yi, R. C., Cheng, X. X., Sie, S. H., Lee, J. L., & Hao, W. K.. (2020). A Relaxed Quantization Training Method for Hardware Limitations of Resistive Random Access Memory (ReRAM)-Based Computing-in-Memory. *IEEE Journal on Exploratory Solid-State Computational Devices and Circuits*, *6*(1). Advance online publication. DOI: 10.1109/JXCDC.2020.2992306

Widjaja, G. (2025). Current threats to cyber security: strategies for protecting personal data in the digital age. *International journal of society reviews, 2*(11), 2245-2255.

Wijekoon, J. H. B., & Dudek, P. (2008). Compact Silicon Neuron Circuit with Spiking and Bursting Behaviour. *Neural Networks*, *21*(2–3). Advance online publication. DOI: 10.1016/j.neunet.2007.12.037 PMID: 18262751

Wikimedia Foundation. (2024). *Explainable artificial intelligence*. Retrieved from https://en.wikipedia.org/wiki/Explainable_artificial_intelligence

WilmerHale. (2024). What are high-risk AI systems within the meaning of the EU's AI Act, and what requirements apply to them? *WilmerHale Privacy and Cybersecurity Law Blog*. Retrieved from https://www.wilmerhale.com/en/insights/blogs/wilmerhale-privacy-and-cybersecurity-law/20240717-what-are-highrisk-ai-systems-within-the-meaning-of-the-eus-ai-act-and-what-requirements-apply-to-them

Wiz. (2025). *NIST AI risk management* ***structure****: A tl;dr*. Retrieved from https://www.wiz.io/academy/nist-ai-risk-management-framework

Woods, N. (2022). Users' Psychopathologies: Impact on Cybercrime Vulnerabilities and Cybersecurity Behavior. In Computational Methods in Applied Sciences (pp. 93–134). Springer International Publishing.

Xavier, K. F., Subashini, K., Vijayalakshmi, P., Selvalakshmi, B., Sudhakar, G., & Pradeepa, K. (2025). Integrating Artificial Intelligence and Machine Learning for Enhanced Cyber Security in Industry 4.0: Designing a Smart Factory with IoT and CPS. *Artificial Intelligence and Machine Learning for Industry*, *4*(0), 267–286.

Xi, B. (2021). *Adversarial Machine Learning for Cybersecurity and Computer Vision: Current Developments and Challenges*. https://arxiv.org/abs/2107.02894

Xu, Q., Wang, Y., Chen, B., Li, Z., & Wang, N. (2023). Firing Pattern in a Memristive Hodgkin–Huxley Circuit: Numerical Simulation and Analog Circuit Validation. *Chaos, Solitons, and Fractals*, *172*. Advance online publication. DOI: 10.1016/j.chaos.2023.113627

Yang, J. Q., Wang, R., Ren, Y., Jing, Y. M., Zhan, P. W., Zhou, Y., & Su, T. H. (2020). Neuromorphic Engineering: From Biological to Spike-Based Hardware Nervous Systems. *Advanced Materials*, *32*(52). Advance online publication. DOI: 10.1002/adma.202003610 PMID: 33165986

Yang, Q., Huang, A., Fan, L., Seng Chan, C., Han Lim, J., Woh Ng, K., Sheng Ong, D., Li, B., Yang, Q., Huang, A., Fan, L., Chan, C. S., Lim, J. H., Ng, K. W., Ong, D. S., & Li Federated, B. (2023). Federated Learning with Privacy-preserving and Model IP-right-protection. *Machine Intelligence Research*, *20*(1), 19–37. DOI: 10.1007/s11633

Yang, Y., & Raine, A. (2009). Prefrontal structural and functional brain imaging findings in antisocial, violent, and psychopathic individuals: A meta-analysis. *Psychiatry Research: Neuroimaging*, *174*(2), 81–88. DOI: 10.1016/j.pscychresns.2009.03.012

Yeo, S., Enoch, M. A., Gorodetsky, E., Akhtar, L., Schuebel, K., Roy, A., & Goldman, D. (2017). The influence of FKBP5 genotype on expression of FKBP5 and other glucocorticoid-regulated genes, dependent on trauma exposure. *Genes Brain & Behavior*, *16*(2), 223–232. DOI: 10.1111/GBB.12342

Yilmaz, E., & Can, O. (2024). Unveiling shadows: Harnessing Artificial Intelligence for insider threat detection. *Eng. Technol. Appl. Sci. Res.*, *14*(2), 13341–13346.

Yin, C., Zhu, Y., Fei, J., & He, X. (2017). A deep learning approach for intrusion detection using recurrent neural networks. *IEEE Access : Practical Innovations, Open Solutions*, *5*, 21954–21961. DOI: 10.1109/ACCESS.2017.2762418

Young, A. R., Dean, M., Plank, J. S., & Rose, G. S. (2019). A Review of Spiking Neuromorphic Hardware Communication Systems. *IEEE Access : Practical Innovations, Open Solutions*, *7*. Advance online publication. DOI: 10.1109/ACCESS.2019.2941772

Yuan, S., Zheng, P., Wu, X., & Li, Q. (2019, December). Insider threat detection via hierarchical neural temporal point processes. 2019 IEEE International Conference on Big Data (Big).

Zahm, W., Stern, T., Bal, M., Sengupta, A., Jose, A., Chelian, S., & Vasan, S. (2022). Cyber-neuro RT: Real-time neuromorphic cybersecurity. *Procedia Computer Science, 213*, 536–545.

Zhang, W., Gao, B., Tang, J., Yao, P., Yu, S., Meng, F. C., Yoo, H. J., Qian, H., & Wu, H. (2020). Neuro-Inspired Computing Chips. *Nature Electronics, 3*(7). Advance online publication. DOI: 10.1038/s41928-020-0435-7

Zhang, W., Xu, M., Feng, Y., Mao, Z., & Yan, Z. (2024). The Effect of Procrastination on Physical Exercise among College Students—The Chain Effect of Exercise Commitment and Action Control. *International Journal of Mental Health Promotion, 26*(8), 611–622. DOI: 10.32604/ijmhp.2024.052730

Zhang, X., Ma, Z., Zheng, H., Li, T., Chen, K., Wang, X., Liu, C., Xu, L., Wu, X., Lin, D., & Lin, H. (2020). The combination of brain-computer interfaces and artificial intelligence: Applications and challenges. *Annals of Translational Medicine, 8*(11), 712–712. DOI: 10.21037/atm.2019.11.109 PMID: 32617332

Zhang, Z., Al Hamadi, H., Damiani, E., Yeun, C. Y., & Taher, F. (2022). Explainable artificial intelligence applications in cyber security: State-of-the-art in research. *IEEE Access : Practical Innovations, Open Solutions, 10*, 93104–93139.

Zhao, W., Gangaraju, K., & Yuan, F. (2025). Multimodal perception-driven decision-making for human-robot interaction: A survey. *Frontiers in Robotics and AI, 12*, 1604472. PMID: 40917482

Zhong, Y., Wu, L., Liu, X., & Jiang, J. (2022). *Exploiting the Potential of Datasets: A Data-Centric Approach for Model Robustness*. https://arxiv.org/abs/2203.05323

Zou, A., Phan, L., Wang, J., Duenas, D., Lin, M., Andriushchenko, M., Wang, R., Kolter, Z., Fredrikson, M., & Hendrycks, D. (2024). *Improving Alignment and Robustness with Circuit* Breakers. https://arxiv.org/abs/2406.04313

Zou, Z., Alimohamadi, H., Kim, Y., Najafi, M. H., Srinivasa, N., & Imani, M. (2022). EventHD: Robust and Efficient Hyperdimensional Learning with Neuromorphic Sensor. *Frontiers in Neuroscience, 16*. Advance online publication. DOI: 10.3389/fnins.2022.858329 PMID: 35968370

Zwolinska, M. (2015). INTERNATIONAL TRANSFERS OF PERSONAL DATA. TOWARDS A GLOBAL CONSENSUS ON DATA PROTECTION STANDARDS TRANSFERENCIAS INTERNACIONALES DE DATOS PERSONALES. HACIA UN CONSENSO GLOBAL EN NIVELES. http://www.derecom.com/derecom/

About the Contributors

Shafiq Ul Rehman is an experienced educator and professional consultant with a background in curriculum development and educational technology. His teaching and research experience spans more than 12 years. Dr. Shafiq has worked with various educational institutions to implement sustainable practices and innovative teaching strategies. Dr. Shafiq received his Ph.D. degree from Universiti Sains Malaysia (USM), Malaysia, in 2017. He was a Postdoctoral Research Fellow at Singapore University of Technology and Design (SUTD), Singapore, from 2017 to 2020. He is currently Acting Dean, College of Information Technology and Chairman Department of Computer Science, Kingdom University, Bahrain. He is also a Senior Assistant Professor with research interests in cybersecurity, artificial intelligence, and the latest emerging IT technologies. He lectures in various Computer Science and IT courses, including developing curriculum and courseware in tandem with current technology trends. In addition to editing 8 books, he has authored over 80 international research publications in the fields of cybersecurity, artificial intelligence, healthcare, IoT, and other emerging technologies. His expertise in these fields extends to academic and industrial consulting, as well as speaking and training at a variety of international organizations, conferences, and seminars.

***

Adetunji Oludele Adebayo is a renowned information security analyst and savvy technology leader who works at the crucial nexus of artificial intelligence and cybersecurity, with a focus on the emerging area of GenAI Governance, Risk, and Compliance (GRC). His knowledge is extensive, encompassing everything from IT audits and third-party supply chain security to operational resilience and risk management. He holds the esteemed CISM and Lead Implementer (ISO 20000, 27001, 22301) certifications. Adetunji Oludele Adebayo, a successful author, conference speaker, and dual MSc degree holder in technology management and cybersecurity, brings a distinct technical perspective to the development of safe and innovative technological futures

Ashraf Alam currently holds the position of Research Faculty at the Centre of Excellence in Public Policy, Sustainability and ESG Research, housed within the Faculty of Law and Policy Studies at Alliance University, Bangalore. Renowned for his transdisciplinary acumen spanning education, technology, and policy studies, Dr. Ashraf has been distinguished as one of the World's Top 2% Scientists by Stanford University and Elsevier, an accolade that highlights the breadth and depth of his scholarly impact. His prolific academic output includes over fifty SCOPUS-indexed publications and more than one hundred conference presentations at esteemed national and international academic forums. His educational trajectory reflects both depth and versatility: a Ph.D. in Education from the Indian Institute of Technology (IIT) Kharagpur, an M.Ed. with a concentration in Mathematics Education, and a B.S. in Computer Science from the University of Delhi. He also holds postgraduate degrees in Public Administration (M.A.) and Mathematics (M.Sc.), supplemented by a suite of postgraduate diplomas in Higher Education, Guidance and Counselling, Educational Technology, Criminology and Police Administration, and Value Education. Dr. Ashraf is an active participant in global scholarly discourse. As Associate Editor of Frontiers in Education, he plays a pivotal role in curating and guiding intellectual contributions across the Educational, Pedagogical, and Learning Sciences. Concurrently, he serves as Founder and Director of Academic Chronicles Private Limited, where he orchestrates editorial board formation and develops strategic frameworks for peer-reviewed publishing in the Social, Behavioural, and Humanistic Sciences. His research has been disseminated through elite academic platforms, including Elsevier, Springer, Taylor & Francis, Wiley, Routledge, Sage, Emerald, and IEEE, and addresses a remarkably diverse array of topics such as pedagogical theories, educational administration, educational psychology, educational sociology, educational policy, technology-integrated learning, mathematics education, educational philosophy, educational technology, teacher education, and AI/ML in learning environments. Dr. Ashraf's scholarly rigor is further demonstrated by his success in qualifying multiple prestigious examinations including UGC-NET-JRF in both Education and Adult and Continuing Education, UGC- NET in Public Administration, and GATE in Humanities and Social Sciences. At the heart of Dr. Ashraf's intellectual ethos lies a steadfast belief in education as a catalytic and emancipatory force capable of engendering social justice, human flourishing, societal progress, and sustainable transformation. His recent explorations into 'Happiness Engineering' and holistic well- being in school ecosystems articulate a vision of education that transcends instrumentalist paradigms, prioritizing emotional intelligence, global consciousness, empathy, and psychosocial resilience among learners. His research agenda seeks to conceive educational praxis through the affordances of inclusive digital learning, gamified instructional design, and artificial intelligence (AIEd), thereby constructing robust, ethically grounded frameworks for 21st century education. At Alliance University, Dr. Ashraf remains committed to architecting pedagogical models that not only cultivate intellectual dexterity and cognitive excellence but also prepare learners for morally responsive leadership, intellectual nimbleness, and responsible global citizenship in an increasingly volatile, uncertain, complex, and ambiguous (VUCA) world.

Kiran R. Dodiya is an experienced Cyber Forensic Expert and Assistant Professor specializing in cyber security and digital forensics. He has taught at prestigious institutions and is currently pursuing a PhD in Biochemistry and Forensic Science. With a strong background in ethical hacking and malware analysis, Kiranbhai is passionate about educating students and contributing to the field of cyber forensics. His expertise includes malware forensic, computer forensics, and data recovery software. Kiranbhai's commitment to professional growth is evident through his participation in workshops, seminars, and research publications. He is dedicated to shaping the next generation of professionals in the field and combatting cybercrimes.

Kapil Kumar is an accomplished forensic scientist and academician with a PhD degree and extensive experience in forensic science research. He currently serves as an Associate Professor in the Department of Forensic Science at Gujarat University, Ahmedabad, India. His academic portfolio reflects a sustained commitment to teaching, research, and scholarly mentorship in areas central to forensic investigations. His multidisciplinary expertise spans traditional forensic domains such as forensic ballistics, questioned document examination, forensic psychology, forensic medicine and digital forensics, as well as emerging intersections between forensic practice and technology. Dr. Kumar's academic leadership integrates rigorous scientific inquiry with practical relevance to criminal investigations and judicial processes, positioning him as a respected contributor to both national and international forensic science communities.

Dipak Kumar Mahida is a distinguished research scholar in the Department of Forensic Science, currently pursuing his Ph.D. in forensic toxicology with a specialized focus on the analysis of poisonous plants and pesticides. With a deep-seated commitment to his field, he has qualified for the National Eligibility Test (NET) for Assistant Professor and secured eligibility for the prestigious National Fellowship for his doctoral studies in India. His academic journey is enriched with the publication of numerous articles in high-impact, peer-reviewed, and indexed journals. Dipak Kumar's expertise extends beyond publishing, as he has presented his research at both national and international conferences, peer-reviewed articles for esteemed journals, and authored chapters for notable publishers worldwide. His focused work in environmental toxicology has also earned him recognition in the scientific community, where he continues to make significant contributions, advancing the frontiers of forensic science.

Ankita Patel, Dr., is an accomplished forensic scientist and Assistant Professor at Gujarat University, Ahmedabad, where she has been shaping the field of forensic science for over a decade. Holding both an M.Sc. and Ph.D. in Forensic Science, her academic journey is marked by a strong focus on bridging science and justice. Dr. Ankita Patel was awarded the prestigious UGC Junior Research Fellowship (JRF) in Forensic Science, a highly competitive fellowship provided by the University Grants Commission (UGC), New Delhi. It supported her Ph.D. research, focusing on the role of forensic evidence in criminal trials. Her expertise spans multiple subfields, including Forensic Toxicology, Environment Toxicology, Analytical Toxicology, Forensic Anthropology, and Criminology, where she has made significant contributions through her research. She has made significant contributions to academia, with numerous peer-reviewed research papers and multiple book chapters on diverse forensic and toxicology topics. Her professional accomplishments are complemented by various prestigious awards, including the Best Performance Award from the Ministry of Home Affairs, Government of India. Dr. Patel's expertise also extends beyond academics, as she frequently participates in conferences, workshops, and seminars, sharing her insights on the evolving role of forensic science in society. Driven by a passion for scientific innovation and justice, Dr. Patel continues to shape the discourse in forensic science through her research, teaching, and community outreach.

Harshini R is a postgraduate student in Forensic Science affiliated to Gujarat University, Ahmedabad. Born and brought in Bangalore. With a passion for reading and writing, the author's area of research focuses on the fields of Forensic Psychology, Criminology, Neurocriminology and Forensic Anthropology. Harshini holds a bachelor's degree in Criminology and Forensic Science, Psychology and Sociology. She is sports enthusiast, who has been a part of few National and University games.

Ravikumar R. Natarajan is an experienced academician with over 12+ years of teaching and research expertise across institutions in India, the UAE, and the Maldives. He currently serves as an Assistant Professor at Marwadi University,

Rajkot, specializing in Machine Learning, Recommender Systems, and AI-driven applications in healthcare and security. He holds a Ph.D. in Machine Learning and Recommender Systems from Amity University, Jaipur, a Master of Engineering in CSE from VMRF University, Salem, and a Bachelor of Engineering in CSE from Anna University. He also has a MiniMBA from the Swiss eLearning Institute. Dr. Ravikumar has authored more than 8+ multiple SCIE/Scopus-indexed journal articles, 25+ IEEE/Springer conference papers, and co-authored a book on Artificial Intelligence. He has also published 9 patents and contributed 10+ book chapters in emerging domains such as Federated Learning, Blockchain, and Digital Twins for IGI Global, Wiley and Springer publisher. He actively mentors students through initiatives like the Research Activities Club (RAC) and Student Research Internship Training (SRIT), promoting innovation and research culture.

Aarthi S is a dedicated Assistant Professor in Computer Science with over six years of teaching experience. She is currently pursuing her Ph.D. at Marwadi University, Gujarat, and holds an M.Phil. and MCA from Bharathiar University, Tamil Nadu. Throughout her academic career, Aarthi has specialized in programming languages such as C++, Java, and C, and contributed to research in recommender systems and AI-related data privacy. She has published journal articles, contributed to book chapters, and actively participated in technical workshops. Known for her student mentorship and engagement in academic events, Aarthi remains committed to fostering innovation and excellence in computer science education.

Shreha S. A is a postgraduate scholar pursuing her M.Sc. in Clinical Psychology at PSG College of Arts and Science, Coimbatore. With a strong academic foundation in psychology, she is dedicated to understanding human behaviour, mental health challenges, and evidence-based therapeutic practices. Her academic journey reflects a deep commitment to developing clinical competencies, including psychological assessment, counselling skills, and intervention planning for diverse populations. Shreha aims to contribute to the field of mental health through research, community engagement, and professional practice. Her interests span cognitive-behavioural approaches, child and adolescent psychology, mental wellness promotion, and neuropsychology. She aspires to work as a clinical psychologist equipped with both scientific knowledge and empathetic care to support individuals facing psychological difficulties. Through her ongoing training and academic exposure at PSG College of Arts and Science, she continues to build a strong foundation that will guide her future contributions to mental health awareness, clinical practice, and psychological well-being.

Saptarshi Kumar Sarkar is an Assistant Professor at Brainware University, dedicated to fostering academic excellence and innovation. With a strong background in artificial intelligence (AI), machine learning (ML), and social networking, he brings deep expertise and a passion for research to his teaching. His scholarly work has made meaningful contributions to the advancement of these evolving fields.

Anupama Sen, an Assistant Professor at Brainware University, is committed to academic excellence. She brings extensive knowledge and experience to her students, with research interests spanning artificial intelligence (AI), machine learning (ML), and social networking. Her contributions have significantly advanced these fields.

Affaan Shaikh is the Founder & CEO of Neuratia Labs. As an AI engineer, researcher and neuroscientist, he develops cutting-edge solutions at the intersection of artificial intelligence, neuroscience, and medical technology. His research spans neurodegenerative disease diagnosis, brain-computer interfaces (BCIs), and AI in aerospace. With over 10 peer-reviewed papers in journals like IEEE and Springer, Affaan is an active contributor to the tech community. He has mentored 20+ aspiring researchers and writers and is passionate about innovation, leadership, and public engagement.

Muhammad Usman Tariq is a strategic higher education leader and scholar with more than 17 years of international experience across academia, research, and industry. He holds dual doctorates, a PhD in Artificial Intelligence and a Doctorate in Business Administration and has published extensively as the author of research articles, case studies, book chapters, and academic texts. His contributions also include several patents, reflecting his applied research in technology, business, and education. He is the Founder and CEO of TheCaseHQ.com, a global hub for professional certification programmes, narrative and video case studies, and digital learning innovation. In addition, he serves as President of the Gulf Higher Education Network (Gulf HE), an initiative dedicated to advancing academic practice, faculty development, and institutional collaboration across the region. He is a Principal Fellow of Advance HE (UK), Chartered Fellow of the CIPD (UK), Senior Fellow of SEDA (UK), and a Senior Member of IEEE, reflecting his standing as both an academic innovator and a global professional leader.

Aparna V B is a B.Sc. student in Neuroscience Technology at Yenepoya School of Allied Health Sciences, Yenepoya University, India.

Index

A

B

C

D

P

R

S

www.ingramcontent.com/pod-product-compliance
Lightning Source LLC
LaVergne TN
LVHW081536300926
849161LV00006B/1452